Health Education in Schools

KING ALFRED'S COLLEGE
WINCHESTER

To be returned on or before the day marked
below:-

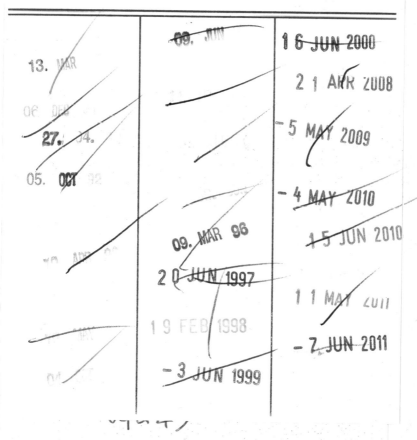

Health Education in Schools

Edited by
James Cowley, Kenneth David and Trefor Williams

Harper & Row, Publishers
London

Cambridge
Hagerstown
Philadelphia
New York

San Francisco
Mexico City
Sao Paulo
Sydney

Harper & Row Ltd
28 Tavistock Street
London WC2E 7PN

British Library Cataloguing in Publication Data
Health education in schools. – (Harper education
    series)
    1. Health education
    I. Cowley, J.   II. David, K.   III. Williams, T.
    613'.07   RA440

ISBN 0-06-318178-9
ISBN 0-06-318179-7 Pbk

Typeset by Inforum Ltd, Portsmouth
Printed and bound by The Pitman Press, Bath

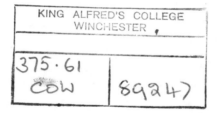

CONTENTS

Abbreviations

The following abbreviations of periodical titles are used in the references to this book:

Am. Soc. Rev.	*American Sociological Review*
Br. Dent. J.	*British Dental Journal*
Br. J. Prev. Soc. Med.	*British Journal of Preventive and Social Medicine*
Camb. J. Ed.	*Cambridge Journal of Education*
Child Dev.	*Child Development*
Curric. Rev. Bul.	*Curriculum Review Bulletin*
Educ. Canada	*Education Canada*
Educ Leader	*Educational Leadership*
Educ. Res.	*Educational Research*
Gift. Child Q.	*Gifted Child Quarterly*
Hlth Educ. Monogr.	*Health Education Monograph*
Hlth Soc. Servs. J.	*Health and Social Services Journal*
Int. J. Hlth Educ.	*International Journal of Health Education*
J. Consult. Psychol.	*Journal of Consulting Psychology*
J. Counsel. Psychol.	*Journal of Counseling Psychology*
J. Curric. Studies	*Journal of Curriculum Studies*
J. Drug. Educ.	*Journal of Drug Education*
J. Educ. Res.	*Journal of Educational Research*
J. Inst. Hlth Educ.	*Journal of the Institute of Health Education*
J. Pers. Soc. Psy.	*Journal of Personality and Social Psychology*
J. Personality	*Journal of Personality*
J. Read.	*Journal of Reading*
J. Saf. Res.	*Journal of Safety Research*
J. Sch. Hlth	*Journal of School Health*
Personn. Guidance J.	*Personnel and Guidance Journal*
Psychol. Rep.	*Psychological Reports*
R. Soc. Hlth J.	*Royal Society of Health Journal*
Sask. J. Educ. Res.	*Saskatchewan Journal of Educational Research*

LIST OF CONTRIBUTORS

John Tomlinson MA, FRSA
Director of Education, Cheshire and Chairman, Schools Council
Foreword
Keith Tones MA, MSc, PhD
Principal Lecturer, Leeds Polytechnic
Affective Education and Health
Mrs Gill Williams MEd
Lecturer in Health Education, London University
David Aspin BA, PhD, DipEd
Professor of Education (Philosophy), London University
The Philosophy of Health Education Related to Schools
Nicholas Dorn BSc, MA
Assistant Director, Institute for the Study of Drug Dependence
A Questioning View of Health Education
Vaughan Johnson BA, MIHE
Deputy Headteacher, Greenleys School, Milton Keynes and former
Disseminator of SCHEP 5–13
Health Education in Primary Schools
Trefor Williams BA, DHe
Director, Schools Council Health Education Projects
Health Education in Secondary Schools
Tim Hull MSc, MIBiol
Deputy Director, Schools Council Health Education Project 13–18
The Contribution of Biology to School Health Education
Mrs Winifred Hart DipEd, DipSociology
Inspector for Health Education, ILEA
Health Education in the Home Economics Curriculum

John Wright MA, DLC
  Principal Lecturer, Nonington College and Chairman of the Physical
  Education Association's Study Group on Health and Recreation
  Physical Education and Health Education
Peter Farley MA (Oxon)
  Schools Council Health Education Project 13–18
  The Contribution of English to Health Education
Ian Birnie
  County Adviser for Schools, Lancashire
  Health Education Through Religious Education
Kenneth David BA
  Freelance Lecturer & formerly County Adviser for Schools, Lancashire
  Health Education and the Pastoral System
Tony Evans Dip. Guidance & Counselling
  Thornes House School, Wakefield
  Classroom Approaches
William Rice MA(Hons), MIHE
  Senior Assistant Director, Teachers' Advisory Council on Alcohol and
  Drug Education
  Discussion, Role Play and Simulation in the Classroom
Jeff Lee BA(Hons)
  Field Officer (Schools), Health Education Council
  Teaching Skills
Ian McCafferty BA, MEd
  Area Health Education Officer, Nottinghamshire
  The Role of Visitors and Area Health Education Teams
James Cowley BA, MEd, MIHE
  Director Health Promotion Services, Government of South Australia
  Health Commission and formerly of the Open university
  The In-Service Education of Teachers in Health Education
Marilyn Stephens BSc(Hons)
  Evaluator, Schools Council Health Education Projects
  Evaluation of Health Education

FOREWORD

Health education has for a long time been a 'cinderella' subject in most British schools. Yet the schools are only reflecting the ambivalent attitude towards health education which is displayed by health professionals, society at large and most individuals. However, there are good reasons for thinking that a change in educational and social attitudes is both necessary and possible.

Much was achieved by the first historical wave of public health action – better public water supply, sewerage and housing standards. These, together with certain medical advances such as vaccination, immunization, obstetric procedures and antenatal and postnatal care, caused a dramatic improvement in the nation's health and especially the life expectancy of children, from the 1850s to the 1950s.

We now need a second wave. Much of the illness, disability and suffering in our society is self-inflicted. Excesses or imbalances of smoking, drinking and eating and lack of exercise damage individuals. Less obviously, but just as surely, these and similar practices also hurt and damage others. We assault our children when drunk, each other on the road and our sexual partners with sexually transmitted diseases. Industrial organizations kill and maim their employees with industrial diseases and injuries, their customers with hazardous products and the community with pollution. Our society and social organizations induce stress in an increasing number of people each year, yet families and firms are ill-equipped with the knowledge or attitudes needed to give effective help or to remedy the causes.

Moreover, having helped, directly or indirectly, to inflict illness on ourselves we make matters worse by failing to perceive the illness and by making ineffective use of health services and health products. As infectious diseases are brought under control, handicapping conditions affect a larger proportion of those who survive and their families must learn how to help to manage the condition. As life expectancy increases, more survive into their eighties and need the help and understanding of their families and neighbours.

It seems obvious that our society has not adjusted to these circumstances and that health education must be a prime way of ensuring that it does. The case for health education is therefore unanswerable. But that does not define what health education needs to be or how it can be provided. Certainly it must be more than just 'giving the facts'. It is clear that direct teaching, whether of schoolchildren or adults, is not sufficient to change attitudes which are culturally deeply ingrained. Moreover, a heavy-handed approach is an assault on individual liberty.

The task of the school must be to ensure that children are given knowledge about human development, good diet, health-promoting habits and ways of organizing families and other social groups which promote cohesion and self-confidence rather than stress and breakdown. This cannot be done by merely adding another 'subject' to an already overloaded curriculum. It depends on all teachers understanding how their subject relates to these aspects of life. And that in turn depends on certain senior teachers in a school being given the responsibility to ensure that the theme of health education gets adequate recognition in the curriculum, and also in the hidden curriculum of attitudes and values which a school transmits incidentally by its organization, teaching methods and relationships.

This book sets out to present a wide view of health education in schools, and I am glad to commend it to teachers. The writers are well known in their respective fields, and the editors are nationally known and respected for their work in pastoral care, health education and curriculum development. From their views teachers will be able to assess their own contribution to health education; that is, to an important aspect of the way in which schools prepare pupils for living in the future.

John Tomlinson
Chairman, Schools Council
Director of Education, Cheshire

INTRODUCTION

In this book we set out to survey the present position of health education in schools in the United Kingdom, and to provide evidence of possible future developments. The book is intended as a basic reader or primer for this wide-ranging and diffuse area of education.

Health education is seldom nowadays seen as a narrow parade of physical matters; it is almost universally understood as an omnibus title for physical and mental attitudes to responsible health for the individual and the community, to well-being within a supportive family life and to lives lived positively and with some contentment. Curriculum terms such as 'personal and social education' correlate closely with this view of health.

We hope that *Health Education in Schools* will, with this wide view in mind, provide support or legitimization for the present endeavours of practitioners in health education working in and with schools, and will offer a framework for consideration by others who are facing the need to systematize work in this area. As John Tomlinson says in his foreword, 'a change in educational and social attitudes is both necessary and possible', and we are quite sure that a planned and co-ordinated approach to health education in schools is bound to develop in future. This book may help in this development, for we feel that the work surveyed here should be seen as part of the basic and in-service training of all teachers, not of specialists only. We also feel that such a survey should be part of the reading of health staff who are associated with schools, and of many medical staff and perhaps parents.

Every educational approach needs to be supported by a philosophy and theory, and this is provided by some of our contributors. We believe, however, that there is a strong practical theme to this book as well, and many of our contributors are concerned with classroom practice as well as with curricular management and development.

In Part I readers will find statements on the theory behind health education. Part II deals with approaches in primary and secondary education, with some emphasis on the Schools Council Health Education Projects. In Part III the contributions of particular academic subjects and of school pastoral organization are reviewed. Although the theme throughout the book is to commend a co-ordinated approach to health education by schools rather than a subject specialism, we need to use the traditional and continuing subject areas in order to transmit the health message.

In Part IV we concentrate on practical approaches to health education within the classroom, and point to the need for informal education skills in the modern view of health education. Part V illustrates the contributions of other services, the necessity for in-service education and the constant need to evaluate our work in this field.

The Appendices to the book should serve as a source of reference of organizations, courses, materials, government reports and books which can support the work of teachers.

This book cannot and should not be prescriptive; it is intended as a source book to provide ideas for those who plan for health education and those who teach it. All schools should have a plan for how they influence children in their health careers, in company with caring parents, but that plan has to be based on that particular school and the personalities within it. We have therefore avoided too much emphasis on particular schemes, in the hope that curriculum planners will seek what their school needs, perhaps from several sources. The formulation of health schemes should only be attempted when set within the specific context of a particular school with its own idiosyncracies and ethos.

We would like to pay tribute to the considerable help given in the preparation of this book by Dee John, Shirley Boyer and Nadine Culshaw. We value also the help of Dr Margaret Jones of the Health Education Council, Mrs Slavin of the Schools Council Health Education Project and colleagues from the Teachers' Advisory Council on Alcohol and Drug Education.

PART 1

THE BASES OF HEALTH EDUCATION

INTRODUCTION

One of the major constraining influences upon the success of health education is the failure to develop and use a methodology appropriate to its needs. Those involved in health education have long recognized the need to go beyond the mere passing on of facts and information, if the aim of helping young people to make choices and decisions relevant to their lives is to be achieved. Keith Tones is well known and respected for his work in this area, and in Chapter 1 he explores the philosophy, relevance and practice of the affective domain generally in health education, drawing widely from research in the field. After reading psychology at Cambridge, Keith Tones taught in a secondary modern school and subsequently lectured in colleges of education until his appointment as principal lecturer in health education at Leeds Polytechnic. He is an honorary lecturer in community medicine at Leeds University and has researched various aspects of health education. He is currently involved in running courses at Leeds Polytechnic for health education specialists, both in schools and in the National Health Service.

Health education, like any educational activity of worth, needs to be underpinned by a sound rationale or deeper philosophy if it is to be taken seriously by practitioners. The essence of philosophic debate lies in asking the right kinds of questions no matter how basic or challenging they might be. This formidable task is undertaken in Chapter 2 by Gill Williams and David Aspin. They ask challenging questions and attempt to provide a contextual framework for teachers to supply their own answers. Gill Williams has wide experience in matters of health education and teacher training, having taught physical education and health education in secondary schools, further education colleges, and colleges of education. After work in Manchester Polytechnic with varied professional training groups, and after taking a master's degree in educational sciences, she became course director of the MSc in health education at Chelsea College, University of London.

David Aspin is professor of education (philosophy) at Kings College, University of London, having previously taught in the universities of Durham, Nottingham and Manchester.

In Chapter 3 Nicholas Dorn, assistant director for the Institute for the Study of Drug Dependence, looks critically at approaches and attitudes in health education, with drug education as a specific example, and he offers a radical viewpoint. He argues that the aims and scope of such education reflect general trends in society and are part of a much broader range of concerns. He uses three examples to support his argument: a Canadian affective education project, an in-service teacher training manual and a discussion of more radical health education. His opinions are challenging and take us well beyond the limits of more conventional viewpoints of what health education implies.

CHAPTER 1

AFFECTIVE EDUCATION AND HEALTH

Keith Tones

> . . . educators must remember that their goal is to produce well adjusted, rational people who can relate and feel, not just non-linear calculating computers . . . (Osman, 1973)

The school curriculum is an amalgam of planned experiences and activities (including content and method of teaching) which describes the ways in which the school attempts to socialize pupils. Curriculum development is the enterprise promoted by educational innovators aiming to change the existing process of socialization. Innovation is necessary because an educational system rarely keeps pace with true social needs; it is rarely completely *relevant*. It frequently ossifies, and unfortunately curators of the curriculum typically resist the onslaught of the innovator. In the words of Benjamin's (1971) witty and allegorical critique of the American education system, the curriculum is often 'saber-toothed'.

The question of relevance assumes a particular significance when the innovator seeks to add to an already crowded curriculum and may require certain existing parts to be removed. The task is difficult at the best of times but even more problematical when the innovation demands not merely new subject matter but a different emphasis or a different approach. Health education is currently searching for recognizable status within a core curriculum in the schools. Its marginal status is recognized by the Scottish Education Department's Curriculum Paper 14 (1974):

> Health education occupies an indeterminate and ambivalent position: it has not yet been accepted as an essential part of the fabric of education. It tends to fall into the no-man's land between the school and the home, or within the school to be everyone's concern but no-one's responsibility. . . . It is often equated with

sex education in the schools' as in the public mind and this itself gives rise to difficulty and confusion.

The problems faced by health education in pressing its territorial claims doubtless have something to do with its ill-defined boundaries and pretensions to be about everything physical, mental and social – a fact which led Goldstein (1975) to comment, '. . . if the study of health is the study of everything, it is the serious study of nothing'. However, the reference in Curriculum Paper 14 to sex education and the schools' anxiety about trespassing on the preserves of the family and the home provides us with a useful insight into the difficulties faced by health education. Schools have tended to be concerned largely with cognitive matters; their function is seen to be that of supplying information and promoting understanding. Health education requires a shift in emphasis from the cognitive to the affective. Although health education has a very important cognitive base, it becomes problematical only when it deals with values and attitudes; it proves difficult when it probes social problems, attempts to increase teacher sensitivities, develops personal and social skills and even attempts to change pupils' behaviours. Part of this problem derives from the fact that teachers are usually ill-prepared to deal with affective issues and are rarely equipped with the teaching methods necessary to handle them. This in turn is doubtless due in part to a belief that such values and behaviours are indeed the province of parents, and in part to a belief that education should focus predominantly on the provision of knowledge and related cognitive skills. The pursuit of rationality should be the school's main contribution to transmitting that which is most worthwhile in society. As Hirst (1969) says: 'If once the central objectives of rationality are submerged, or are given up so that . . . other pursuits take over, then I suggest the school has betrayed its educational trust no matter how successful it may be in these other respects, and no matter how laudable these other ends may be in themselves.'

It is worth drawing attention to the fact that such an approach is at odds with the preventive aims of health education in the National Health Service (Tones, 1976), which tends to consider that the school has a tougher part to play in the fight to promote preventive medicine. Various government reports would seem to adopt this viewpoint (see Appendix IV).

My own belief is that the school cannot reasonably avoid committing itself to affective health education, and this stems partly from the view that supplying knowledge about healthy living seems to have little to do with actually living healthily. It is naive to assume that knowledge leads to rational choice. To view education as providing knowledge and understanding as a basis for free choice of behaviour is to ignore the fact that free choice is illusory, a point McKeown (1976) made forcibly in connection with smoking: 'It is said that the individual must be free to choose whether he wishes to smoke. But he is not free; with a drug of addiction the option is open only at the beginning, so that the critical decision to smoke is taken, not by consenting adults but by children below the age of consent. The question confronting society is not therefore whether smoking by addicts should be prohibited; it is whether it is acceptable to induce children to become addicts at an age when they neither know nor much care about the associated risks.' However, somewhat surprisingly, what is normally considered to be affective education may be essential to providing pupils with the foundations upon which *genuine* free choice may be based. This will be discussed later.

In this chapter the various affective approaches which the school may choose to adopt will be discussed, and I shall consider the implications of such decisions in relation to teaching approaches and the use of particular teaching techniques. Let us first, however, recognize that the provision of a sound knowledge base for health decisions is essential for successful health education. Let us also recognize that health education is not the only curricular subject which is committed to affective education; 'social' education and the various 'creative' and aesthetic subjects are also concerned with non-cognitive aspects of education. Paradoxically, with the prospect of a possible 'silicon chip revolution', these subjects, together with health education, may prove to be of greater significance for society than our more prestigious and traditional school disciplines.

Attitudes and Values: To Change or Merely to Explore?

There are several options open to the teacher of health education and he may decide to select all or just a few of these. His choice – if it is not determined merely by unthinking precedent – may depend on his own educational philosophy and professional ethic. It will also be governed by political factors (if we accept the definition of politics as 'the art of the possible') as well as by what is desirable. These options may well be located on a kind of continuum ranging from the cognitive through the affective to the behavioural domain of health education. I have already mentioned that although the possession of knowledge may be a necessary prerequisite for action, it is certainly not usually sufficient for behavioural change.) People may know, for instance, that contraceptives are available and even accept that their use is desirable, but might fail to put knowledge and belief into practice. A man may recognize intellectually that he is stressed and may know that stress is unhealthy but might find it impossible to take any remedial action. (Accordingly health educators may feel that they should venture from the cognitive into the affective domain and employ persuasive tactics in order to modify attitudes and change values) In some instances, of course, the use of persuasion may be omitted and a direct onslaught made on behaviour. For instance, the teacher may shape a child's behaviour by the selective use of reward and punishment: praise for being good, tidy, clean or obedient and scolding for antisocial or unhealthy activities. On occasions the teacher's approach may not differ markedly from the token reward system used in training the mentally ill or the techniques employed by the psychologist B. F. Skinner in training laboratory pigeons to play ping pong; it will merely be less efficient! *Fig.* 1.1 describes the options open to the teacher.

Fig. 1.1

Cognitive	Affective	Action
1. Provision of facts and information	5. Exploration and clarification of values	8. Developing skills and routines
2. Promotion of understanding	6. Development of approved values	
3. Development or modification of beliefs	7. Changing of undesirable values and attitudes	
4. Development of decision-making competence		

The nature of the cognitive options needs little explanation. It will be seen that they are ranged hierarchically from '1' to '4'. (The provision of facts and information is a relatively simple operation but has least value and applicability for the learner. On the other hand, it is more difficult to modify beliefs and develop general capabilities such as decision-making.

However, the benefits accruing from these teaching activities are potentially much greater. The nature of health beliefs will be discussed below. Now let us consider the affective options.

All health educationists would recognize the importance of the four cognitive options referred to above, but many would go further and insist that the values underlying behaviour and related to cognitive processes are of such importance that they cannot be ignored. They might claim, for example, that an understanding of sexuality – the 'facts of life' – should not be taught without reference to relationships and the moral issues and value judgements implicit in sexual behaviour. They might however be reluctant to impose their own values or the values of any particular class or culture in the community. For them the value clarification (VC) approach might be recommended.

Value clarification

In recent years in the USA the VC approach seems to have acquired almost cult status. Some indication of this approach is best provided by one of its chief proponents, Sidney Simon (Simon et al., 1972; Simon, 1974): ' . . . too often the important choices in life are made on the basis of peer pressure, unthinking submission to authority or the power of propaganda.' 'The values clarification approach does not aim to instil one particular set of values' but as a result of the VC process, '. . . students become . . . less apathetic, less flighty, less conforming, less over-dissenting. They are more zestful and energetic, more critical in their thinking and are more likely to follow through on decisions.'

Raths (1966), a pioneer of value clarification, claims, 'If children are helped to use the valuing process . . ., we assert that they will behave in ways that are less apathetic, confused, and irrational and in ways that are more positive, purposeful, and enthusiastic.' He goes on to quote Gardner (1964), making a point which is significant in the light of our discussion of socialization below. 'Instead of giving young people the impression that their task is to stand a dreary watch over the ancient values, we should be telling them the firm but bracing truth that it is their task to recreate those values continuously in their own time.'

The VC process is defined by Simon as a hierarchy of seven subprocesses:

PRIZING   1 Prizing and cherishing
                2 Publicly affirming, when appropriate
                3 Choosing from alternatives

CHOOSING 4   Choosing after consideration of consequences
          5   Choosing freely
ACTING   6   Acting
          7   Acting with a pattern, consistency and repetition.

Two points are worth making at this stage: first, the VC approach is by no means value-free. Rationality, zest and vigour are, for example, obviously highly prized. The second point is that if we take the seven subprocesses at face value and pursue the approach to its logical conclusion, we may have to face an outcome which would be unacceptable to most teachers.

The pupil, after having explored and clarified his beliefs and values and demonstrated that he is sensitive to the implications of his actions, would proceed to 'prize' his values and develop an integrated and consistent value system. It would not apparently matter if this system resulted in all kinds of 'antisocial' and 'unhealthy' behaviour! As Forcinelli (1974) pointed out, '. . . an educational system can produce a dishonest and potentially dysfunctional product and then merely say these are legitimate expressions of individual preferences. . . . It is possible to conceive of one going through (value clarification procedures) and deciding that he values intolerance or thieving.'

Goodlett (1976) also recognizes the problematic nature of 'pure VC' work, but emphasizes the need to teach 'responsibility' 'In order to make personally satisfying and *socially responsible* decisions . . . (children) . . . must have a good understanding of self; what one values; *what society values*; the valuing process; the effects of peer pressure; risk taking behaviours; the strategies used in making decisions; the necessary information, and the ability to identify alternatives and the consequences of behaviour.' He goes on to suggest an appropriate procedure for clarifying values, taking account of the impact of actions derived from those values on other people.

1   Encounter a problem
2   Seek help and gather information
3   Know what you want and be honest with yourself regarding your values and feelings
4   Look before you leap
5   Write down all your alternatives and identify the consequences – for and against – of each
6   Anticipate the reaction of others

7   Choose one alternative after weighing up your values
8   Try it out on someone
9   Accept the consequences
10 Evaluate your decision.

Value clarification and the question of neutrality

Implicit in the value clarification approach is the relatively neutral stance adopted by the teacher. His role is neither to promote a particular set of values nor to change attitudes. This was the approach taken by Stenhouse in the Humanities Curriculum Project (Schools Council, 1970). The project was established in 1967 to offer 'stimulus, support and materials appropriate to enquiry-based courses which cross the traditional boundaries between English, History, Geography, Religious Knowledge and Social Studies'. It was avowedly concerned with controversial issues.

Fraser (quoted in Stenhouse, 1969b) defines a controversial issue thus: 'A controversial issue involves a problem about which different individuals and groups urge conflicting courses of action. It is an issue for which society has not found a solution that can be universally or almost universally accepted. It is an issue of sufficient significance that each of the proposed ways of dealing with it is objectionable to some section of the citizenry and arouses protest. The protest may result from a feeling that a cherished belief, an economic interest, or a basic principle is threatened. It may come because the welfare of organisations or groups seems at stake.'

There is clearly a considerable difference between those issues about which there is little consensus and which therefore involve a variety of value judgements, and those issues about which there is a social consensus. It is the former type of issue with which Stenhouse was concerned. I shall argue that the latter type of issue may well require more than mere value clarification. We have so far defined a range of options open to the teacher. Let us now consider the options open to the teacher on this more specific question of handling controversial issues. One approach would be for the school to determine its policy about a particular issue and then instruct teachers to toe the line. This would rarely happen and although something of this sort might occur implicitly as part of the 'hidden curriculum', any overt statement of intent on controversial values would be avoided. In fact a common solution would be to avoid controversy wherever possible. The inadequacy of this approach is well stated by Stenhouse (1969a) when talking about a teacher's response to the question, 'Do you meet the problem of pregnancy often with your pupils?' To quote Stenhouse, 'Her reply was: "Almost never, and you'd be surprised the number who get pregnant in the year after they leave school." She said this with satisfaction. If we are to move from this attitude of custodial containment to the desire to help pupils to cope with life after they have left school, we must at some time wean them from dependence on our authority.'

A second approach is to face up to controversial issues but to allow the teacher to present his own views, at least when they are solicited. This seems reasonable at first, but Stenhouse's view was that the very nature of the teacher's authority role and the relatively authoritarian structure of the school militated against the development of independent thought and affective decision-making capabilities in the 'student'. In fact even where group discussion and enquiry-based learning are used, there is a danger that the discussion might degenerate into '. . . a guessing game about the mind of the teacher'. And as Stenhouse remarks, 'A "guessing game" is merely disguised instruction.'

For these reasons the Humanities Curriculum Project adopted not only a discussion-based, interdisciplinary approach which promoted enquiry, but defined the teacher's role as that of a 'neutral and impartial chairman and resource consultant'. The teacher's aim is not of course to teach neutrality but rather to foster *responsible* commitment in the pupil. This role will be examined later when we consider the kind of group methods which affective education demands.

Before considering those issues which may require a committed stance, it should be noted that apart from being difficult and even painful for some teachers, the neutral role may be considered to have the same miragelike qualities as health itself – worth pursuing but impossible to achieve. White (1969) challenges the concept of neutrality, pointing out that it may not only be difficult to achieve but may even run counter to the principles of true education: 'Bias is inescapable as long as one assumes that gobbets of information are going to be fed into the discussion, as described. . . . Even the "neutral" chairman-teacher has to select which gobbets to feed in and when. The rational way to minimise bias is to give children a thorough critical grounding in the background factual disciplines – social history, economics etc. so that *they* are in a position to select the relevant data against which these moral issues are to be assessed, or, at least, to evaluate the data which others introduce.'

The question is one about which teachers must decide for themselves, while taking into account the practicability of the various courses of action. In any case I shall suggest later that the approach advocated by Stenhouse may well make a major, more indirect contribution to health through the development of 'self-empowerment' in children.

Responsibility and the 'considerate way of life'

We may now consider the sixth option listed in *Fig.* 1.1, that is, the deliberate promotion of health values rather than their exploration or clarification. If the child does not value his life and health, should we not attempt to develop in him this kind of value? We would normally talk about 'responsibility' in this instance. A person should take responsibility for his health and the health of kin and community, but does this not imply some conflict with the belief that an individual should be free to choose his own pathway to health or self-destruction once he has been given the 'facts' and clarified his values? Goodlett (1976) has perhaps already offered a solution when he talked about social responsibility. There can be little question that in a democracy a school, like any other agency of socialization, has a duty to foster the belief that freedom of choice should be restricted as soon as it can be shown that exercising this freedom of choice in some way harms someone else.

It is difficult, therefore, to avoid the conclusion that the school should, in its health teaching, promote this 'considerate way of life'. In fact this rationale underlies McPhail's moral education project, *Lifeline* (McPhail et al., 1972). The project's aims are to '. . . help young people . . . in the 13–16 age range, adopt a considerate style of life . . . to take other people's needs and feelings into account as well as their own'. That this approach is consistent with Goodlett's comments is clear from a further comment by McPhail: '. . . boys and girls . . . (should) . . . see themselves as people who have a contribution to make in their community, without at the same time telling them what kind of adults they ought to be or what system of values and beliefs they ought to have'.

Living Well and the 'Considerate Way of Life'

McPhail, in addition to producing the project described above, was responsible for one of the more recent curriculum projects in health education. This is the Health Education Council Project 12–18, *Living Well*, designed for children aged twelve–eighteen (McPhail, 1977). Like the Humanities Curriculum Project, *Living Well* is a value clarification approach which asks the teacher to avoid pressing his own opinions on his pupils. He is not, however, expected to adopt the same degree of neutrality as Stenhouse's 'chairman'. McPhail also supplies evidence for discussion and role play in the form of photographs, cartoons and case study material. However, *Living Well* offers rather more specific guidelines for discussing the issues raised by the stimulus material which was derived from interviews with 480 adolescents. It also has a clearly stated aim of improving adolescent health.

'The aim of this project is to promote healthy living . . . to help adolescents and those with whom they come into contact to a better quality of life, a fuller and more satisfying experience of healthy living.' Through discussion and role play, it is argued, adolescents will develop an insight into social relationships and behaviours, and will increase not only their verbal competence but also their decision-making ability and, most importantly, will develop empathy. We have therefore moved away from neutrality and are now concerned with responsibility. It is hoped that by putting themselves '. . . in others' shoes', pupils will '. . . apply what they learn from the experience to their treatment of others'. In other words the project, like its predecessor *Lifeline*, takes as its starting point the value system we have called the 'considerate way of life'. Good health has been defined as that state which exists when an individual's mental, physical and social potential have been actualized, and for this reason self-actualization is seen by many health educationalists to be an ideal worth striving for. However, as Bandura (1969) rightly says, '. . . self-actualisation might be equally questioned on moral grounds, particularly by innocent victims of self-actualised despots or less notorious but selfish, self-directed persons'.

So it is important that the values underpinning the 'considerate way of life' are promoted by health education. Such a principle may serve as a fundamental premise and framework for those who are concerned about promoting their own value system or intervening in individual freedom to choose life or death; health or illness. *Living Well* clearly pursues this goal, although McPhail (1977) may be overoptimistic when he says that '. . . when there is a conflict between a reasonable and unreasonable reaction to behaviour, the reasonable reaction is likely to be the more influential because it is more considerate of the individual's interest and so more attractive to him'.

In fact, the project's 'healthy' message is presented clearly enough in the various scenarios portrayed in the discussion material. The discussion arising from this material will doubtless reveal that the disco noise depicted on one of the cards will indeed impair hearing; that 'a little of what you fancy' will probably not do you much good; that 'just sitting there all day in the office' is not a very healthy or interesting occupation; that high heels and a tube dress are not the best equipment for either walking or foot health; and that groping for the light socket in the dark is apt to be a shocking experience. These situations are just a few of those presented in 'And How Are We Feeling Today?' In a companion set of materials entitled 'Support Group', pupils are asked to devise means of providing support for individuals in a variety of health predicaments. The message is a positive one: responsibility is to be fostered. But what about those who are irresponsible? What about those who ignore the rational course of action or who shun the considerate way of life? Should the teacher employ his affective weapons and progress to the seventh option offered in *Fig.* 1.1 to modify values and life styles and go all out for attitude change? McKeown's (1976) comment about the involvement of behaviour in health is worth reiterating at this point. 'Our habits commonly begin as pleasures of which we have no need and end as necessities in which we have no pleasure. Nevertheless we tend to resent the suggestion that anyone should try to change them, even on the disarming grounds that they do so for our own good.'

Do we then try to change attitudes for people's own good? As we shall see this question is somewhat naive and it is important to consider just what is actually involved in determining the kind of decision a person may make (or fail to make) to protect his own (and other people's) health. If we do this we may discover some ways of promoting rational and healthy decision-making without having recourse to coercion, manipulation and persuasion which may, like attempts to shift deep-seated values and behaviours, probably be beyond the scope of school health education. If an alternative approach exists it will probably be concerned with the process of 'self-empowerment' referred to above.

Affective Education and Preventive Health Decisions

It is possible to think of three major systems contributing to an individual's intention to follow a particular course of action. One of these may be termed a belief system, the second could be called a motivation system while the third describes the effect of a variety of social pressures ranging from general social norms to pressures exerted by small groups or powerful individuals. For instance, before an individual adolescent develops an intention to act considerately by, say, dissuading a friend from riding his motorbike under the influence of drink, he must have developed certain beliefs about the dangers of driving and drinking; he must value the health and welfare of others and be able to resist the jeers of his peer group. *Fig.* 1.2 below describes this 'health action model' (Tones, 1979), whose systems we will now consider in more detail.

First, we shall examine the belief system. A belief has to do with subjective probabilities. It defines the way in which an individual views the

Fig. 1.2   A health action model

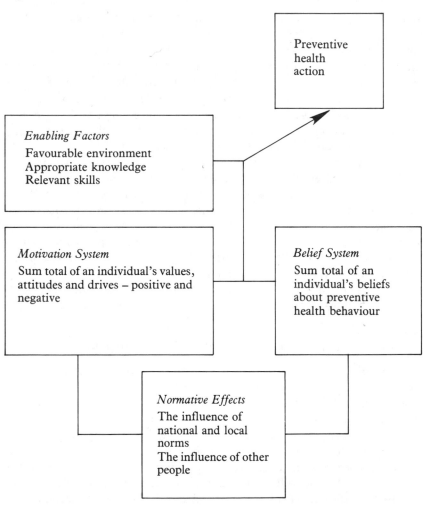

relationship between some object and its attribute, for example the relationship between exercise and health, or between smoking and lung cancer. It is common sense that unless a child is reasonably convinced that there is a high probability that walking to school will make him feel better, he is unlikely to have the slightest inclination to do so, especially when it is far more comfortable to travel by bus. Consider too the case of a teacher who is attempting to persuade her class not to take up smoking or to give it up if they are already smokers. Suppose she uses an approach which suggests that boys will not like kissing a girl whose mouth smells like an ashtray. Clearly the girls will have to accept the probability that the statement is true before they are likely to change their behaviour, and it is more than likely that their own experience and observation may be the reverse of what the teacher has claimed. In fact, if we take account of Bynner's (1969) findings that girls take up smoking in pursuit of precocity and sophistication, it is very likely that the smokers may be seen to enjoy greater sexual success than the non-smokers.

Let us consider too a typical approach to dental health education which promises caries-free experience if the child cleans his teeth regularly and zealously adheres to a diet which is free from refined carbohydrates. Obviously the child, or his parent, must believe that statement. What happens when children who do follow these precepts still find that they need fillings at the dentist and note that some children who frequent the school tuck shop seem to have perfect teeth?

The importance of health beliefs has been emphasized for many years in the 'health belief model' (Becker, 1974), which claims amongst other things that individuals will only take preventive health action if the following conditions are fulfilled:

1   The individual believes that he is *susceptible* to the health hazard; for example, he must believe that the motorbike accident *will* happen to him unless he enrols for the local authority training scheme.
2   The individual believes that ill health is *serious*; for example, he must believe it is important to have an extra few years of life and die at seventy-five rather than sixty-five.
3   The individual believes that the recommended health action is *effective*; for example, he must believe that brushing his teeth will really prevent tooth decay.
4   The individual believes that there are minimal *disadvantages* or costs involved in the recommended 'healthy' behaviour; for example, he

must not believe that being helpful and kind to other children will
result in his being labelled 'weak' or 'teacher's pet'.
5   The individual needs some 'general health motivation'; he must value
health in a positive way.

Let us now consider the motivational system shown in *Fig*. 1.2. It is
obvious that children may well believe that smoking is unhealthy or that
certain diets will be 'better for them', but that in the last analysis they may
not *care*. In other words, an individual must not only believe what he is told
but must be motivated to do something about it. Beliefs are relatively easy to
produce but motivation is notoriously difficult to achieve, especially where
this demands a change in some cherished practice or deep-seated value.
However, before we investigate the motivational system further, we should
first consider how values and motives are created through the process of
socialization.

Socialization and the Formation of Values and Attitudes

We have already referred to the school as a socialization agency. However, it
would be a mistake to assume that the teacher is necessarily the first or most
important educational influence on the child. Children bring to the school
already formed beliefs and attitudes (for instance, to alcohol, smoking and
sexuality); they are not 'attitudinal virgins'. The Jesuits affirmed, 'Give me
the child until he is seven and I will give you the man.' Proverbs 22:6
claimed, 'Train up a child in the way that he should go: and when he is old,
he will not depart from it', and the same wisdom is contained in the 'law of
primacy' which claims that primary socialization is more powerful than
secondary socialization. In other words the influence of parents, family and
home on the child during the preschool years is potentially much more
powerful than any attempts the school or other secondary socializing agencies may make to transmit values or attitudes. It is therefore apparent that
where the primary socialization process has been thorough, attempts to
resocialize (to change existing behaviours, values and attitudes) will either
meet with little success or require the use of behaviour change methods
which are likely to be viewed as unethical. The socialization process is well
illustrated by the notion of health career which is described with reference
to nutrition in *Fig*. 1.3 below.

The importance of good nutrition for health is widely recognized,
whether it be in relation to specific diseases or to general well-being. It is

Fig. 1.3   A nutrition career

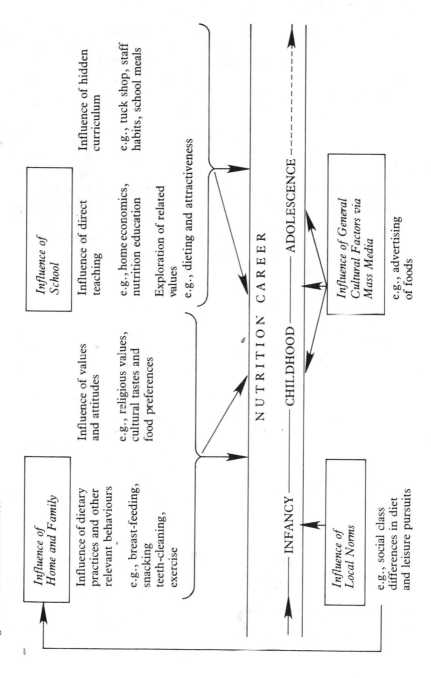

perhaps not so obvious that apart from possibly helping to minimize the risk of coronary heart disease in her offspring when they are middle-aged, the mother who breast-feeds her child may inadvertently teach to her older children the acceptability of this practice and thus make it more likely that *they* will breast-feed their children when *they* become parents. Moreover, as a kind of bonus, the mother may make a contribution to her children's sex education by creating more frank and open attitudes to sexuality and nudity. The parent who takes regular exercise and encourages his children to do so is establishing a norm which may well reduce the chance of his children becoming obese in later life. The development of a taste for foods high in dietary fibre may also have a preventive function just as the inadvertent creation of a 'sweet tooth' may have harmful effects such as dental caries and a weight problem.

I have so far referred to primary and secondary socialization and described how parents, schools, peer groups and other agencies promote health-related values and attitudes. They also produce knowledge and beliefs relating to these values which help to buttress these values against attack from any outside agencies intent upon producing some change in attitudes or life style. Such knowledge is not necessarily transmitted formally; in primary socialization parents would 'teach' their children informally and may well get it all wrong, as the many 'old wives' tales' relating to sex and childbirth clearly demonstrate. These values, attitudes and beliefs are internalized by the child, who draws on this affective reservoir and uses it as a basis for decisions, both during childhood and later in adult life. When exhorted by the health educationalist to modify her diet, say, or view cancer with less apprehension, her decision about what to eat or whether to have a cyto test may be largely determined by previous socialization. We should therefore consider critically the stance adopted by some educationalists who believe that it is unethical or uneducational to do more than provide clear information and leave the individual to make a free and informed choice. As we said earlier, in many instances such free choice is illusory. It may be necessary to make informed decision-making genuinely possible; we may need to support our information with persuasion so that the individual is in a better position to make a more unbiased choice, although as we shall see there may be another way – the way of 'self-empowerment'.

In all this we must remember that there is an all-pervasive, secondary socializing influence operating throughout the health career: the influence of the general or local cultural climate, often transmitted via the mass media. It is beyond the scope of this chapter to discuss the function of the mass media, but it is worth commenting on the naive faith which many seem to have in the power of, say, television to influence attitudes and behaviour. It is argued that if only health education had at its disposal sufficient funds to lavish on spectacular media advertising, the health product would be sold to its apathetic consumers. Nothing could be further from the truth; where people are neither committed to nor ready for change, the mass media may indeed produce a significant change. However, where the message which is presented involves the expenditure of effort, reduces pleasure or produces some degree of suffering, which is precisely what much health education requires of its client, then the media will have a negligible effect. As Murrow (1963) said, 'Propaganda is limited by prevailing interests, social trends, and prejudices; it is encouraged by ignorance of the facts.' However, 'the propagandist can retard or accelerate a trend in public opinion, but he cannot reverse it'. If we wish to promote values and stimulate behaviour, it is to primary socialization that we must turn.

There are of course several instances where an individual adopts behaviours which do not seem to have been socialized in him during his early years or at a later stage by any distinguishable agency such as the school. People seem to acquire values and adopt behaviours in anticipation of some future role: as adolescents they act out what they perceive to be an appropriate adult role; as future mothers they play the part prescribed for them; as they approach retirement they may adopt what they perceive to be appropriate behaviours for the elderly and the pensioner. This phenomenon is often referred to as anticipatory socialization, and may also be illustrated by reference to individuals who adopt life styles and norms which are characteristic of some 'reference group', that is, a group to which they do not in fact belong but to which they aspire, probably because they covet the material benefits, status or prestige of such a group. It might be argued that the tendency for immigrant minorities to bottle-feed their infants is due to their adoption of a behaviour which symbolizes the material advantages of Western society. If we believe that one of the school's more important functions is to provide its pupils with an 'outfit for life', then it must play an important part in the anticipatory socialization of children; it must prepare the adolescent for his adult role. Indeed, the term 'family life education' gives a clear indication of its anticipatory function. One of the more obvious tasks of health education is to explore and clarify the values and norms underlying the behaviours which are implicit in many adult roles and reference group activities, together with the implications of those values and behaviours.

Let us now reconsider *Fig*. 1.2(Health education may, as we have seen, be concerned with the development of accurate and appropriate beliefs. It may be concerned with the development of values, and we have suggested that the most important and generally acceptable value may well be the one underlying the 'considerate way of life'. It may also be concerned merely to explore existing values and clarify their implications, and perhaps check them against the basic criteria of 'responsibility' and the 'considerate way of life'. Should the school, however, go further and attempt to change existing values where they are seen to be 'unhealthy'? Should the inconsiderate and antisocial pupil be resocialized, always supposing that it is possible to reverse the influence of primary socialization? Before taking this question any further, let us note the third main component in *Fig*. 1.2: the set of influences described in terms of normative effects. We must never forget how important other people are in affecting an individual's health decisions. One part of a person's belief system will be a cluster of beliefs about how other people will react to any given action. For instance, 'What will mother, dad, my school friends or other significant people think if I smoke?', 'How will my parents react if I tell them that my Home Economics teacher thinks the food we eat at home is unhealthy?' These beliefs are important but will of course only influence the health decision if the individual is motivated to take account of them; if, for instance, they are at all bothered about what their parents, teachers or friends may think.

Arguably the general influences of national norms will have less effect on the individual than immediate local expectations, while the close network of immediate family and family friends will be most powerful of all. The influence of the immediate environment on an individual's health career is especially significant when we take into account the well-documented social class gradient in health (Stacey, 1977). There is a consistent improvement in virtually every health measure as we move from social class V to social class I. A similar phenomenon may be observed in the use made of health services (with the exception perhaps of social services), a fact which led Hart (1965) to coin the term 'inverse care law', signifying that those who least need the services make most use of them. The social environment will perpetuate these differences by influencing values, attitudes and routines, often by providing bad examples. Consider, for instance, the different rates of smoking in different social classes. In 1976 29% of social class I males were smoking compared with 52% of social class V males. In the same year, 24% of social class I women smoked compared with 43% of social class V women (Cappell, 1978).

It is evident that one of the functions of health education will be to examine this kind of influence in the context of value clarifying discussion. For example, what are commercial advertisements trying to do and how are they seeking to do it when they invite appeal to emergent feminism in selling cigarettes for newly liberated women? What should we do when the gang whose 'machismo' you admired expect you to steal and smoke? Is male toughness really related to hard drinking and smoking; is it really good to be sophisticated?

A variety of possibilities for health education are shown in *Fig.* 1.2. Any one input may be sufficient to trigger some appropriate health-related decision. In terms of 'enabling factors', an individual may well believe that contraception is necessary to prevent unwanted pregnancies and may actually subscribe to the set of values we have labelled 'the considerate way of life'. However, he may lack the specific knowledge about where to seek family planning advice, or perhaps more importantly the social skill needed to purchase over-the-counter contraceptives! The question which each health education teacher must face is how far he is prepared to go in promoting change. Typically the greatest uncertainty will be about whether it is feasible or desirable to actually change values. In considering this, the teacher should bear in mind that the motivation system consists of an aggregate of both positive and negative values and attitudes. The strength and direction of the motivational 'push' will be the result of the sum of all these separate components, as indicated in *Fig.* 1.2.

Some of these components will be especially powerful and are usually termed 'drives'. For instance, unsatisfied hunger and thirst would be particularly powerful and outweigh less powerful values and interests. Although drives of this nature are not likely to concern educators in Western society, the drives of sexuality, or such 'acquired' drives as alcohol addiction or smoking, have an obvious influence on much health-related behaviour. Few teachers would feel that it was either appropriate or ethical to try to change religious values, even if such values militated against the teacher's heart-felt conviction about the importance of promoting family planning. Similarly a determined attempt to modify the cultural values and beliefs of ethnic minorities about, say, diet or clothing, would be unacceptable to many.

However, what about that most significant of values – self-esteem? We accumulate a whole set of beliefs about ourselves, such as how other people regard us, how intelligent or likeable we are, what kind of body we have and how attractive it is to the opposite sex. This amalgam of beliefs is the self-concept. The extent to which we value and respect our self-concept is usually described in terms of self-esteem. It is usually considered that a positive self-image and high self-esteem are conducive to good mental health. It is also reasonably well established that high self-esteem provides an individual with a degree of independence that allows him to resist pressure from, say, peer groups, and have the courage of his convictions. It could well prove to be the case that to modify an individual's self-esteem would enable him to resist many antihealth pressures from individuals and shrug off the blandishments of the media to smoke or consume alcohol, for example. Changing this particular value might be one of the single most effective health education measures at our disposal. Is it ethical to do so? I suspect that few teachers would have any objection to changing this kind of value from negative to positive.

Self-Empowerment and Health

The question of self-esteem leads directly to the broader issue of self-empowerment. The term is vague and emotive but of potentially great significance for health education. Earlier in this chapter reference was made to a major dilemma which health educationalists had to face. We may feel that it is unethical to use any degree of coercion to oblige individuals to modify their manifestly unhealthy behaviour. We would wish to avoid this kind of paternalism and would prefer people to make an informed choice of behaviour once they are in full possession of the facts (provided of course that they adopted the 'considerate way of life'!).

However, despite our concern to protect individual freedoms, we have pointed out already how people are rarely in a position to choose freely; their addictions, their socialization and the social pressures they face all conspire to bias their decision-making and their choices. Self-empowerment is a process designed to restore decision-making capabilities and to equip individuals with a belief in their autonomy, together with the skills necessary to enable them to decide what to do about their own health, their family's health and the health of the community. Hopson and Scally (1981) argue strongly that the school should provide a kind of self-empowering 'survival and growth kit for an age of future shock. . . . a school should provide a basic survival kit for young people . . . they need to be taught skills like value clarification, decision-making, how to cope with crises, intellectual and emotional problem-solving, helping, assertiveness, relationship building, how to find appropriate information and use personal and physical resources which are available in the community. They need to be made more aware of themselves, others and the world around them, in order to become more self-empowered people.'

Approaches such as decision-making and value clarification have been mentioned already. I would now like to consider four important and related elements which are involved in the self-empowerment process. They are the development of deferred gratification, the promotion of self-esteem, instruction in key social skills and the development of internal locus of control.

Deferred gratification

A common factor in many health education messages is an exhortation to young people to avoid certain behaviours because they will damage their health. The exhortation may typically be accompanied by a threat, overt or veiled, that something unpleasant may happen. Alternatively health education may offer a prospect of some reward, such as good health, fitness or the prospect of a longer life. In both cases reward or punishment are scheduled for some dim and distant future time, so distant in fact as to be meaningless. The problem is compounded by the fact that the behaviour to be changed may be intrinsically rewarding, either physically or socially, and the new behaviour may demand effort or even be unpleasant or exhausting! In other words the young person may be asked to defer present gratification for some future long-term reward. Now clearly if one of the major values in an individual's motivation system involves such deferred gratification, then the health measure proposed will appear much more attractive. To possess such a deferred gratification capability is clearly self-empowering.

Various investigators have demonstrated that techniques of child-rearing differ from one social class to another, as do the emotional climate of the home and parental approaches to discipline. It is very probable that an acceptance of the importance of deferring gratification for a better, long-term pay-off is built into children during the process of primary socialization. It is perhaps suggestive that the adoption of health measures, such as jogging and non-smoking, to combat premature coronary artery disease is primarily a feature of middle-class groups. It would not be surprising if the deferred gratification value was largely responsible. The teacher who is concerned with promoting self-empowerment must therefore ask whether he has at his disposal techniques to develop a deferred gratification value where none has been previously socialized.

Self-esteem

Self-esteem is more obviously associated with health; it is generally accepted that high self-esteem is a component of mental health. The individual who is high in self-esteem is happier and copes better with the various stresses and strains of life. Less obvious perhaps is the fact that people who enjoy high self-esteem seem to be more capable of autonomous thought; not only do they form their own opinions but they have the courage of their convictions (Coopersmith, 1967). As we have already indicated, the individual is exposed to many antihealth influences during his health career; he is under pressure from both the mass media and his peer group to adopt behaviours which may be unhealthy or antisocial. For all of these reasons, it is clear that the promotion of self-esteem is an important feature of health education, a fact which the Schools Council Health Education Project 5–13 (Schools Council, 1976) clearly recognizes:

> The second idea which has influenced our thinking very much is our belief that the way in which children see themselves is important in deciding how they might behave in a variety of circumstances. . . . Do they come to school predisposed to achievement and success or to under-achievement and failure? Children will have developed many different perceptions about themselves and their abilities which can be thought of as invisible tags which accompany them everywhere. . . .

Education to foster self-esteem involves several processes (Hamachek, 1971; Samuels, 1977). First, it is important to deal with the cognitive, belief element, to have the child develop a realistic self-concept, that is, a set of beliefs and 'images' which defines the individual's subjective assessment of his real self. Obviously it is not at all beneficial to create a realistic self-concept if the reality is unsatisfactory. It is therefore important to try to modify the child's actual self so that he becomes more competent, more acceptable to his peers and generally worthy of esteem. Again SCHEP 5–13 suggests ways of doing this which require the teacher carefully to plan activities for the child which he can achieve, albeit with difficulty, thus enhancing self-esteem.

Social relationships are of great importance in self-esteem education. Apart from the obvious parental influence on a child's self-esteem, his classmates will play a major part in determining his level of self-respect. The teacher's task is therefore twofold: first, to sensitize children to the ways in which they can affect other children's well-being – which is all part of the promotion of a 'considerate way of life'; and secondly, to equip the individual child with actual social and personal skills which will make him or her more genuinely accepted. We must not forget, of course, the ways in which the teacher himself may improve or damage the child's self-esteem, usually inadvertently. The effect of the whole ethos and structure of the school on children's self-esteem is also well documented, for example the negative effect of streaming on those in lower streams and the labelling process which Hargreaves (1967) aptly described in his identification of a 'delinquescent' subculture of recalcitrant drop-outs in the secondary school.

Social skills training

Social relationships are therefore important in the development of self-esteem. They are also an important element in their own right for the promotion of social health and self-empowerment. We may identify two main features in social skills training: the first has to do with improving techniques of interacting with others. For instance, assertiveness training would be useful in increasing social competence (Galassi and Galassi, 1977). Training in the social techniques involved in relating to the opposite sex would be valuable for the adolescent in fostering his heterosexual develop-ment and his self-confidence; it would fit well into an integrated scheme of sex education and education for personal relationships. Perhaps more important, however, are those social skills referred to in connection with self-esteem: the sensitivity training designed to help individuals react to the needs of their peers, their parents and, later, their children. Brown (1978) has shown convincingly how the ability to communicate on an affective basis with a spouse or friend is an important 'immunizing' factor against depressive illness. It is difficult to imagine the potential benefits for the health of society which could be derived from teaching 'everyday counsel-ling' skills to children in school.

Locus of control

Social relationship teaching is correlated with the promotion of self-esteem, and self-esteem is itself correlated with the fourth of the main elements in self-empowerment – what has been called 'locus of control' (Fitch, 1970). Like self-esteem, locus of control is significantly related to health behaviours. The concept of locus of control is derived from Rotter's (1954) social learning theory. As *Fig.* 1.2 indicates, health decisions result from motivation and beliefs; for instance, an individual must have the motivation to lose weight but must also believe that it is possible for her to do so. Rotter argued that people differed in the extent of their belief in the possibility of achieving their goals and desires. Some people believe that they are masters of their own destiny and their locus of control was said to be internal. An internal locus of control is clearly therefore self-empowering.

On the other hand, those having an external locus of control are more likely to believe that goal attainment is under the control of powerful external forces such as luck, fate or powerful others. Various researchers have demonstrated that external locus of control is associated more with sickness, while internal control is associated with non-smoking (James et al., 1965), reduction or cessation of smoking (Strickland, 1973), greater likelihood of contraceptive practice (Lundy, 1972), weight loss (Jeffrey and Christensen, 1972), seatbelt usage (Williams, 1972) and preventive dental care (Dabbs and Kirscht, 1971). Of particular importance to health educators at a time when the importance of self-reliance and self-care is being emphasized is Seeman and Evans' (1962) finding that 'internals' knew more about their medical condition, were more inquisitive with doctors and nurses and indicated less satisfaction with the amount of information received in hospitals.

An illustration of the nature of these beliefs is provided by items from the 'Children's Health Locus of Control Scale' described by Parcel and Mexer (1978). The letter (I) indicates internal locus of control, (P) indicates external locus of control in which the individual believes he is controlled by powerful others (e.g., significant others in *Fig.* 1.2 or 'authority' generally), while (C) refers to beliefs in control by chance or fate.

I can do things to keep me from getting sick. (I)
If I get sick, it is because getting sick just happens. (C)
My mother must tell me how to keep from getting sick. (P)
Only a doctor or a nurse keeps me from getting sick. (P)
When I am sick I can do things to get better. (I)
If I get hurt it is because accidents just happen. (C)
Other people must tell me what to do when I feel sick. (P)
The teacher must tell me how to keep from having accidents at school. (P)
Other people must tell me how to stay healthy. (P)
There are things I can do to have healthy teeth. (I)

We mentioned earlier the link between self-esteem and locus of control, and equally significant is the link between locus of control and deferred gratification. Phares (1976) reports on several studies demonstrating this association. The importance of deferred gratification has already been mentioned, but it is worth reiterating Phares' words, 'To attain control over one's environment, to achieve competence, or to reach positions of power and influence generally, all require that the individual eschew the lure of the present for the greater promise of the future.' To this list we should add the achievement of health.

Methods and Resources for Health Education

Although this is not the place for a detailed discussion of health education methodology, some mention of methods is essential since any involvement in affective education, whether it be concerned with attitude change, value clarification or self-empowerment, demands the adoption of methods which may well differ from those ordinarily employed. These methods will also demand more from the majority of teachers.

Attitude change techniques

Analyses of successful attitude change ventures usually focus on one or more of four factors: audience factors, message factors, source factors and method factors. Teachers are of course familiar with the need to take account of the characteristics of their pupils, certainly in relation to cognitive aspects such as intelligence or developmental stage. Those engaged in the business of attitude change would, however, need to adopt the adage of 'different strokes for different folks' and to carefully choose a method appropriate to their audience. For example, they may adopt different tactics or construct a different message for 'internals' as opposed to 'externals', who might be expected to respond better to an appeal to authority. Authority is clearly a source factor of some significance. Most people are well aware of the ways in which commercial advertising carefully chooses an attractive or authoritative sponsor for its product. In the context of teaching we should not forget the possible influence of a teacher's personality on a child's attitudes and beliefs, in spite of what the teacher actually says or teaches. This point is made strongly by Curriculum Paper 14 (Scottish Education Department, 1974):

> . . . information loses its credibility if the teacher is known not to practise what he preaches. . . .
> . . . possibly nothing does more to obscure the clarity of the anti-smoking message than the blue haze which emanates from the staff room.

We have already mentioned the effect of the 'hidden curriculum' on attitudes, and a teacher's personality and behaviour are inextricably entwined with the 'hidden curriculum'. The relevance of this for the neutral stance referred to above is obvious. There are those too who would argue that if the school is serious about promoting responsible and healthy decision-making, it may only achieve this goal by actually allowing children to make decisions and exercise responsibility!

Before focusing on methods, it is worth commenting on message factors in attitude change. Once again advertising exemplifies the attention given to the careful structuring of a persuasive message. Health educators should perhaps learn from the advertisers who go to great lengths to avoid generating anxiety and fear. There is clear evidence that the arousal of fear is frequently counterproductive. But how often do teachers use fear appeal in order to deter drug taking and stamp out smoking?

If we are to look at the study of persuasive communications for advice on attitude change methods, then we would learn first that any methods used should be interpersonal, as opposed to the use of film or mass media. There are two kinds of interpersonal method which concern us here: face-to-face counselling and the use of small groups. Clearly role play, an important tool in affective education, may be employed in either of these two situations.

Everyday counselling

The importance of source factors has already been mentioned, and this principle is further developed in the theory and practice of counselling. The term 'counselling' is still somewhat vague, but would usually not be used to describe persuasion attempts although some of the skills of the counsellor may well put him in an influential position. A discussion of counselling is beyond the scope of this book, so I will content myself with suggesting that key counsellor skills should be part of the repertoire of any teacher working in the affective domain. These skills also merge imperceptibly with those of the successful group leader.

In the first place the teacher should be sensitive, in other words he should be capable of picking up subtle gradations of feeling from his client; he should be skilled in interpreting non-verbal communication. A second feature of the counselling situation which is of significance in many persuasion attempts and which needs careful handling, is that of self-disclosure. The client/pupil will inevitably reveal many of his values and feelings, and it is clearly important that he should not regret doing this. This in effect means that the teacher must carefully control self-disclosure and ensure that the prevailing climate is warm and accepting. It is perhaps for this reason that the 'holy trinity' of counselling has been described as 'respect, empathy, and genuineness'. The counsellor should possess these qualities, which also characterize the successful supportive group. Let us note in addition that a recently formulated recipe for successful attitude change has been described as involving the promotion of self-disclosure followed by 'quasi-unconditional positive regard' (Janis, 1975). In other words providing respect, empathy and genuineness, but only on condition that the client makes an effort to modify his unhealthy behaviour!

Before considering the group as an instrument of affective education, let us recall a point made earlier. If one of our aims in self-empowerment education is to promote a variety of social skills – and a 'considerate way of life' – then we are certainly concerned with promoting the very skills which we have said the teacher needs to be an effective 'everyday' counsellor (see, for instance, Carkhuff, 1973). Perhaps children should be taught the 'life skill' of counselling. I must emphasize that the kind of counselling to which I have referred is not the trouble-shooting, therapeutic variety, except in the very broadest, primary preventive sense. The former kind needs special training; the latter kind might well be provided by a relatively short period of in-service training. Such training would inevitably involve the same sort of value clarification process involved in the kind of health education already discussed.

Work with groups

The use of group discussion in changing attitudes has been well documented and derives from the classic work of Kurt Lewin in the 1940s (Lewin, 1947). Lewin and his collaborators used a technique which is now called group discussion-decision, to modify attitudes to such practices as infant feeding and meal preparation. The critical element in successful group work of this kind seemed to be connected with the group reaching a decision in the context of a climate of general agreement. More recently Bond (1958) demonstrated the superiority of this approach in persuading women to carry out breast self-examination as compared with a more didactic, lecture-type approach. Affective education in school, however, is likely to be concerned not with changing attitudes of this kind but with the exploration of values and questions of health and responsibility. Before considering this approach in more detail, let us note now that for genuine understanding of issues of any kind, the evidence for the superiority of group discussion is overwhelmingly strong. The problem is that the technique is costly in terms of time, especially since membership numbers of between twelve and sixteen are usually recommended.

Group work and the neutral chairman

The question of authority and source characteristics was mentioned above. The Humanities Curriculum Project (HCP), as we have seen, specified the role of a neutral chairman to deal with this difficulty. Let us consider briefly what happens in a typical HCP session. First, the teacher will help his group to explore controversial issues in a non-didactic way. His duty is to foster continuity of discussion, represent alternative or minority views, challenge consensus and complacency and try to minimize the effect of individual dominance. He will use a pack of stimulus materials in order to introduce 'evidence'; these materials include pictures, cartoons, newspaper reports, extracts from literature, tape recordings and film. In this way he will avoid introducing his own biases and will ensure that all issues are explored. He will habitually clarify, summarize, question and reflect back upon questions raised within the group. The relationship with his pupils will be democratic; pupils are, revealingly, termed 'students'. Out of this process it is hoped that rationality, sensitivity, imaginativeness, tolerance and co-operation will emerge. As we shall see there is some evidence that this may indeed be the case.

The issues with which McPhail is concerned are perhaps less controversial and the pursuit of the 'considerate way of life' is more obvious. Neutrality is not sacrosanct and the development of sensitivity and empathy is a major aim. The dialectical flavour of *Living Well* is revealed by the kind of questions which guide the use of the pictorial 'evidence'. For instance, pupils are asked to discuss what 'A' is saying to 'B' in a particular picture. Pupils are asked to imagine how they would feel in 'A's position and in 'B's position. How would other people other than 'A' and 'B' be affected by the exchange? The move towards the development of social skills is implicit in the question, 'Can you suggest better ways of handling the situation?' Discussion leads naturally to simulation and provides an opportunity for emotional involvement and the development of empathy and, perhaps, decision-making skills.

Group work and personal growth

So far we have examined group discussion-based approaches which have explored health issues generally and, perhaps incidentally, have been concerned with other health-related factors such as the promotion of decision-making skills or the fostering of self-esteem. Certain other approaches seek to use the group experience to develop various personal attributes in the pursuit of what might be called mental or social health. One such approach was developed by Button (1974) with youth workers and later applied to secondary schools. Button quotes Ottaway's (1966) description of developmental group work as 'the normal man's therapy'. He himself sees group work as a process concerned with '. . . building the social competence of the individual so that he becomes more capable of dealing with his own problems'. Developmental group work should also encourage self-reliance and self-discovery, and its relation to self-esteem and education for responsibility is self-evident. More particularly, developmental group work involves 'an examination of . . . feelings towards authority and the nature of authority, and into an exploration of friendship, of loneliness and of a wide range of other relationships. Some will examine sexual relationships and feelings and may need basic information about sex, and others will be concerned with parents and family, their own childhood and themselves.' (Button, 1974). This last comment serves to remind us that even where there is emphasis on group processes, the cognitive element is still important. The main focus, however, is on relationships and the dynamics of social interaction.

Grainger (1970) describes a related approach which has much in common with sensitivity training or T-groups, whose main function is to examine human interaction and group life by experiencing it and observing it. Grainger's aim was to '. . . extend the principle of free discovery into the realm of personal relationships, and to help children to discover themselves and to discover a morality by which to live'. The prospect of this kind of involvement will be threatening to most teachers, even to those who are committed to affective education. Grainger claims that the risks taken are nonetheless justified, given that children should experience personal relationships rather than just talk about them: '. . . unless we, as adults, will risk being personally involved in the moral education of children, such education is likely to remain an affair of the head without ever touching the heart'.

Let us remind ourselves of what we might hope to achieve from using group work and then consider if it is possible at all to minimize threat and reduce risk. Apart from discussing health issues and the various values and behaviours underlying these issues, we are hoping to develop in children certain characteristics and skills which will facilitate genuine free choice of action and promote responsibility and, ultimately, improve health. In particular we would hope to promote self-esteem as a significant feature of well-being and as a factor related to self-empowerment. We wish to potentiate the deferring of gratification and develop an internal locus of control, as these factors will better equip an individual to make rational health choices. We wish also to improve social relationships and sensitivities as the former seem to be important to most people's well-being and the latter essential to considerate and caring behaviour. The group approach, together with related activities (not forgetting the influence of the 'hidden curriculum'), seems to offer the best chance of achieving these goals. Given some degree of training in sensitivity and counselling, most teachers would be capable of using this approach. They will, however, do so more readily if they have at their disposal a variety of structured experiences to feed into group work and use rather like the stimulus material supplied as 'evidence' by the Humanities Curriculum Project and *Living Well*. Hopson and Scally (1981) have described a range of such techniques. The Schools Council Health Education Project 5–13 suggests, in addition, the use of a game designed to foster sensitivity and facilitate self-esteem. In this, children are asked to discuss a particular issue while wearing labels of which they themselves are ignorant. The group is told to follow the instructions on the labels, such as 'Ignore me', 'Treat me with respect'. Subsequently the children discuss their feelings and may become more aware of the way in which their behaviour may affect other people.

Self-awareness may also be promoted by playing card games which reward risk-taking with bonus points. For instance, the risk involved in asking group members to say what they most admire about the individual playing the card. Hoeper et al. (1974) describe a whole series of such 'awareness games' which are designed to stimulate various characteristics: social interaction, group roles and pressures, empathy. There are also exercises to develop self-assertion, which has an obvious link with internal locus of control. Thayer (1976) suggests some fifty strategies for experimental learning designed, amongst other things, to promote awareness of self and others and develop affective communication skills.

Evaluation

We have considered a range of approaches to affective education which centre on group techniques and involve various structured experimental learning situations. In all this the importance of the teacher possessing certain basic counselling skills has been stressed. It is important of course to know how well these approaches actually work. How successful is affective education, especially when compared with the impact of the primary socialization function of home and family? Unfortunately it is rare for any approach in education to be evaluated in an objective way. However the Humanities Curriculum Project is an exception to this rule. The development team administered a battery of some twenty-one objective tests in addition to the usual more intuitive evaluation of curriculum projects.

In brief, statistically significant shifts were demonstrated in intelligence, conscientiousness, adventurousness, self-sufficiency, comprehension, vocabulary, reduced hostility, awareness of social problems and two measures of self-esteem. It will be apparent that several of these measures relate to the self-empowerment dimension already discussed. Of particular significance was the observation that these objectively measured benefits were only noticeable in schools in which teachers had been trained in the proper use of the group approach; where untrained teachers employed the materials, the results were no different from those of the control schools.

To return finally to the options available to teachers of health education, teachers must decide whether they are to limit themselves to a more traditional cognitive function in health education or whether they will venture into the more difficult but rewarding affective domain. They have to decide just how far they will venture into the interior; whether they will restrict themselves to crossing the frontier and exploring values or whether they will involve themselves with the kind of group work and structured experiences which are designed to foster personal and social growth in their pupils. Whatever they do, it is important that they are well prepared. Teacher education and training in the necessary skills are the essential ingredients of success in this field.

Summary

The affective aspects of education pose particular problems for the school and this is reflected in the difficulties faced by health education in its efforts to gain access to a crowded curriculum. While the provision of health information and the promotion of decision-making skills present little challenge, controversial issues, values and attitude change strategies all offer a threat to the equanimity of teachers. Nonetheless affective education may prove to be the major benefit which schools might bestow on their pupils.

While deliberate attempts to change health attitudes might not be the concern of school health education, the exploration and clarification of health values as a basis for decision-making are of great importance. Although the adoption of a neutral stance in values education has much to recommend it, teachers cannot realistically avoid subscribing to certain key values related to the acquisition of responsibility and a 'considerate way of life'.

In order to operate effectively and coherently within the affective domain, teachers must understand the ways in which beliefs, motives, interpersonal influences and other sociopsychological factors govern an individual's health decisions. They must also be aware of how the process of socialization influences the formation of values and attitudes and gives rise to a kind of health career. Only through an understanding of the dynamic interplay of all these factors can the school determine the ways in which it might most effectively develop affective education. However, even if a school undertakes the difficult task of exploring and promoting values, it will not have done enough to enable pupils to make genuinely informed and responsible health decisions. In order to do this the goal of self-empowerment must be pursued; children must be taught 'life skills', their self-esteem must be enhanced, their capabilities improved and their belief in their capacity to control their own lives must be strengthened.

If affective education is to be successful, conventional teaching methods will need to be supplemented. Teachers will need to acquire group teaching skills and the strategies of everyday counselling. Moreover, they will need to recognize and control the manifold influences of the 'hidden curriculum'.

References

Advisory Committee on Alcoholism (1977) *Report on the Prevention of Alcoholism*. London, DHSS.

Bandura, A. (1969) *Principles of Behaviour Modification*. London, Holt, Rinehart & Winston.

Becker, M. H. (1974) 'The health belief model and personal health behaviour'. *Hlth Educ. Monogr.*, vol. 2, no. 4.

Benjamin, H. (1971) 'The saber-tooth curriculum', in Hooper, R. (ed.), *The Curriculum: Context, design and development*. Edinburgh, Oliver & Boyd.

Bond, B. W. (1958) 'A study in health education methods'. *Int. J. Hlth Educ.*, vol. 1, no. 1.

British Nutrition Foundation, DHSS and Health Education Council (1977)

Nutrition Education (joint report). London, HMSO.

Brown, G. W. (1978) 'Depression: a sociological view', in Tuckett, D. (ed.), *Basic Readings in Medical Sociology*. London, Tavistock.

Button, L. (1974) *Developmental Group Work with Adolescents*. London, Hodder & Stoughton.

Bynner, J. M. (1969) *The Young Smoker*. Government Social Survey. London, HMSO.

Cappell, P. J. (1978) 'Trends in cigarette smoking in the United Kingdom'. *Health Trends*, vol. 10, pp. 49–54.

Carkhuff, R. R. (1973) *The Art of Helping, An introduction to life skills*. Amherst, Mass., Human Resource Development Press.

Coopersmith, S. (1967) *The Antecedents of Self Esteem*. Oxford, W. H. Freeman.

Dabbs, J. M. and Kirscht, J. P. (1971) 'Internal control and the taking of influenza shots'. *Psychol. Rep.*, vol. 28, pp. 959–962.

Department of Health and Social Security (1977) *Fit for the Future* (The Court Report). Report of the Committee on Child Health Services. London, HMSO.

Expenditure Committee (House of Commons) (1977) *Preventive Medicine*. First Report 1976–1977. London, HMSO.

Fitch, G. (1970) 'Effects of self esteem, perceived performance, and choice on causal attributions'. *J. Pers. Soc. Psy.*, vol. 16, pp. 311–315.

Forcinelli, O. (1974) 'Values education in the public school'. *Thrust*, March 1974.

Galassi, M. D. and Galassi, J. P. (1977) *Assert Yourself! How to Be Your Own Person*. New York, Human Sciences Press.

Gardner, J. W. (1964) *Self Renewal*. New York, Harper & Row.

Goldstein, M. (1975) 'Defining and studying health at the college level'. *Int. J. Hlth Educ.*, vol. XVIII, no. 4, pp. 241–253.

Goodlett, D. E. (1976) 'Values clarification – where does it belong?' *Hlth Educ.*, vol. 7, no. 2, March–April.

Grainger, A. J. (1970) *The Bullring: A classroom experiment in moral education*. Oxford, Pergamon Press.

Hamachek, D. E. (1971) *Encounters with the Self*. London, Holt, Rinehart & Winston.

Hargreaves, D. (1967) *Social Relations in a Secondary School*. London, Routledge & Kegan Paul.

Hart, J. T. (1965) 'The inverse care law', in Cox, C. and Mead, A. (eds), *A Sociology of Medical Practice*. West Drayton, Middx, Collier Macmillan.

Hirst, P. (1969) 'The logic of the curriculum'. *J. Curric. Studies*, vol. 1, no. 2, pp. 142–158.

Hoeper, C., Kutzleb, U., Stobbe, A. and Weber, B. (1974) *Awareness Games*. New York, St Martin's Press.

Hopson, B. and Scally, M. (1981) *Lifeskills Teaching*. London, McGraw-Hill.

James, W. H., Woodruff, A. B. and Werner, W. (1965) 'Effect of internal and external control upon changes in smoking behaviour'. *J. Consult. Psychol.*, vol. 29, pp. 184–186.

Janis, I. (1975) 'Effectiveness of social support for stressful decisions', in Deutsch, M. (ed.), *Applying Social Psychology*. New York, John Wiley.

Jeffrey, D. B. and Christensen, E. R. (1972) *The Relative Efficacy of Behaviour Therapy, Will-power and Non-treatment Control Procedures for Weight Loss*. New York, Association for Advancement of Behaviour Therapy.

Lewin, K. (1947) 'Frontiers in group dynamics: concept, method and reality in social science; social equilibria and social change'. *Human Relations*, vol. 1, no. 1, pp. 5–42.

Lundy, J. R. (1972) 'Some personality correlates of contraceptive use among unmarried female college students'. *J. Personality*, vol. 80, pp. 9–14.

McKeown, T. (1976) *The Role of Medicine: Dream, mirage, or nemesis?* London, Nuffield Provincial Hospitals Trust.

McPhail, P. (1977) *Living Well*. Health Education Council Project 12–18. Cambridge, Cambridge University Press.

McPhail, P., Ungoed-Thomas, J. R. and Chapman, H. (1972) *Moral Education in the Secondary School*. London, Longman.

Murrow, E. (1963) In Brown, J. A. C. (ed.), *Techniques of Persuasion*. London, Penguin.

Osman, J. (1973) 'A rationale for using value clarification in health education'. *J. Sch. Hlth*, vol. XLIII, no. 10.

Ottaway, A. K. C. (1966) *Learning Through Group Experience*. London, Routledge & Kegan Paul.

Parcel, G. S. and Mexer, M. D. (1978) 'Development of an instrument to measure children's health locus of control'. *Hlth Educ. Monogr.*, vol. 6, no. 2, pp. 149–159.

Phares, E. J. (1976) *Locus of Control in Personality*. Morristown, N.J., Silver Burdett.

Raths, L. E., Merrill, H. and Simon, B. S. (1966) *Values and Teaching*.

Wembley, Middx, Merrill.

Rotter, J. B. (1954) *Social Learning and Clinical Psychology*. Englewood Cliffs, N.J., Prentice-Hall.

Samuels, S. C. (1977) *Enhancing Self Concepts in Early Childhood*. New York, Human Sciences Press.

Schools Council (1970) Humanities Curriculum Project. London, Heinemann.

Schools Council (1972) *Humanities Curriculum Project Evaluation Report*, no. 6, April 1972.

Schools Council (1976) Schools Council Health Education Project 5–13. London, Nelson.

Scottish Education Department (1974) *Health Education in Schools*. Curriculum Paper 14. London, HMSO.

Seeman, M. and Evans, J. W. (1962) 'Alienation and learning in a hospital setting'. *Am. Soc. Rev.*, vol. 27, pp. 772–783.

Select Committee on Violence in the Family (1977) *Violence to Children*. First Report 1976–1977. London, HMSO.

Simon, S. B. (1974) *Meeting Yourself Halfway*. Niles, Ill., Argos Communications.

Simon, S. B., Howe, W. L. and Kirschenbaum, H. (1972) *Values Clarification: A handbook of practical strategies for teachers and students*. New York, Hart.

Stacey, M. (1977) *Hlth Soc. Servs J.*, 3 June, 1977.

Stenhouse, L. (1969a) 'Open minded teaching'. *New Society*, 24 July, 1969.

Stenhouse, L. (1969b) 'Handling controversial issues in the classroom'. *Educ. Canada*, December 1969.

Strickland, B. R. (1973) *Locus of Control: Where have we been and where are we going?* Montreal, American Psychological Association.

Thayer, L. (ed.) (1976) *Effective Education*. La Jolla, Cal., University Associates.

Tones, B. K. (1976) 'The organisation of community health education: a case for strategic integration'. *Hlth Educ.*, September/October 1976.

Tones, B. K. (1979) In Sutherland, I. (ed.), *Health Education: Perspectives and choices*. London, Allen & Unwin.

White, J. (1969) 'Open minded society'. *New Society*, 31 July, 1969.

Williams, A. F. (1972) 'Factors associated with seat belt use in families'. *J. Saf. Res.*, vol. 4, no. 3, pp. 133–138.

CHAPTER 2

THE PHILOSOPHY OF HEALTH EDUCATION RELATED TO SCHOOLS

Gill Williams and David Aspin

Introduction

In the daily life of the teacher in school there is always so much to do which is directly concerned with the practical teaching situation, and so little time in which to do it. It is not surprising, therefore, to find that theoretical problems such as those concerned with the philosophy of education are often put to one side, either to await that distant day when there may be time to spare or, alternatively, to be consigned to the care of 'experts' or 'theorists' whose time is thought to be relatively free from the constraints of 'real' problems. In this chapter we hope to show that not only is the philosophy of health education a crucial and inescapable part of the teaching of the subject (and thus one of the bases and perspectives which the teacher of health education needs to acquire), but also that the conclusions which are reached as a result of philosophical considerations have *practical* consequences for developing curricula in health education.

Philosophy is often thought of as 'vague, urbane and cultivated sermonizing about the nature of reality and the place of man in the world', a kind of 'what's it all about' enterprise, where one person's 'philosophy' is as good as anyone else's and where, therefore, no firm conclusions (let alone prescriptions for action) can be drawn. Let us be clear that we are not dealing with this kind of model of philosophy in this chapter. Nor do we intend to go to what some people would call the 'other extreme' of philosophy, namely that of a highly technical and rigorous exercise of analysis and criticism directly but solely concerned with the meanings of words, such as is exemplified in the writings of philosophers like Ayer (1936) and Austin (1962). These models and others, such as, for example, 'political philosophies' like Marxism, have a long tradition and much to commend them. They illustrate, however, that there is no such thing as one 'true version' or a single, 'correct' version of philosophy; the choice of an appropriate model will depend, as it does in subject teaching in schools, upon the desired aims and outcomes.

Thus, in attempting to provide a model of philosophy for health education we need to be clear about what we hope will result from our efforts. Our own experiences lead us to think that there are at least three important questions which ought to be examined and which are concerned both with the teaching of health education in our schools and with health education in its widest sense, that is in the community at large. The first question is about the *nature* of health education itself; the second is concerned with the grounds on which the enterprise of health education can be justified; the third with the ethics of intervention. In other words, what is health education? Why do we concern ourselves with it? Why should we set about it in certain cases and circumstances?

In attempting to show how one might go about finding answers to these questions – or at least delineating approaches to some of them – we shall be drawing upon the insights offered by the models already referred to and to other 'kinds' of philosophy too. For example, the deeply held beliefs, attitudes and values to which we are all committed are often hidden from others and only become explicit, or 'public', through our expressed preferences, ambitions, political and moral views, and through our general behaviour or commitment to a certain 'form of life'. It is, however, those hidden, underlying presuppositions which are crucial in terms of their influence not only upon our health behaviour but also upon the aims of the kinds of programmes offered by health educators. One element in our version of philosophy, therefore, will need to be an attempt to *elicit and analyse* the fundamental presuppositions which underpin and serve to define the 'form of life' within which we believe the enterprise of health education most properly takes place. Such analysis is not undertaken simply for its own sake, but for particular reasons. It is undertaken in an attempt to promote clarity of theoretical understanding. This is a task which we see to be of crucial importance for it is clear that one cannot promote clarity of thought and rational decision-making in our pupils if we, as teachers, are unaware of those elements, principles and concepts which form the basis of decision-making about our own work and which, in turn, are not self-evident but need to be publicly justified (a point to which we will return later). Such analysis is also undertaken in an attempt to provide us with the second element in this study, which is to endeavour to construct a theoretical framework against which present-day health education programmes could be measured in an attempt to see how the practice matches the principles. In this way we would discover where the areas of weakness lie and would thus be able to show what amendments, refinements or even wholesale restructuring might take place in order to achieve a closer 'match'.

We see, then, two main characteristics in the kind of philosophy which we intend to advocate here: first, the need for rigorous analysis of those concepts which are crucial to the enterprise of health education, together with an examination of the presuppositions which underpin them. (This type of activity has been described by Strawson (1958) as 'descriptive metaphysics'.) In this form our philosophy has much in common with the linguistic analysis to which we have already referred. Secondly, however, we are strongly inclined to believe that there is a 'practical pay-off' or 'creative' element, which is concerned with prescriptions about what, logically, ought to follow such analysis. In this respect, ours is a form of philosophy which owes much to the notion of philosophy as a species of 'problem-solving' (Popper, 1973).

Some Prerequisites

Before going on to examine health education in this way it is important to be clear about the nature and status of such a philosophical examination. It does not purport to provide *the* answer; indeed, it would not be a philosophical enterprise if that were to be its intention. The very analyses we offer and engage in presuppose criteria of correctness which are themselves not immune from further scrutiny. Our willingness to advance hypotheses and conjectures which propose to criticize or refute the views of others is based upon the expectation that these will, in turn, be subjected to logical criticism. Any conclusions which we draw only stand until such time as they can be refuted by further relevant and rational argument; such is the nature of philosophy. However, because such an analysis of health education can only be seen as provisional in nature, it does not mean that it is unimportant or pointless. Any enterprise which attempts to influence the lives of others needs to be publicly justified if it is to be accorded any weight or acceptance, whilst the presuppositions upon which such justification is based ought, too, to be open to scrutiny rather than be hidden or unexamined. It is this public examination of such presuppositions, and the consequent extraction of implied prescriptions for action that is, we believe, the job of the philosopher.

In philosophical language, the three basic questions about health education to which we have already referred (What is it? Why do it? On what basis do we set about it?) resolve themselves into four problems: definition, epistemology, ethics and metaphysics. In the rest of this chapter we will try to deal with these issues and to come to some conclusions which might form a soundly based philosophy for health education.

Definition

It is with the question of meaning that the problems of the philosopher of health education begin, for if we cannot easily understand the terms being employed in our discourse about the subject then we cannot proceed further to any examination of the validity of arguments employing them. Thus the definition and analysis of terms become a prior stage in conceptualization, for it is upon them that all that follows will depend.

Health educators will understand the difficulty in attempting to define health education. Although one might expect other teachers to lack understanding of this subject, which is a relatively recent development in the school curriculum, it appears that there is not even consensus about the definition of the subject among health educators themselves. A cursory examination of the syllabuses offered under the title of health education will confirm this. The lack of clear definition is also illustrated by the considerable pressure which has been exerted during at least the past two decades to relabel the subject. The reasons for such pressure to change the name are wide-ranging. They include the claims that a new label for the subject would encourage a move away from its old image of being solely concerned with hygiene and exercise, to something which is thought to be a more accurate description of the present scope of the subject. Arguments are also offered to support a change of name based on the belief that such relabelling would improve the status of the subject within the school curriculum, whilst yet others claim that the title is dull and should be changed to something which stimulates interest.

Such relabelling has been strongly resisted by some people on the grounds that to call the subject, say, social education, health studies, personal development or whatever, gives an inaccurate picture and misses the fundamental features and key characteristics of what they see as 'health education'. If this is, indeed, the case, then it is necessary to spell out just what those characteristics are, for it is on such grounds that claims for it to be a 'subject area' (or what Hirst (1965) might call a 'field of knowledge') depend.

Definitions which are offered in an attempt to obtain conceptual clarity are of various kinds, but perhaps the most important thing to keep in mind in reading this section is that there are, in our view, no such things as uncontentious definitions; the very fact that there is a need to define at all implies a lack of agreement about meaning. Of the various types of definition which are offered four kinds are regularly met, particularly in connection with health education: reportive, descriptive, persuasive and programmatic definitions, all of which are, philosophically speaking, open to severe criticism.

Reportive definitions are best exemplified by those definitions drawn from dictionaries or wordbooks of etymological derivation; descriptive definitions simply set out the main ways in which a word is used by language users of that culture in their common communications. There are powerful objections, and these can be briefly summarized thus: just because a particular word happens to be used in a particular way in a particular cultural climate at a particular time, there is no reason why we should ourselves derive any norms from that as to the way(s) in which we should use such words. The only criterion of meaning and intelligibility in public discourse employing such terms is the way in which people employ them; 'the meaning of a word is its use in language' (Wittgenstein, 1953). Thus, to define health education we need to look at the present circumstances of its use in discourse and at the interest and intentions of those who participate in such discourse.

Persuasive definitions are those which seek to put forward norms, values or prescriptions under the guise of analysis, while programmatic definitions are those which urge a whole programme to be followed under the heading of the term so described (many definitions of 'education' function in precisely this way). Often such definitions function as little more than slogans; that is, they provide a rallying call to those who share similar convictions which, on fuller examination, proves to be empty of content and capable of 'meaning' almost anything which the persuader wishes to claim. An example often used to illustrate such absence of specific meaning may be found in the use of the word 'democracy'. To those who claim to be supporters of democracy the use of the word as a label for a political system or institution immediately suggests that the object of the labelling is a 'good' thing, worthy of praise, support or whatever. But the word itself tells us nothing about that object in the absence of further clarification, and one has only to look at the ways in which the label is applied to see that a variety of interpretations can be placed upon its use. The word 'democracy', for example, is often used to describe the political system which operates in Great Britain (though the appropriateness of such a label for our system is fiercely disputed by some of its citizens and by outsiders, too). It also appears to be legitimately used to describe not only the political systems of many Western European countries, but also those of Canada and the United States, although these systems and their constituent institutions show distinct and different features. It might, of course, be claimed, that some of the shared features which such systems may be said to exhibit justify the legitimacy of a claim to the correctness of such labelling, but this, of course, illustrates the need for further definition of the sort to which we have already referred. At the same time even the presence of such shared features might be difficult to discuss when one extends such a term to the description of the political system of the German Democratic Republic, the People's Republic of China and so on.

Clearly, in cases such as these, the use of definitions which are persuasive in character does little to promote clarity of conceptualization, in the absence of further support. It will, we think, be readily recognized that some uses of the word 'health' operate in a similar fashion; health foods, health farms, healthy minds, healthy habits, healthy bank balances and so on all appeal to the general value which we place on 'health', though much further information needs to be acquired before the terms make sense. In a similar way the idea of putting health education in the school timetable is likely to receive support from those already committed to the subject; those who know little or nothing about it will require a great deal more information and a more sustained attempt to reach an agreed definition about what it is before committing themselves to its support.

These persuasive definitions often appear under the guise of authoritative definitions. In such cases the criticisms already made against persuasive definitions are equally applicable but there is, too, an additional factor. For not only is there an assumption of shared value ('we all know health is a good thing') but there is covert (and, often, overt) pressure to accept such a definition because it is thought to come from 'an authority'. The dubious character of such definitions is epitomized by the definition of health made by the World Health Organization. This illustrates not only the tendentiousness of such statements but may help us to counter the many claims which teachers of health education meet with in the process of their work and which ought not to be accepted at their face value, however much they are supported by some sort of 'authority'.

The Constitution of the World Health Organization (1946) includes the following statement:

> Health is a positive state of mental, physical, and social well-being and not merely the absence of disease or infirmity.

This definition was welcomed with great enthusiasm by workers in the field of health and health education for here, at last, seemed to be the definitive statement which would clarify what had always been a rather vague area; furthermore it had been laid down by a group of people whose credentials might reasonably be thought to confer on them the right to make such statements. It did, in fact, serve a useful purpose for it emphasized the necessity to take into account factors beyond the physical (hence the mental and social aspects) in any consideration of health problems. What, then, is wrong with it? There are, we think, several aspects of this definition which will not stand up to critical scrutiny, for whilst the definition avoids the fallacy of negative definition (health defined as 'not being ill' is totally uninformative), it raises a whole range of other issues which require further examination. To define health as a 'state of . . . well-being', for example, is to commit a blatant *petitio principii*; its opposite, 'illness as a state of ill-being', illustrates this. Further, to use the word 'state' to describe someone's condition implies some terminal, fixed and static end which can be attained and then 'sunk into'; to predicate such a logical category for the 'health' of organic beings whose condition is fundamentally dynamic is, in our view, to make a mistake. Equally so it suggests the *presence* of something, and to some degree (implied by the word 'positive'). The fundamental weakness of such a definition can be shown if the following questions are asked: what is it that is present if health is 'not merely the absence of disease', and what is it to be 'positive'? What degree of whatever it is must there be present for the WHO to admit that the organism is healthy?

Now these sorts of questions have *not* been asked, nor criticisms made, of the World Health Organization's definition, merely as an exercise in complaint. The problems of that definition are important, we believe, for two reasons. The first concerns the right of the 'authority' body in question to make such pronouncements which are binding and coercive not only on future word usage but upon vast schemes of public policy based upon and incorporating a definitional base of such dubiety. The mere fact of labelling a group such as this as the 'World Health Organization' may be an administrative convenience or politically desirable, or may even show that it is representative of world medical opinion; it does, however, give the impression of that group having what we might call a 'hot line to truth'. Such a group is as likely to be fallible as any other committee, however, in the definitions which they make, which will be influenced by their need to compromise or to offer blanket prescriptions which are meant to cover a host of individual situations.

Their claim, too, to be 'representative' of the whole spectrum of opinion (on which their legitimacy rests) is limited, in turn, by the perceptions and consequent selections of those in whom the responsibility for deciding membership of such committees is invested. Thus although all members may share a knowledge and interest in the particular area in which they are thought to be experts, it does not necessarily follow that these are the people who ought, logically, to be able to pronounce authoritatively upon it. It is not necessarily the case, for example, that doctors (or politicians, or health economists or whoever) are authorities on the definition of 'health' (Culyer, 1976) any more than, say, teachers (or parents, or members of the local education committee) could be said to be *the* authority who should produce *the* definition of education. The problem here is twofold: first, how can we ensure that a truly 'representative' group speaks for the whole community of interest in that field (and, in turn, how can we know the criteria by which such a group could be judged to be 'representative' so that we would know when we had 'got it right'). Secondly, as in all committees, any joint statement is likely to be a compromise between the parties contributing to it, and this says nothing about whether such a joint statement in any way resembles either individual beliefs or a 'correct definition'.

The second reason why we have spent so much time in trying to show some of the weaknesses of authority definitions of the kind offered by the WHO is that they admirably illustrate the absurdity of blanket definitions such as 'Health is X' or 'Education is Y'. It seems to us that it is not merely a question of people 'not having got it right *yet*', a view which assumes that, given a sufficient amount of time and an adequate amount of thought, the answer is there, somewhere, and will eventually be found. What we are claiming is not only that there is no such *one thing* as 'health', but rather that although the different uses of the word bear certain resemblances to each other (what Wittgenstein (1953) called 'family resemblances'), the 'meaning' is relative to the context in which the word is used. If this were not to be so we would find ourselves in the invidious position not only of having to match each individual and his word usages of 'health' against a set of quite arbitrary criteria (and, because of the nature of the dynamics of human development, maturation, or ageing, of finding most of them 'wanting'), but also of changing, equally arbitrarily, the common usages of the word 'health', thus denying the fact that language *is* a function of the ways in which it is used.

What seems to make sense in this debate is that *any* claim to health will need to take into consideration a wide range of other variables such as age, sex, previous history and so on. The label 'healthy', it seems to us, is meaningfully applied to those people whose functioning comes within and between certain acceptable parameters which set up limits, and it has been shown that crossing to the other side of these can be deleterious, and possibly even terminal, to our normal state of human being. Thus, when our condition comes within these parameters we are 'healthy'; when it transgresses any of them we are not. This is no new idea, as can be seen from the words of William Farr (1839):

> To accuse the human race of perpetual malady is as ridiculous as to attribute with some theological writer, unremitting wickedness of the human heart; but if every alteration of the multiplied parts of the human body, every transient tremble of its infinite movements, every indigestion in man and every fit of hysteria in woman, were reckoned, few days of human life would remain entirely clear. . . .

There is little to suggest in recent years, in spite of attempts to claim the contrary by bodies such as the WHO, that we are any nearer to a single definition of health than was William Farr. The most that can be said is something like 'In this situation (or context) I take "health" to be . . .' – a statement which will be based on such knowledge as is available and relevant and which will, in turn, be open to critical reconsideration and redefinition in the light of new evidence and rational debate.

Similarly the term 'health education' has many meanings, and we believe that to solve the problem of reconciling the various inconsistencies between them, the only kind of acceptable definition is a stipulative one of the kind: 'in this situation (scheme of work, school, project, or whatever) I take health education to be as follows . . .'. We should then spell out what the particular characteristics of the enterprise in that particular context are to be – the ones to which we shall attach greatest importance and on which we shall base our practical policies. It goes without saying, of course, that the basis for such stipulation is open to public appraisal and must be capable of being rationally defended, for we are concerned here with an enterprise in which, we believe, we are publicly answerable for our decisions and actions and which ought not, as a matter of morality (or professional ethics), to be based on some private or idiosyncratic whim. The question now arises, then, as to what sorts of considerations ought to be taken into account when making rational decisions about what will constitute an individual teacher's definition of health education.

Epistemology

At this point the scope of our inquiry shifts from the problems of meaning to those of cognition. For what we must now consider is the epistemological character of health education; that is to say, the nature and scope of those forms of thought and awareness that give the enterprise its whole identity and purpose, and which give us grounds for claiming that there are certain features and characteristics that make health education what it is and such that it could not be subsumed under any other label. What, to use the language of Wittgenstein (1953), are the relevant 'universes of discourse' that constitute this 'form of life'? Or, to use the language of Hirst (1965), upon which of the various forms of knowledge does that field of knowledge which we may call health education draw in order to work out answers to its particular practical problems? These are not the only issues in this particular field of epistemology, for we also have to decide which criteria we will use in order to judge one kind of answer as being the correct one in preference to another. A glance at the range and complexity of the various kinds of problems concerning criteria for selection of the cognitive bases of curricular subjects, such as can be found in the work of such figures as Hirst (1965), Barrow (1976) and White (1973) in England, and Phenix (1964), Tykociner (1964) and Schwab (1964) in America, will serve to underline the contentiousness of the selection of any criteria of demarcation in this area. At the same time one has only to look at the differences between, say, Popper (1949) and Kuhn (1962), or Winch (1959) and MacIntyre (1967), on the issue of the status of scientific paradigms to see that the whole attempt to give any account of the cognitive character of health education is fraught with difficulties.

Yet it is perhaps here that we do have some means of assessing such speculations, some 'principle of corrigibility'. For Hirst (1973) is surely right when he suggests that the whole point of any educational theory is that it is, ultimately, an enterprise of a *practical* kind. By this Hirst means that it is an undertaking that sets out to give practical answers to questions such as 'What ought we to do?' or, in our case, 'What ought we to do in order best to educate our children (or fellow adults) with particular reference to the safeguarding or improvement of their health?' The epistemology of our field thus becomes orientated towards the production of practical policies and the exercise becomes one of a problem-solving kind concerned with questions of the kind: 'What sorts of "health behaviour" enhance or diminish health?'; 'What sorts of knowledge do people need in order to be able to make rational decisions about their own health behaviour?'; 'How relevant are the existing educational methods which we use in order to help people to make rational decisions concerning their health?'; 'What sorts of factors need to be taken into consideration when planning a health education curriculum?'; 'What will constitute a successful outcome to such a curriculum, and by what means is success to be evaluated?'

These, and other similar questions, are ones which have been exercising groups such as the Schools Council Health Education Project teams, the Health Education Council, the Teachers' Advisory Council on Alcohol and Drug Education and others, as well as many individual teachers of health education. Indeed, this book is an attempt to help teachers to examine just such problems. Its contents could be said to be a reflection of the views of the editors and authors as to the range of subjects which, when taken together, form the basic curriculum for health education. In our view it should, at the least, draw upon such disciplined forms of understanding and analysis as the scientific, the mathematic, the historical, the philosophical and, above all, the modes of judgement and appraisal which we believe are its prime determinants and chief underlying bases – moral belief and judgement and interpersonal understanding.

At this stage it might be a useful philosophical exercise for the reader to examine the contents of this book to see whether the kinds of questions which he or she thinks are important in health education have been tackled. If there are gaps between the reader's expectations and the contents of this book, he might find it interesting to speculate as to the kinds of explanations which might be offered for such differences of opinion. One possible explanation might be found in differing definitions of health education between reader and writers (or between the different contributors to the book too). Alternatively it may be that, whilst basic definitions are shared, the criteria upon which epistemological choices are made are not. Thus, for example, we may agree in our definition of what health education is but disagree about the kinds of knowledge which are seen to be crucial parts of such an enterprise. One has only to look at the arguments concerned with the relative importance of biological knowledge compared with interpersonal knowledge in what the media refer to as 'sex education' to recognize that major and often protracted disagreement persists about what constitutes relevant content.

There is, too, a third area where there is lack of consensus, and this is the moral or ethical aspect of health education. For whilst one might agree with others about the definition of the subject and about the modes of cognition which are central to it, it is nevertheless possible to disagree about the ethical basis on which health education is offered. The problem here concerns not only the means which would constitute a moral way of going about the enterprise but also, and more importantly, whether health education should be offered at all.

Ethics

One of the most compelling moral problems in the field of health education is that of intervention, and its justification. This is a problem of normative ethics on two levels – the general and the particular. In the first case this involves asking whether, as a matter of policy, we ought to attempt to influence or alter attitudes and health behaviour *at all*, rather than allowing people to make their own choices and cope with the results in their own way, for it might be claimed (and, indeed, often is) that such interference takes away a person's autonomy and influences the person to follow *our* preferred life style rather than his own. For to decide to attempt health education *at all* presupposes that we think we *ought* to, and that entails being prepared to justify the intervention constituted by such an attempt in terms of reasons which are public, that is to say impartial, and such that any person could understand and, in principle, make his own. Having once decided that, however, we arrive at the second level of the problem in the normative sphere: what particular strategies of intervention ought we to adopt and adhere to, not only in general but in particular cases too? Is it sufficient, for example, to present 'the facts' and leave the pupils to make up their own minds? How justifiable is it to set out to influence attitudes and behaviour so that pupils come to act in accordance with what we believe to be 'good' or 'right' on the basis of evidence which *we* accept? And what of cases where one child, say, out of the whole school responds to our teaching in an adverse way, where the outcome of one educational programme is the opposite to the one desired? In such cases are we to be judged on the grounds of our good intentions or on the outcome of our policies and teaching and, if the latter, is it the 'nearly one hundred percent success' that counts or the 'less than one percent failure' that will give us cause for concern?

The very fact that we pose such moral questions as those above clearly rests upon, and presupposes, a whole framework of value judgements about what it is to be a 'full human being' or 'person'. To draw out what might be the major elements of such judgements is not an easy task, for they are often unstated or unexamined. Further, to conclude that some of these values should be changed, or even rejected, is something which is likely to meet with resistance, particularly in those cases where such refinement may involve altering a person's whole approach to their work or even lead to changes in the whole curriculum of a school, or to the ways in which we plan for community projects.

There are, in addition, ethical questions which need to be raised about the particular kinds of programmes offered, and the teaching methods which are employed. It is often suggested, for example, that certain desirable health habits could best be inculcated in our pupils through conditioning processes of the kind advocated by B. F. Skinner. In terms of learning efficiency, such claims may appeal. Others advocate the use of fear to induce behavioural change though, in terms of effectiveness, there is some doubt about its use despite its long tradition as a means of control in both home and school and, for that matter, in society at large too. On the wider scale there are those who advocate the withdrawal of facilities as a means of ensuring desirable health behaviour (as, for example, those who claim that there would be a drop in the numbers of people smoking or of people driving carelessly if NHS facilities were denied to those who smoked or were involved in road accidents). Others claim that what is needed is legislation to remove temptation from those who cannot resist it; thus the sale of cigarettes would be banned, motorcycles or fast cars would be outlawed and, presumably, food rationing would be introduced as a means of preventing obesity and so on.

Leaving aside the problem of whether such methods of inducing desirable health behaviour would actually work in practice, it is likely that such ideas would meet with a mixed reception on moral grounds. For some this kind of control may be regarded as an acceptable means to an end, whilst for others it will be totally abhorrent. Such divergence of views rests not only upon the individual's beliefs about what constitutes a moral way of dealing with health education but also, in turn, upon the metaphysical basis of such moral views, namely the whole range of individual beliefs about the nature of man and of his relations to his fellows. For clearly, if one takes the

Skinnerian view that man differs from animals only in the degree of his sophistication, and that talk of morality, freedom and human dignity is merely a convenient fiction, then the consequences of such a belief in terms of how we behave towards our pupils (or other recipients of our health education programmes) will be very different from those prescriptions for action which would follow from, say, adherence to the Kantian principle of not treating persons as means to an end but always as ends in themselves.

In this way it seems to us that health education exemplifies the philosophical problems both of concepts of human nature *and* moral values for there will be, conceptually, all the difference in the world between the sorts of programmes devised in an attempt to encourage personal autonomy and those in which it is thought to be simply a matter of inculcating the 'right' attitudes or the 'correct' response to stimuli. Similarly there will be a vast difference between the evaluation of programmes put forward by those who believe that each individual is of crucial importance and those for whom some 'casualties' or 'failures' are an acceptable cost in the cause of 'the greater good'.

In practice, does this mean that any programme of health education based on the individual beliefs of teachers will do? For some philosophers (and for teachers of health education too) such fundamental disagreements of moral standpoint are to be accepted as a matter of course. Atkinson (1965), for example, describes the logic of moral judgement thus: 'Take any moral position and its opposite can be maintained without logical error or factual mistake.' Hare (1952), by contrast, contends that it would be perfectly possible for two moral agents to follow the 'rules' of moral deliberation and both be right in their conclusions, even though they came to mutually contradictory conclusions. Such a view is sharply rebutted by other philosophers. For example, Foot (1958) remarks:

> How 'X is good' can be a well founded moral judgement when 'X is bad' can be equally well founded it is not easy to see.

Moreover, there will be many teachers and philosophers who would support her when she asks:

> How can questions such as 'What does it matter?' 'What harm does it do?' . . . and 'Why is it important?' be set aside here?

In Foot's view it is not the case that in moral matters *anything* goes; for her, as for Warnock (1967), there *are* some incontrovertible 'facts of life' in moral matters. No-one would disagree that to lose a limb was a horror to be avoided or that a life of a quality in which humans could be seen as 'flourishing' was an end to be desired and promoted.

It is likely that some teachers will be found who support the views of Hare and Atkinson, whilst others will find themselves in sympathy with the views of Foot. What *is* important for teachers of health education is that they are aware of this dichotomy in our delineation of our 'moral facts of life' and, further, of the need to acquaint themselves with the arguments which are claimed to support each view. For it is from this area that many questions about the content and methodology of health education often arise, and it is then necessary to be able to offer a rational defence of the system of moral values which has been influential in our personal selections and judgements of ultimate moral worth (Hudson, 1972).

Conclusion

At the beginning of this chapter we said that in our view the philosophy of health education was such a radical and fundamental part of the theoretical framework of the subject that the skills of the philosopher were those which all teachers of health education need to acquire. On this basis every teacher of health education is a philosopher of health education for, as Scheffler (1973) demonstrates, subject X presupposes a philosophy of X; indeed without such an ineliminable basis, the whole foundation of our teaching would crumble. So far we have attempted to show the kinds of philosophical questions which form this ineliminable basis for health education and some of the answers which may be offered on the basis of different underlying presuppositions. Clearly it is not possible here to do more than simply indicate where some of the problems might lie. Indeed a glance at any book list concerned with some of the concepts which we have mentioned here ('epistemology', 'education', 'ethics' and so on) will show very readily how superficial our approach has been. If, however, it causes any readers to question the basis on which they plan their own work, set aims and objectives and attempt to evaluate it, or, alternatively, causes them to question our own presuppositions then we will feel that our efforts have been worth while. It must be admitted, however, that in the manner of all teachers we set our sights high and hope that some will feel stimulated (or irritated) enough by our assumptions to read more philosophy and then attack us on our own ground.

Two things were claimed to characterize the kind of philosophy which we have employed here. The first is an attempt to elicit and analyse the concepts which are crucial to health education, and we have attempted to show how one might set about this with reference to certain concepts which we selected on the basis of what we see to be their central importance, though there are others which would benefit too from such analysis (for example 'evidence' and 'evaluation', to name but two). Our second claim was that such analysis necessarily leads to a practical pay-off in indicating certain prescriptions for action, and we have already made reference to these in terms of the metaphysical beliefs about the nature of the person and consequent behaviour, in terms of teaching processes, towards him. But we make no claim to a monopoly of insight or truth in this matter; teachers are equal partners and of equal standing in the truth-seeking activity that is philosophy. 'It is for the teacher to show his pupils the ropes,' as Ryle (1966) cogently remarked, 'but it is for the pupil himself to climb them.' Or, to change the metaphor, we hope that having brought you this far, we can 'pull up the ladder' (Wittgenstein, 1923) and encourage you to go ahead *on your own* and ask these sorts of questions, make these critical evaluations and systematically build a coherent and self-consistent philosophy of health education.

Summary

There are many features of health education which are ill-defined, muddled and open to dispute. In this chapter we have selected three areas: the nature of health education, its justification and the ethics of intervention, which we feel need consideration and clarification if health educators are to be able to argue for the subject to be included in the curriculum.

Two beliefs underpin this chapter: first, that philosophy has something practical to offer in that it provides a framework for thinking about the subject, and in turn, a logical basis for curriculum decisions; secondly, that it is teachers who are best placed to undertake such an exercise since they are the people with knowledge of both pupils and subject. It is clear that in order to undertake this kind of thinking, teachers will need to develop their philosophical skills, and we try to show how this might be done in relation to health education.

References

Atkinson, R. F. (1965) 'Instruction and indoctrination', in Archambault, R. D. (ed.), *Philosophical Analysis and Education*. London, Routledge & Kegan Paul.

Austin, J. L. (1962) *How to Do Things with Words*. Rev. ed. Oxford, Clarendon Press.

Ayer, A. J. (1936) *Language, Truth and Logic*. London, Hutchinson.

Barrow, R. (1955) *Common Sense and the Curriculum*. London, Allen & Unwin.

Culyer, A. J. (1976) *Need and the National Health Service*. London, Robertson.

Farr, W. (1839) 'Vital statistics', in McCulloch, J. M. (ed.), *Statistical Account of the British Empire*. London, Longman.

Foot, P. (1958) 'Moral arguments'. *Mind*, vol. LXVII, October 1958, p. 502.

Hare, R. M. (1952) *The Language of Morals*. London, Oxford University Press.

Hirst, P. H. (1965) 'Liberal education and the nature of knowledge', in Archambault, R. D. (ed.), *Philosophical Analysis and Education*. London, Routledge & Kegan Paul.

Hirst, P. H. (1973) 'The nature of educational theory II', in Langford, G. and O'Connor, D. J. (eds), *New Essays in Philosophy of Education*. London, Routledge & Kegan Paul.

Hudson, W. D. (1972) *Modern Moral Philosophy*. London, Macmillan, p. 320ff.

Kuhn, T. S. (1962) *The Structure of Scientific Revolutions*. Chicago, Ill., University of Chicago Press.

MacIntyre, A. (1967) 'The idea of a social science'. *Proceedings of the Aristotelian Society*, supplementary volume.

Phenix, P. H. (1964) *Realms of Meaning*. New York, McGraw-Hill.

Popper, K. R. (1949) *The Logic of Scientific Discovery*. London, Hutchinson.

Popper, K. R. (1973) *Objective Knowledge*. London, Oxford University Press.

Ryle, G. (1966) 'Teaching and training', in Peters, R. S. (ed.), *The Concept of Education*. London, Routledge & Kegan Paul.

Scheffler, I. (1973) In Doyle, J. F. (ed.), *Educational Judgements*. London, Routledge & Kegan Paul.

Schwab, J. J. (1964) 'The structure of the disciplines', in Elam, S. (ed.), *Education and the Structure of Knowledge*. Chicago, Ill., Rand McNally.

Strawson, P. F. (1958) *Individuals: An essay in descriptive metaphysics*. London, Methuen.

Tykociner, J. T. (1964) 'Zetetics and areas of knowledge', in Elam, S. (ed.), *Education and the Structure of Knowledge*. Chicago, Ill., Rand McNally.

Warnock, G. J. (1967) *Contemporary Moral Philosophy*. London, Macmillan, p. 52ff.

White, J. P. (1973) *Towards a Compulsory Curriculum*. London, Routledge & Kegan Paul.

Winch, P. (1959) *The Idea of a Social Science*. London, Routledge & Kegan Paul.

Wittgenstein, L. (1953) *Philosophical Investigations* (trs. G. E. M. Anscombe). Oxford, Blackwell. (Section 43).

Wittgenstein, L. (1923) *Tractatus Logico-Philosophicus*. London, Routledge & Kegan Paul (concluding remarks).

CHAPTER 3

A QUESTIONING VIEW OF HEALTH EDUCATION

Nicholas Dorn

The Unhealthy Conservatism of Affective Education

Elsewhere I have offered some comment and evidence on the efficacy of three drug educational strategies (Dorn, 1977). Substance-focused approaches, concerned with facts about the drugs, are quite often thought to have been proved ineffective or counter-productive, and person-focused, affective or values programmes have been proposed as replacements. Significantly the trend towards affective approaches has gone hand in hand with a tendency to propose that younger and younger age-groups should be educated. One useful (to the affective camp) result of this is that evaluation becomes almost impossible; the affective programme is supposed to have its central effects so many years after teaching that follow-up and evaluation become difficult.

Both substance- and person-focused programmes, however, share an assumption which reduces their relevance to pupils' real needs in relation to legal and illegal drugs. The assumption is that initial experimentation results from an internal state of the individual (knowledge, attitude, value or motive) and is highly questionable. Most initial experimentation is preceded by a belief and intention not to experiment, but this intention is not called into play in the choice situation, because the choice situation is unlike the situation in relation to which the belief/intention was formed. In order to be relevant to the choice situations (offer situations) which children are most likely to face in their futures, rather than being relevant to the existing antidrug ideologies which they already share with adults, education must place facts and feelings within the context of a discussion of choice situations. Hence we have situational education, an example of which was evaluated in a recent Anglo-Danish study (Dorn, 1977; Dorn et al., 1977).

However, situational education of a realistic kind faces many obstacles. It obliges us to face the realities of social life and the situations which occur in it. Basically the choice is between ignoring social realities (as purely substance-focused education may do) or acknowledging their existence (as situational education attempts to do) or telling lies about life (as, I shall attempt to show, affective education may do).

Affective education may appear to be concerned with real life, but it often tells lies about life. Released from the obligation to talk about 'facts', it is able to tell lies not directly, but by allegory and analogy. In order to illustrate this, let us take as an example the recent Canadian affective programme *The Hole in the Fence* (Non-Medical Drugs Directorate, 1975). This is designed for children under ten years old, and has three medium-term goals which are supposed to contribute to a longer-term goal. The three medium-term goals are: to develop self-confidence and self-esteem; to develop awareness of self and others, and to stimulate interpersonal skills. 'In so doing, the programme would prepare the child, in the long-term, to cope with drug-use decisions.'

To understand the concerns of the producers of *The Hole in the Fence*, we have to examine the materials themselves. The 'creative concept' of the materials was originally entitled *Vegetable Farm*. When, as a result of further development, the creative conceptualization was finalized in 1975, it was re-titled *The Hole in the Fence*. In addition to those themes which one might associate with the stated objectives of the programme, two others may be found in the materials. These themes are 'authority', and 'the pusher' and the nature of the drugs he sells.

Authority in *The Hole in the Fence*

There are three distinct authority figures in the programme. These are the good figure of the liberal state, the psychopathic figure of the bully and the racist figure of the conservative.

Mr Cabbage 'is the leader of the garden. He is big and strong and kind. Mr Cabbage knows about a lot of things and everybody likes and respects him.' In case there is any confusion, it is made clear that Mr Cabbage is not an elected representative, but a permanent institution. When the garden is visited by *Chinese Cabbage*, an election is held to determine who will go to visit China (a land of dragons, birds, chopsticks, fireworks and celebrations). Mr Cabbage is not a candidate; he runs the election. He is the permanent leader of the garden, and as such is concerned only that the other vegetables act in the interests of their own welfare. There are two other authority figures. *Mr Cauliflower* is the picture of defeated conservatism and a racist to boot, discriminating against the dark-skinned *Eggplant*. He only manages to influence the vegetables for a short time. *Cucumber* is a bit of a psychopath, always kicking the smaller vegetables. He gets his come-uppance when they turn on him and throw him in the pond. The rest of the vegetables are, with the exception of *Mushroom*, just ordinary folk. They laugh and cry, have doubts and uncertainties which they overcome, and develop their personalities just like you and me.

These characters live in a world divided into three parts. Inside the fence is *reality*; you have your ups and downs, but you pull through to have fun tomorrow. It is a world without work and without the problems associated with work, or with anticipation of it or of its absence; problems which will face children in their teens, when they will be expected to apply some of the lessons learnt in the programme. Instead of production, consumption is a theme. When you are too young to vote, you can get satisfaction from 'all the ice cream and chocolate cake you can eat'. Outside the garden, there are foreign parts (e.g., China, from which Chinese Cabbage comes, or an unidentified country from which Eggplant brings his unusually coloured flesh and drug-induced *unreality* where 'even when it rained, it seemed that the sun shone every day. It was as if candy floss grew on trees and the water turned to soda-pop.'

This then is the view of the world which the producers wish children to internalize, and within which the following drug-specific themes occur.

The pusher in *The Hole in the Fence*

The Hole in the Fence is far from being a 'non-drug' programme. The pusher is present in the shape of Mushroom, who lingers by the hole in the garden fence, just as pushers have traditionally hidden behind bushes or lurked outside the school gate. Mushroom offers his magic potion as a compensation for any upsets and as a way of forgetting problems and of feeling better in general. He is the only source of drugs and 'you always have to pay'. In addition he cheats you, since the drugs have no effects apart from encouraging over-confidence.

Now it is clear that this programme is simply telling lies about drugs and about the circumstances in which pupils are most likely to meet them. Most children will be offered a drug – either legal or illegal – for the first time by one of their peers or parents, and not by a pusher who makes them pay. The programme encourages totally unrealistic expectations of drug choice situations. The existence of the programme demonstrates that the hoary old tale of pushers preying upon ordinary kids at moments of weakness, which would appear hack and misleading if told in a straightforward way, becomes acceptable if disguised.

Furthermore, contrary to the storyline, drugs do have effects, as any child who observes his peers or listens to them, or experiments himself, will know. The programme will be discredited on this score as soon as the child comes across alternative sources of information. One would have thought that programme designers were now beyond the stage of trying to wish drug effects out of existence.

The programme is most interesting if looked at as a demonstration of the continuing concerns of the state. Foreigners and people with different coloured skins are a part of social reality now, and the racist-conservative element that opposes them is on the decline. We still have bullies and psychopaths but the moral indignation of the people can defeat them. The liberal state oversees elections, is always in the background to help people when they are frightened, offers advice and is concerned about their welfare, but it does not intervene physically against Mushroom. This is yet another distortion of the real world, in which pushers are hounded.

A simple choice of social worlds is offered to children: 'In my garden you can escape from the world', says Mushroom. 'In ours', says Mr Cabbage, 'you can enjoy living in it. We'd like you to stay, but it's your decision. You must choose.'

But the choice offered is a rigged one. The choice is not necessarily between non-drug 'reality' and drugged 'unreality'. We say 'not necessarily' because if the programme and other such information sources were to succeed in convincing children that drugs = unreality, then an unpleasant self-fulfilling prophecy might operate. Currently, most drug experimentation is not motivated by 'the desire to escape problems', however much that motivation might be fantasized, extolled and projected by those who see themselves as psychoanalytic counsellors and therapists. Certainly, the desire to help deviants in ways which make us feel better about ourselves, is understandable. But there is considerable danger of offering to the deviant an iatrogenic model of his or her own deviancy. At this moment, most drug experimentation is casual, episodic and without significant harm, partly because of the positive expectations, situational clues and subcultural supports which are available. It would indeed be damaging if the interpretive framework offered by programmes like *The Hole in the Fence* became dominant. The programme says, in effect, 'here is something which people with problems do'; let us hope that children do not believe them! Is this what is meant by 'preparing the child to cope with drug-use decisions'?

If the real Mr Cabbage is listening, he will do well to stop telling this sort of story. Or, if *The Hole in the Fence* is to be properly evaluated, then the evaluation should include investigation of the hypothesis that the programme promotes dependency or expectations of dependency following experimentation. It would have been preferable, of course, had the programme been evaluated before being generally released to the Canadian school system.

Who needs their values clarified?

One English observer of the drug scene in the 1960s used to distinguish between 'the drug problem' and 'the drug-problem problem'. This is a valuable distinction as long as one goes on to observe that a large part of the drug problem is caused by the drug-problem problem; it is not so much drugs that cause casualties but the way in which people use drugs and react to others who use them. Drug education ought to be concerned with this issue, but not in a way which exacerbates social reaction to users and encourages their labelling and self-labelling as 'sick'.

No education is going to reduce drug experimentation much; therefore one has to ask what its impact will be on the style and consequences of drug experimentation. We have to ask ourselves how we want experimenters to interpret the significance and meaning of their experimentation during and after the event. Should we really seek to make them interpret their state of intoxication and feelings during the following days and weeks in terms such as problem evasion, dependency, inadequacy, unreality, etc. I would say that we should not. However, programmes stressing values, social attitudes and psychological development *may*, if positioned within a strategy which recognizes the real world, have a very valuable contribution to make in education. But in order to make this contribution, their sponsors will first have to engage in a little value clarification themselves.

It would, however, be wrong to say that there was a simple choice to be made between pro-dependency propaganda, on the one hand, and pro-health education on the other. The actions of educators, like the actions of children, are explicable only within the situations in which they occur. Educational and social programmes are made to serve a number of purposes and to solve a number of problems. It is not just a case of individual programme producers projecting their own personal concerns and problems onto educational materials. On the contrary, the concerns apparent in drug education are concerns shared by *many* people, especially those in the welfare agencies who are concerned with the proper socialization and work readiness of young people. But it is questionable whether health education should be made a vehicle of these concerns to the extent that its efficacy *qua* health education is undermined. Let us ask that question, and then discuss the pros and cons: should drug education be made a vehicle of welfare agency concerns about the socialization of youth?

The question could be given several sorts of answers. First, there is the straightforward, common-sense answer, which asserts that drugs have such power, and threaten such disaster that they threaten not just the socialization of youth but also the whole basis of social life as we know it. To give this answer, one has either to ascribe a strange power to chemicals, or else to ascribe a strange weakness to social life as we know it today, or both (perhaps one belief implies the other). In either case, it follows that drug education cannot be a central weapon in the preservation of 'civilization', since more severe measures against drugs are both justified and necessary. If drugs are so seductive and powerful, then Mr Cabbage's liberal counter-measures are too mild; we must resurrect the authoritarian leader Mr Cauliflower, who will use firm measures in driving this menace, and other menaces, out of the garden. This is the paranoid conservative solution to social problems.

If, on the other hand, one feels that the *inherent* dangers of drugs have been exaggerated (as several governmental commissions have come to feel having examined the medical and historical evidence), then one would believe that drugs as such probably cannot destroy the garden, though they might make it better or worse for its inhabitants, individually and/or collectively. The question then becomes: does making drug education a vehicle for such wider concerns do more good in relation to drugs and in relation to those wider concerns, than it does harm?

Let us ask what are the wider concerns of Mr Cabbage and his creators? Apparently, the 'reality' of the garden excludes two particular issues – *sex* and *work* (cf. the Garden of Eden). Childhood must be kept free of these adult problem areas. The implicit assumption seems to be that children will only develop into properly sexed and work-ready adults as long as their *innocence* in relation to these adult problem areas is prolonged. The reality that is judged appropriate for children is a quite different reality to that in which adults live, yet is one which is supposed to smooth the path to the adult world, where sex and work join consumption and leisure. The wider, non-drug concerns of such education would therefore appear to include *the enforcement of the innocence of childhood*. Also, the broader concerns of such education would seem to include the inculcation of an unreserved love for the permanent, non-elected leader of the garden: 'Mr Cabbage is so great. I wish I could be like him.' Do these themes fit together? Are innocence of sex and of work, on the one hand, and an unquestioning adoration of the leader, on the other hand, mutual prerequisites? Or does Mr Cabbage think they are? There is an unpleasant political philosophy hidden behind the liberal surface of this propaganda.

We cannot, for reasons of space, follow that discussion through to its conclusion. We must simply note that different people would place different values upon the innocence of childhood, some calling it 'normal development' whilst others would call it something else. In any event, the extent to which an educational programme does achieve broad social or asocial ends of this kind, and the extent to which it achieves more limited (but connected) ends of increasing or decreasing problem-motivated drug use, will lead one to characterize it as, on balance, good or bad. I call it bad.

The end of drug education and of the drug problem

It is hoped that some aspects of current approaches to drug education have been successfully called into question by the argument offered here. But the path forward is not without ambiguity. Such ambiguity cannot be resolved at a stroke, but can be dealt with as we progress along the path if we have a clear view of our long-term goal. The long-term goal that I favour is the abolition of the drug problem; that is, the abolition of all the beliefs and practices of individuals and agencies that cause drug experimentation and use *to be associated with a higher rate of social and negative harm than need be.* Drug education and other social practices which achieve short-term goals that might be valued for themselves, but which make the longer-term goal of abolition recede, ought not to be encouraged. Such a stance may lead us to adopt unusual positions; for instance, I have argued elsewhere (Dorn, 1980) that certain approaches to cannabis law reform should be opposed in the interests of a longer-term solution of the broader drug problem. Similarly, although it might be argued that liberal policy reforms which seek to label drug users or other deviants as 'sick' rather than 'criminal' might appear preferable on 'humanitarian' grounds, such reforms have grossly undesirable political and individual effects. Such issues, or the fudging of them, find their echoes within drug education, within health education generally and within broader social policy areas.

Perhaps the greatest, hidden failure in evaluating contemporary drug education has been our rather naive acceptance that it has primarily to do with drugs and the socialization of schoolchildren. Perhaps the main significance of much of contemporary drug education lies in its role as a tool for the resocialization of the *adult socializers* and for the production of a *professional consensus* about the desirability of a modern, liberal, pathologizing perspective on drug use and on social deviance generally. After all, teaching something to others (e.g., to children) is one good way of learning it oneself. Perhaps tomorrow's educational and social welfare experts will look back on today and be appalled at the way in which, unable to prevent social deviancy, educators convinced themselves and each other of the need to strip it of meaning and purpose. Preferring social pathology to social diversity, drug education, together with the professional ideologies it supports, deserves an early death. Devising a suitable manner to ensure its demise and non-replacement is not a simple or self-contained task. It will require us to make connection not only with the broader field of health education, but with contemporary developments of theory and practice across the whole front of social reproduction and control.

The Tendency to Subvert any Radical Alternative

This section of the chapter reports briefly upon some aspects of the recent evaluation of a prototype in-service teacher training manual. The manual was produced in response to the unsurprising finding, in a preceding evaluation of the classroom materials *Facts and Feelings About Drugs But Decisions About Situations*, that teachers who were judged to be more understanding of and sympathetic to this 'situational' approach taught more successfully than those who were not. The training manual, jocularly entitled *Psst . . . want to try some drug education?*, was produced in order to explore the possibilities of increasing teachers' understanding and commitment. It was placed in the hands of various training agencies in England and Denmark, who agreed to use it as the basis for running short in-service courses. These courses (five in England and two in Denmark) were the object of the evaluation exercise. It was hoped that interested trainers and trainees might subsequently become involved in a revision of both the pupil and teacher-training materials, and that they might then be published. In the event, the evaluation ran into stormy waters, the research team became indisposed and dispersed, and revision of the materials was delayed. The full reasons for this would have to be analysed in terms of the material and moral forces at play in and around the agencies concerned, and this task is not attempted here. What is attempted is a brief clarification of the possibilities for a radical health education, and of the problems that may arise as both conservatives and radicals come to agree on the proposition (in my view, a false one) that radical health education may be viewed simply as an opposition to conservative values.

In order to develop this discussion, some more details have to be given about the prototype 'situation' classroom and training materials. The classroom materials focused upon a pupils' booklet, designed to be used for several lessons totalling five to ten hours. It had two main components: 'Facts and Feelings About Drugs' and 'Decisions About Situations' which corresponded to its two main goals of increasing factual knowledge and enhancing decision-making skills. The knowledge goal has three subgoals, concerned with basic facts about legal and illegal drugs (alcohol, aspirin, cannabis, coffee, sedative pills, cigarettes, etc.); facts about immediate effects (and dose, mood and situational factors involved in the construction of these effects); and facts about the acquisition and effects of habits. The facts set out in the pupils' booklet were scrupulously accurate, with none of the dark lies, ambiguities and silences characterizing much drug education. The evaluation found that the course was substantially successful in increasing knowledge for all subgroups of pupils (boys and girls, experimenters and non-experimenters, medium and lower social class, etc.). (Evaluation was by use of specially designed questionnaires in a matched control-groups post-test design, plus various qualitative measures of process and outcome. See the reports published by the Institute for the Study of Drug Dependence and the Health Education Council for details.)

The decision-making skill goal of the pupil materials was less straightforward. Starting from the proposition that education which deals only with facts about substances (cognitive, substance-focused approach) and/or with feelings about self (affective approach) is simply irrelevant to choice-making in which the significance of such facts and feelings are reconstructed in the light of the person's negotiation of the meaning of the choice situation as a whole, it becomes evident that education has to include realistic discussion about possible and probable real-life choice situations. The decision-making skills goal had three subgoals. First, that pupils should be able to show that they realized that choices take place *in situations* which structure the process and outcome of decision-making. Secondly, that pupils should have *realistic anticipations* of possible future choice situations. They should realize, for instance, that the vignette of the pusher with a syringe in one hand and candy in the other, standing by the school gate, is unlikely to correspond to the offer situations they are most likely to meet. Thirdly, pupils should be able to *apply* factual knowledge to possible choice situations, and to predict possible outcomes of specific choices. In the pupils' booklet, various strategies and exercises for teaching towards these goals were employed.

Direct observation of some classes, scrutiny of teachers' diaries and debriefing interview records suggested that these strategies were only partly successful as teaching techniques. The moralism and conservatism of many pupils (who are often deeply involved with dramatic cultural myths that 'unprepare' them for real-life problems), and of some teachers, helped to produce a situation in which, as the evaluation showed, only slight enhancement in decision-making skills (as defined above and measured three months after the end of teaching) occurred. This small shift away from fantasy was achieved, however, without any increase in levels of experimentation with any legal or illegal drugs (as predicted by the situational approach, according to which experimentation results from opportunity and from exposure to and negotiation of choice situations, and not from abstract knowledge or attitudes). The course was evaluated in Danish as well as in English schools (twenty English schools and ten Danish schools), and the findings were substantially the same in both countries. Considering that this was the first course in the drugs/alcohol area to have any of the following features – clearly stated goals, a reasonably long teaching time and an evaluation (using relevant instruments, a tight design and a delayed post-test) – the project seemed relatively encouraging. This is not, however, to deny the serious problems of underlying theory and practical application. (For an early acknowledgement of *some* of these problems, see Dorn et al., 1977, ch. 3.)

The training manual project was an attempt to explore the problems that might be involved in convincing and equipping teachers to teach 'situationally'. The project proceeded through several stages: planning; writing a six-unit manual; placing it in the hands of various training agencies; evaluation of course processes and outcomes. I shall in no way attempt to summarize all aspects of the evaluation, but shall focus upon two aspects of the manual – its tightly programmed structure and its rather 'mixed' theoretical tendency – which together proved to be the major source of problems for trainers and trainees. The tightly programmed structure of the manual instructed the trainers to present particular topics in particular ways, and in a particular order. The theoretical tendency consists of (1) exposition of the situational approach (based on an interactionist social psychology); (2) an exposition of the forces that socially construct and define 'youth dependencies' as forces of moral panic, and recommendation of an abolitionist approach to dissolving this moral panic (this was based on a critical and structural sociology); and (3) a practical discussion about how to deal with concrete and immediate drug/alcohol problems as they might present themselves in schools (this was based on a common-sense appreciation of the role strains and pressures confronting teachers). The common thread to these diverse and only partially connecting expositions was an insistence that drug/alcohol education should aim to reduce moral panic, iatrogenic stereotypes, habits and casualties, *rather than* speaking against experimentation, as drug education has traditionally and ineffectively done. An abandonment of experimentation prevention was presented as an essential prerequisite for working out a strategy for reducing *casualties*. It was the obligation to present this argument that caused difficulties for some of the trainers.

The key to understanding what happened in the five courses now follows. The training manual (TM) had been written as a programmed text, with clear instructions to trainers on how, minute by minute, they should run six-session training courses for school teachers (trainees). But the manual (and the pupils' booklet to which it referred) were brought into play in complex situations also involving:

- trainers with particular characteristics, concerns and social resources;
- trainees with particular characteristics, concerns and social resources;
- course organizers (sometimes overlapping with trainers or evaluators) and venues (with various physical and social characteristics);
- the principal investigator, the two evaluators and the circumstances obtaining in and around their London and Copenhagen offices;
- the broader political, educational and social contexts.

The main conclusion about the use of the manual in these circumstances is that it is improper to talk of the manual alone having simple effects on trainees. The combinations of manual, trainees, trainers, course organizers, venues and evaluators were different in each of the five courses; what really occurred was different in each course and, in some cases, did not correspond to the intentions of the manual author (sometimes being in direct contradiction to those intentions); and trainees' learning outcomes were highly variable.

It has already been established that the prototype situational classroom teaching material is suitable only for a proportion of secondary schools. What the evaluation of the manual has done is to confirm that the manual is, similarly, suitable for use with only some training agencies and some teachers. The evaluation sharpened our perceptions of the similarities and differences between the manual's situational and partially radical approach, and the approach of some trainers which is oriented towards conservative approaches involving affective teaching methods for 'prevention of experimentation' (backed up by rationales involving the teacher's duty rather than the efficiency of the teaching). The manual's distinction between prevention of experimentation and minimization of casualties was sometimes unacceptable to trainers and/or to trainees, and when this occurred all parties experienced strain and adopted various strategies for relieving the situation.

Other trainers and trainees, however, were positively oriented towards the manual's intentions, and this was particularly true of the two 'Southtown' (England) trainers (health education officers), and of the Danish trainer at 'Danetown' (Kirsten Hvidtfeldt), who had earlier been involved in the development of the situational pupils' materials. In these circumstances, the courses were happier, yet the trainers' commitment to make the manual work allows us to pinpoint some ambiguities and shortcomings in the manual that could be resolved. These fall into three categories: in the first place, there are changes and improvements that could be made within the present framework of the manual. Secondly, there is the question of whether such a tightly programmed, trainer-spoken manual is most appropriate, and whether (given a restriction of the manual to sympathetic trainers and trainees) the manual ought to be recast as a group self-training manual to be used by teachers to whom the trainer relates as a co-ordinator, consultant and resource-person. Thirdly, there is the question of the need for clarification of the theoretical/political/educational position of the manual, which contains within itself a number of conflicting elements. The manual is, indeed, caught between an individualistic model involving personal decisions (within choice situations) and a sociostructural model involving arguments about the 'abolition of the drug problem' (in respect of production of drug casualties). What is missing is the intermediate level of cultural, subcultural and institutional practices and values which provide the context for choice situations (i.e., which 'connect' individuals into social structure).

A full revision of the training manual would therefore involve:

1   Theoretical developments designed to 'fill in' the gap between the situational, personal, decision-making and abolitionist policy-making aspects of the manual, with material related to institutions, subcultures, etc. This would, in turn, require some changes in the situational and abolitionist models, as they are brought together.

2   Consideration given to recasting the manual as a group self-training manual, using trainers as guides and consultants and resource-persons rather than as parrots. (This possibility was actually considered at the beginning of this project but, probably mistakenly, not pursued at that time.) These groups might stay in mutually supporting contact for extended periods.

3   Since the manual is largely keyed to the prototype pupils' classroom materials, the rewriting of the manual should ideally both inform and be informed by the rewriting of the pupils' materials. This would result in a package consisting of a teachers' group self-training manual, a brief teachers' classroom guide and pupils' materials. This package could be produced either for Denmark or for England, or for both countries.

However, such a revised prototype training manual and classroom materials would still have to face the major problem that some trainers and teachers, who are committed to an antidrug stance of speaking against experimentation, are unable to differentiate experimentation from habit and/or casualty, and are unable to adopt a casualty reduction approach. Their prior commitment to the conservative approach of confirming that experimentation = harm leads them to seek ways of subverting the situational/abolitionist approach. An easy way of doing this is to hand: since, for conservatives, one has to be either antidrug or else pro-drug, they translate the manual's refusal to take up an anti-experimentation position into a charge that it is pro-drug.

This characterization of the manual deals with the radical, casualty reduction challenge to conservative anti-experimentation ideology simply by declaring the manual author to be 'beyond the pale', by projecting onto him the very imagery which he is concerned to dissolve. This is one way of neutralizing any radical alternative in health education – by employing the same discrediting, oppressive and destructive techniques which are generally employed against 'deviants'.

But it is not only conservatives who may subvert the radical approach to casualty reduction. There is also the danger that some radicals in health education may fall into the trap of equating radical health education with a strategy involving some positive encouragement of drug use. This tendency may be particularly tempting to those who, sickened by the self-righteous pronouncements and stigmatizing strategies of conservative health education, react in a purely oppositional manner. Whereas the more conservative trainers and trainees attacked the manual as encouraging drug use, thus identifying drug use with radicalism, radicals may fall prey to the same tendency also identifying drug use with radicalism, but this time approving the couplet; for them oppositional patterns of drug use can be used as part of a life style of political resistance. If authority opposes drug use (or any other 'deviancy') then the radicals, according to this 1960s philosophy, should take it up. This conception of radicalism has been devised by the antiradicals.

Yet the conception of radical health education underlying the writing of the training manual was different from the one discussed above. At no time was drug use championed, nor does the radicalism of the manual lie simply in its failure to condemn and stigmatize drug experimentation (that is quite a liberal, integrationist position, in keeping with the theory and attempted practice of many international and national authorities). Rather, radical health education is concerned with the maximization of health by means of the abolition of the structural and institutional conditions that produce it. This was the 'radical' concern of the training manual, and to conflate this concern with the 'radicalism' of oppositional life styles is to subvert the possibility of a radical drug education in the same way and just as effectively as was done by some of the trainers and trainees in the project. In order to avoid such traps we need to grapple with the problem of the position of health education in contemporary society.

Prospects for Radical Health and Social Education

Since the war the United Kingdom and most capitalist countries have passed through successive periods of relative boom and apparent consensus (the 1950s), times of resurrection of conflicts in the industrial, moral and gender-role spheres (the 1960s and early 1970s) and times of generalized crises of economy, social legitimacy and reproduction (the late 1970s and early 1980s). The socioeconomic conditions have brought to the fore social science paradigms that we can call consensus theory, conflict and conspiracy theory, and social reproduction theory respectively. Consensus theory focused upon the re-integration of the supposedly maladjusted deviant into the supposed consensus of freely agreed norms. This is the assumption of nostalgically conservative approaches to health education, such as value clarification and resocialization. The following period of overt social conflicts, and the conflict and conspiracy theories which arose out of it, turned consensus theory on its head; social control was a bad thing because it presupposed a consensus and it oppressed, labelled and stigmatized the weak. Whilst pretending to help them it mystified them and destroyed their ability to demand social justice.

Such a radical inversion of consensus theory, whilst it has some value as an exposé of and as a warning against the labelling procedures of welfare agencies and professions, oversimplifies the real situation. It overestimates the degree with which the powerful ones (classes, professions, men, etc.) in society do actually act without constraint, in their own best interests, thinking totally rationally and outside the constraints of any ideology. It generally underestimates the ways in which the 'powerless' can, within particular material circumstances (e.g., school), resist, renegotiate or transform the meanings and activities thrown at them. When this 'relative power of the powerless' is acknowledged within conflict theory, it is often romanticized and celebrated, instead of its full effect being analysed. A radical health education guided by this theoretic tendency might concern itself with the possibilities of 'f . . . in the streets', reading subversive literature whilst 'high' and other such resistance rituals. I would not wish to preach against such a theory and practice, only to locate its historical apotheosis (the 1960s), to question its adequacy and to consider its place in a fuller and less one-dimensional strategy of social-health reform.

In sexual politics, it is now commonplace to assert that 'the personal is political'. By this it is meant that, as distinct from those (radical and conservative) philosophies which separate private and public life, our personal and political lives have to be understood as articulated together; to reform one, we have to reform both. Hence the importance to the person who works for sexual equality in public life of reforming his or her sexism in personal relationships. Equally so, it is little help being non-sexist in this sphere, if we advocate a type of politics which cuts across substantive equality. Further, the distinction between public and private life is neither a watertight nor an objective or universal division; it developed from the early history of capitalism and is now shifting. Education about personal behaviour cannot be abstracted from political education without reducing itself to nostalgia and mystifying its clients. Antidependency education (the broader source of antidrug education) cannot continue without critical scrutiny in a situation when governments are responding to economic crises with measures which reduce the labour market and hence prevent individuals achieving socioeconomic independence. Radical educators cannot simply acclaim the prototype male role of rationality through independence when a progressive alternative is needed (Dorn, 1980).

So, decision-making education about personal behaviour (sex, psychotropics, etc.) cannot be divorced from education about production and about the state's handling of the economy and of social life. The prospect is for a social health education which starts with the pupils' material situations – in the family, in school, out of school, about to make the transition to work, training, education, marriage, childbirth, unemployment, etc. – and discusses with them how these situations come about. Only then can the children have a chance of working out collective strategies for changing these material situations, instead of acting within the range of options which they currently present. The present circumstances supply us with the necessity, and can help us towards the means, for reforming health and social education in this way.

Summary

Health and social education about alcohol and other drugs can be divided into three types, depending on whether it focuses on the chemical substances, upon the developmental psychology of the potential drug user, or upon the situation in which opportunities for and offers of drug experimentation occur. Currently it is affective approaches, based on notions of healthy and unhealthy psychological development, which are in the ascendancy. The first part of this chapter attacks one particular affective programme, characterizing it as telling lies about drugs, as putting forward unrealistic ideas about life and as being potentially dangerous to health. Such affective health education, the author concludes, must be regarded as part of the problem, and is worthy of abolition.

The second part of the chapter reports briefly on an evaluation of a prototype in-service teacher training manual. The manual was designed to enhance teachers' understanding of and commitment to, and ability to use, the ISDD's prototype classroom materials for teaching 'situational' decision-making skills in relation to alcohol, cigarettes, cannabis and other legal and illegal drugs. The evaluation pointed out several basic problems with the training manual, and also illuminated the dangers of a pseudo-radical tendency to romanticize social deviance. The third part explores some problems and prospects for a radical health education, that is, a health education which achieves its aims by going beyond its consigned boundaries. This discussion attempts to place health education within the broader context of post-war problems of social welfare, reproduction and control.

The chapter as a whole moves from the conservative level of analysis which concerns itself with the supposedly deviant person and/or act, through a consideration of the dangers of adopting the sort of 'radical' position (romanticizing or championing deviancy) which is prepared for us within and by current health education and other social welfare ideologies, and towards a new theory and practice of radical and effective social-health education. The aim is a theory and practice that works, because it engages with the real problems inside and outside schools.

References

Dorn, N. (1977) *Teaching Decision-Making Skills About Legal and Illegal Drugs*. London, Health Education Council/Institute for the Study of Drug Dependence.

Dorn, N. (1980) 'The conservatism of the cannabis debate', in Clarke, J. et al. (eds), *Permissiveness and Control*. Proceedings of the National Deviancy Conference. London, Macmillan.

Dorn, N., Thompson, A. and Hvidtfeldt, K. (1977) *The DEDE Project*. London, Health Education Council/Institute for the Study of Drug Dependence.

Non-Medical Drugs Directorate (1975) *The Hole in the Fence*. Copies available in the libraries of the Health Education Council, Teachers' Advisory Council for Alcohol and Drug Education and Institute for the Study of Drug Dependence.

The author wishes to acknowledge the work of Anne Thompson and Kirsten Hvidtfeldt, and of Steve Butters, drawn on in the second part of this chapter.

PART II

THE SCHOOL CONTEXT

INTRODUCTION

The nature, place and scope of health education in the context of the school curriculum is a vital yet beguiling issue which can easily be submerged by the pressures and constraints of the day-to-day activities of a school. Part II therefore focuses attention on the major issues which will face a school contemplating the introduction or further development of health education into the curriculum. What is health education? What are its contents and purpose? What part should it play in the overall life of the school? Should it be treated as a separate subject or as a cross-curricular activity? If the latter, how is it to be organized and co-ordinated and who is to do this? In what way is health education related to other areas of study which contribute to the personal and social curriculum, such as social education, moral education and political education? What teaching methods are appropriate to health education? These and many related issues are discussed in Chapters 4 and 5.

The ethos and traditions of the primary school, rich in the philosophy and practice of child-centred education, would appear to offer a sound pedigree for the development of health education teaching. There is also, however, a very strong tradition of thematic and incidental teaching which could run counter to the need in health education for a carefully planned programme for every school. Vaughan Johnson considers recent thoughts and developments in the philosophy and practice of primary education, as a background to his powerful argument for the need to see health education as an essential and integral part of it. He is at present deputy head of Greenleys Middle School in Buckinghamshire, and was for some years a team member and project disseminator of the Schools Council Health Education Project 5–13. He has visited most of the country in that capacity, and writes from a wide experience of schools and from extensive contact with teachers.

The secondary schools, labouring against the constraints imposed by subject divisions and demands of examinations, present a different set of problems to the initiator of health education. Trefor Williams discusses ways in which health education can play a more important role in the secondary school. From his discussion emerges the need for the careful preparation of a school co-ordinator for the many tasks involved in what should be viewed as school-based curriculum development, and an investment in professional training.

Ten years' teaching in secondary schools, four years as an area health education officer, seven years' teaching in a college of education and three years as head of the school of studies in community care in a college of higher education, have provided Trefor Williams with a considerable and varied background of experience in health and social education. From 1973 to 1980 he was director of the Schools Council Health Education Projects 5–13 and 13–18, now based at the Health Studies Unit of Southampton University. He has also acted as adviser, since 1973, to the television series *Good Health* which is broadcast to junior schools.

CHAPTER 4

HEALTH EDUCATION IN PRIMARY SCHOOLS

Vaughan Johnson

Primary Schools Today

Towards child-centred education

Observers of primary education may be forgiven for feeling that there has been a major change in the nature and purposes of primary schools over the past few decades. The reaction to major government statements such as the Hadow and the Plowden Reports (Board of Education, 1931; CACE, 1967) suggests a rate of change almost unbelievable in its speed, and totally unbelievable if one has any experience of working against years of tradition in education.

John Blackie (1969), formerly an HMI and Chief Inspector for Primary Schools, writing at about the same time as the Plowden Report was being published, tells of the growing influence of colleges of education and HM Inspectorate, of in-service training courses and of the Hadow Report itself which 'gave respectability to ideas which had hitherto been thought of as cranky or idealistic'.

One of these 'cranky' ideas concerned a challenge to the emphasis on subjects at the junior level: 'Teaching by subjects is a mode of instruction which, although it may be appropriate for the older boys and girls, who have themselves developed specialist interests and who are ready to follow the major intellectual pursuits of mankind along the lines of their logical development, does not always correspond with the child's unsystematized, but eager interest.' (Board of Education, 1931). However, by the late 1930s, as Blackie (1969) goes on to comment, 'the number of junior schools which had been substantially affected was very small, and even in the infants' schools, which had started earlier and moved faster, there was still a solid block of conservatism'. The Report's plea in 1931 was for 'activity and experience'; statements were made such as 'the school subjects should not be isolated and labelled in separate compartments of the time-table, but should be treated in close relation to the child's concrete experience', yet, as Razzell (1969) comments in similar vein to Blackie: 'little progress was made in improving the majority of the junior schools. The seed planted by Hadow was to lie dormant for many years.'

Quite clearly the pace of change had not been as fast as many people in the education world had hoped (or feared!), nor had it necessarily taken the directions which the writers of such reports had suggested. In fact the Plowden Report suggested that approximately one-third of the schools studied by HM Inspectors in 1964 had been substantially affected by change in outlook and method, another third somewhat affected and the remaining third very little affected.

The Plowden Report itself (CACE, 1967) did much, however, to consolidate the case for child-centred education, which in many respects had been pioneered by Hadow. Indeed several paragraphs expand quotations from the earlier report such as: 'The curriculum is to be thought of in terms of activity and experience rather than knowledge to be acquired and facts to be stored.' (para. 529). The Plowden Report legitimized the move towards more informal education. It argued against rigid subject divisions, encouraged flexibility and stressed the importance of the children's choice of activity and the integration of their school work, with teachers guiding and stimulating children to learn rather than telling them exactly what to do and when to do it.

> A school is not merely a teaching shop, it must transmit values and attitudes. It is a community in which children learn to live first and foremost as children and not as future adults. In family life children learn to live with people of all ages. The school sets out deliberately to devise the right environment for children, to allow them to be themselves and to develop in the way and at the pace appropriate to them. . . . Not all primary schools correspond to this picture, but it does represent a general and quickening trend. (para. 505)

The Report was advocating a move away from a more 'traditional', teacher-centred, subject-based teaching system towards a more 'progressive', child-centred, discovery method-based learning system. But did this major fundamental shift ever take place? Was it really a trend?

So near and yet so far

Most writers, mainly of course passionate believers or even practitioners on either side of the traditional-progressive debate, seem quite understandably to suggest that enormous changes *have* taken place in large numbers of primary schools. Sir Alec Clegg (1971) (formerly Chief Education Officer of the West Riding of Yorkshire) asserted that such changes were fairly widespread.

> Within a few years there were not two schools out of a thousand working this way, but a score or more, and today (1972) it is hard to find a school that is not influenced in some way or another by the new ways.

The rapid spread of such innovation has certainly been cited by many of its opponents as being the major cause of the decline in standards in our primary schools. So the more critical commentators, including 'Black Paper' authors such as Stuart Froome (1970), talk scathingly of 'learning by stealth', following the 'chance whims and fancies of little children . . . abandoning the timetable and detailed syllabus of work . . .', following 'ineffectual and unprofitable courses' in which the child may 'through interest teach himself, and the teacher watches benevolently from the touch-line'. The foreword to his book *Why Tommy Isn't Learning* addresses it to the 'millions of parents whose children are being handicapped by present day fashionable teaching methods' and the 'thousands of teachers . . . who have been misled for years by educators . . .'.

Without entering into the debate on the rights or wrongs of formal versus informal education, one should nevertheless question the accuracy of these contentions and the degree to which this change in fact occurred. Was it indeed such a 'general and quickening trend'? As little as one year after the publication of the Plowden Report, Razzell (1969) wrote, 'Although the wind of change is blowing through our junior schools there is reason to believe that in some instances it is simply blowing the dust and cobwebs from an archaic structure. The language and motions of modernity are present, but the heart that beats at a deeper level is still pre-Hadow.'

The Plowden Report itself looked back at the slow pace of progress, recognizing 'the force of tradition and of the inherent conservatism of all teaching professions . . .' (para. 509). This more realistic assessment has been borne out by several recent studies. For example, Bennett (1976) suggests that less than 10% of schools fit the Plowden definition (as compared with Blackie's 30% and 30% moving towards it), and a 'generous estimate is that 17% of teachers teach in the manner prescribed by Plowden, while at the other end of the teaching continuum approximately one in four teaches formally'. He asserts that the vast majority of teachers use mixed teaching styles incorporating elements of both formal and informal practice. Bassey (1978) suggests that while 'primary teachers have a great deal of freedom in deciding what children do . . . they use their freedom in highly traditional ways'.

Perhaps most significant of all in this context is the report of HM Inspectors, entitled *Primary Education in England* (DES, 1978), which describes the surveys of seven-, nine- and eleven-year-olds in 1127 classes in 542 representative schools.

> In the survey classes about three-quarters of the teachers employed a mainly didactic approach, while less than one in twenty relied mainly on an exploratory approach. In about one-fifth of the classes teachers employed an appropriate combination of didactic and exploratory methods, varying their approach according to the nature of the task in hand, and could not be said to incline to either approach.

One thing about which all these sources seem to agree is that the move towards real 'child-centred', 'progressive', 'informal', 'exploratory' education can barely be described as a trend, let alone a general trend.

What is primary education trying to do?

The Plowden Report underlined the difficulty of stating aims. Nevertheless, it did so itself implicitly in discussing the practice and outlook of schools. In the final paragraph of the short chapter on aims, the Report states: 'Children need to be themselves, to live with other children and with grown ups, to learn from their environment, to enjoy the present, to get ready for the future, to create and love, to learn to face adversity, to behave responsibly, in a word, to be human beings.' However, it continues, 'Decisions about the influences and situations that ought to be contrived to these *ends* must be left to individual schools, teachers and parents. What must be ensured is that the decisions taken in schools spring from the best available knowledge and are not *simply dictated by habit or convention*.' (para. 507, author's emphases).

It is pertinent to ask how this can be done without a systematic consideration of the aims of the school and its teachers. Is it not essential that schools consider in some detail what it is that they are trying to do, before setting out to refine and develop the ways in which they do it? If not confusion may reign or habit and convention determine what goes on completely unchallenged.

The work of Ashton and her colleagues (1975) on the Schools Council Aims of Primary Education Project is of immense value in this context. This showed very clearly that, while teachers may have difficulty in stating aims, they certainly possess them. Moreover these aims seem to be closely linked to the fundamental beliefs which teachers have about the broad purposes of education. Two major groupings were identified: 'individualistic' teachers – those mainly concerned with developing individual talents and interests; and 'societal' teachers – those mainly concerned with equipping children with skills and attitudes appropriate to the society to which they belong.

Not unnaturally, these two patterns of opinion were often seen to be in opposition, and, as Ashton concludes,

> What they appear to show is not an evolution of thought in education, but the reaction of one tradition against another. The individualistic pattern seems not so much to have developed from and built upon the societal one as to have relegated it to a place of significantly less importance. (p. 90)

The danger in such a situation is that fashions may be seen to change with the swing of the pendulum, often aided and abetted by media pressures, as opinion and unjustified assertion hold sway for a relatively short period of time. But real innovation may not have taken place at all. It is of paramount importance that teachers consider their aims very carefully and relate these to the many conflicting demands made upon them and their pupils, particularly in the wake of the 1978 HMI Report. If such a process is carried out well it should provide a firm basis from which to choose the methods and practices most appropriate to the current needs of the children, the demands of society and the skills, interests and concerns of members of staff. Such a well-founded platform should be better able to resist the wilder blandishments of educational theorists and curriculum innovators, yet at the same time provide a secure and fertile ground for a small number of new and important developments to be tried and developed where appropriate.

Curriculum priorities

In the final paragraph of his 1971 collection of writings on the changing primary school, Sir Alec Clegg wrote:

> . . . whatever the 'method' there is always hope if the teacher can answer with conviction the question 'Why are you teaching what you are teaching in the way you are teaching to this particular child at his stage of development?'

As we have already seen, it is unlikely that many schools and teachers will indeed pose this question sufficiently often. The 1978 HM Inspectors' Report shows the following percentages of schools with 'written guidelines' or 'schemes of work' for individual subjects: 88% maths, 85% language, 72% RE, then 43% science and 17% health education, the same as for dance, less than games (26%) and swimming (19%), but more than French (15%) and humanities (9%).

With the exception of the special legal requirement for an approved religious education component, is this perhaps a guide to curriculum priorities, or does it represent a division between those areas for which planning guidelines are deemed essential (cf. only 43% for science) and those areas which form a more incidental unstructured part of school life or perhaps are not considered at all. Who suggests that certain elements should be planned and co-ordinated, and how do schools arrive at establishing their curriculum priorities? Are they still arrived at through 'habit and convention'? Indeed, even the majority of these schemes and guidelines would show, on closer inspection, a major concern with the 'what' of Clegg's question rather than with the 'why' or the 'how', and their existence in no way indicates that individual teachers are even following them, let alone thinking about their appropriateness.

Following the publication of various reports and papers on education during the period 1976–1978, there has been a great deal of discussion of the trend 'back' towards a concentration of the 'basics'. This has been hailed by traditionalists, the vast majority of whom never really moved away from that end of the continuum, as a welcome return swing of the pendulum to counteract the alleged progressive drift of education over the past few decades. The 1978 HMI Report says categorically, however, that this emphasis is already there: 'High priority is given to teaching children to read, write and learn mathematics.'

The Report underlines the need to extend and enrich curriculum provision in order to build on these basics, stating that these will also directly benefit thereby:

> . . . the effective application of skills, including their use in practical activities is important. The teaching of skills in isolation, whether in language or mathematics does not produce the best results. (p. 112)

It also states unambiguously that:

> Curricular content should be selected not only to suit the interests and abilities of

the children and to provide for the progressive development of the basic skills, but also because it is important in its own right. (p. 113)

So what then do we expect to see in primary schools? A mixture of formal and informal settings and teaching styles, with the emphasis on more formal didactic methods, but often without any clear guidelines except in mathematics and language work? And what are those priorities likely to be? Again in the words of the HMI Report:

> While all would presumably agree that it is essential that children are taught to read, write and calculate, few would regard this as sufficient. It is currently accepted that in the primary school, children are taught to behave in socially and morally acceptable ways, to extend their spoken and written language and appreciation of literature, to comprehend mathematical and scientific ideas, to participate in a range of aesthetic and physical activities and, through their religious, moral, historical and geographical studies, to begin to see their own situation in a broader social context. (p. 16)

Implications for the method and timing of curriculum innovation in health education

Despite the apparent emphasis on 'progressive' primary school education, we must be prepared to accept that the pace of change in education is exceedingly slow; habit and tradition are extremely strong forces which must be recognized and challenged if we are to prevent curriculum innovation from foundering without due consideration.

We cannot assume that the majority of teachers are already 'child-focused' and therefore automatically receptive to practical work, based on the assumption that the child's needs and interests are the first priority. Moreover, we cannot assume too high a level of timetable flexibility nor the freedom or preparedness of teachers to allocate such time as is required to pursue broader aspects of their work as far as we might wish, or even as far as they might wish.

We must realize that many headteachers may not agree with the establishment of health education in its own right in the timetable, and we cannot yet look for much support for this from major general reports on primary education (except in so far as the Plowden Report specifically mentions sex education, and elements of the 'Science' and 'Social abilities' schedules adopted by HM Inspectors in the 1978 Report clearly include major parts of a broadly defined health education programme). Discussion with headteachers must therefore be an important part of the health education curriculum innovator's work.

In the current educational climate we must therefore look to those trends and arguments which can be seen to support our case; for example, the reports and policy of those national and local bodies and organizations which repeatedly stress the importance of health education. We must be prepared to use arguments such as those mentioned in the Primary Inspectors' Report; in other words to extend basic skills to some purpose, in many cases a vital one, by reinforcing and enriching other aspects of the curriculum, using health education as a vehicle for teaching the 'basics' if this is what the current public clamour in education is for. We can find some additional support for health education in demands for a broader social context for education in general. Often this must be linked with better established areas of the curriculum such as religious, moral, social or environmental studies.

It is essential, therefore, that school staff be given an opportunity and actively encouraged to discuss and develop their ideas together, to review what already goes on in the school curriculum and to plan and develop their programme in a manner which will ensure that it is carried out by the majority of colleagues with similar aims and intentions and using similar methods. Without such a process of review and development the work that actually goes on in neighbouring classrooms in the same school may well lead children in totally different directions and may also be at odds with the wider aims of the school.

However, we must be prepared to accept that some schools, particularly those which are thinking through or have thought through their basic aims and philosophy, may be currently engaged in reviewing or developing other aspects of the curriculum. While not denying the importance of health education, they may have neither the time nor the energy to consider it in detail at this particular point in time.

Why Primary Schools Should Do Health Education

The needs of children in the primary school age-range demand some response

Children aged between about five and eleven are growing and developing extremely rapidly, not merely of course in physical terms but also socially, intellectually, emotionally and morally. Their *physical* growth and development may be the most noticeable; enormous changes in size, shape and weight, growing physical strength, new and finer skills, greater co-ordination and, particularly in girls aged about ten and over, their increasingly rapid sexual development. All children are interested in, and many are concerned and need reassurance about, their particular rate of development and what is in store for them.

They are also beginning to form *social* relationships with others of the same sex, in gangs, clubs or societies and later with those of the opposite sex. In some cases they may have difficulty in making these friends and need the help and support of adults to overcome or compensate for this. More positively, peer groups themselves will offer an opportunity to the primary school child to learn to play and live in harmony with others. He will have to compete, to control his feelings, to establish roles and learn social techniques.

There may also be problems of different rates of *intellectual* development and this, of course, is something of which teachers are very well aware. Furthermore, when working with children in this age-range we see their zest for information, their enjoyment of learning and their excitement. Razzell (1969) captures a great deal of this feeling in the use of the phrase 'children at the flood'. By this Razzell means:

> Children from 7 to 12 are delightful people to live and work with. Noisy, energetic and above all eager and full of zest. . . .

> There is little doubt that the most successful schools are those who take these children at the flood and lead them on. (pp. 22, 23)

Closely tied to the children's social and intellectual development is their *emotional* growth. Children are learning throughout the primary age-range how to handle and express emotions. The Plowden Report (1967) comments:

> A major role of the school is to help the child to come to terms with these feelings and not to suppress them, but to understand them and thus to discover how to deal acceptably with them. His experiences with other children give him essential experience in handling relationships. (para. 68)

Is this something which is generally accepted as being a legitimate role of the school? Should teachers specifically think through ways of helping children to come to terms with their emotions?

Finally, let us consider the child's *moral* development which, once again, is closely allied to the other aspects of his development. The Plowden Report describes the stages through which children pass:

The child forms his sense of personal worth and his moral sense from early experiences of acceptance, approval, and disapproval. Out of an externally imposed rule of what is permitted arises a sense of what ought to be done and an internal system of control: in every day terms, a conscience. The very young child, limited in understanding, acts according to strict rules, even though he often breaks them. What is right and wrong relates closely to what his parents say and to the situation arising in the home. Later, as the child develops intellectually and lives with others, his sense of right and wrong derives from a wider circle and becomes more qualified; the rules of a game are seen to be arrived at by consensus, and therefore, modifiable by common agreement. . . . (para. 73)

In summary then, as children of primary school age are growing and developing so rapidly during this period, it is of crucial importance that their potential for healthy growth and development in *all* these dimensions is recognized, encouraged and fostered by, amongst others, those concerned with education. Traditionally, health education has been mainly associated with 'matters physical'. The sorts of problems facing us today clearly demand an extension of this concept to consider these other dimensions outlined above, particularly the social and emotional areas which are often the most important ones when it comes to real decisions about our health and well-being.

Children in the primary school age-range are open to many other 'educational' pressures

A second major reason for providing health education for children in this age-range is that they will receive a certain amount 'willy-nilly'. Consider, for example, the attitudes developing as a result of the eating patterns and choices at home, at school, in the playground or 'at Granny's'!; the exciting smoking, risk-taking or aggressive behaviour observed in older brothers and sisters, more venturesome peers or as seen, and probably admired, on television; the fact of nudity at home, in the showers, in newspapers and books, together with graffiti, fable and fantasy shared in the toilets, at camp or on the way home. Not all of these influences may be significant, not all of them may be negative, but it would seem reasonable, nevertheless, to suggest that together they will in many cases provide young children with an incomplete, misleading or occasionally false set of expectations and assumptions in substantial areas of health behaviour.

So, a variety of educational mechanisms, harmful misunderstanding of context, general confusion about possible courses of action and incorrect knowledge may lead individual children to assume that there is no alternative to smoking, drinking too much, taking risks, being promiscuous and so on, if they are to achieve the 'normal' status and achievements of adolescence or adulthood as they understand it.

This idea can usefully be expressed and clarified by using the sociological term 'career' to develop the notion of health careers. Let us take the example of smoking. Research by Bewley and her colleagues (1973) has shown that one in three children in the final year of primary school have experimented with smoking, and nearly 7% of boys in the sample were 'regular smokers'. Several teachers working with the Schools Council Health Education Project (SCHEP) 5–13 in its early stages also pointed to the fact that many young children (aged five–seven) have well-developed notions of smoking behaviour – buying cigarettes in a shop, emptying ashtrays, drawing cigarettes, etc. – as a mark of recognition for an adult. It is most important, therefore, that we recognize the cumulative effect of various media, family, informal school and peer group pressures upon children and the stages which may precede the actual smoking of tobacco.

A typical child may be well launched on his 'smoking career' by the age of ten. However, ignoring the early development of attitudes towards smoking and children's early experimentation with tobacco, our health education in the past has frequently been applied at the stage when the habit is already formed, and when there remains little time in terms of formal schooling to continue educating and supporting the child. A programme of education aimed at children in the primary school age-range should reach most children before their attitudes have hardened and their habits become ingrained.

This notion of health careers can valuably be applied to other health problems where today's life style is all too often conducive to the transmission and acceptance of norms of behaviour which tend to lead to ill-health, for example in terms of food consumption, dental health and obesity, or over consumption of alcohol, medicines and other drugs. As well as these easily recognizable, personal ill-health habits there exist many other less tangible ones; for example, stress, insensitivity, prejudice and, increasingly, aggression are seen by many observers as endemic in our present society. The attitudes and situational responses associated with all these states will be transmitted to young children whether we like it or not.

If we accept that these influences do come to bear on children of primary school age, then what alternatives are there? We can do nothing, and allow their 'education' in these matters to go by default, or we can wait until a 'problem' occurs, leaving discussion until children are actually in the situation, faced with a choice, or already 'experimenting', or we can recognize the strength of such early influences and try to provide opportunities for them to consider, discuss and learn about other facts, standpoints and possible courses of action *before* these 'other' educators have their main effect and children are faced with having to make 'crisis' decisions.

Many writers have stressed the value of work with younger children. For example, Williams (1976) strongly argues the case for working with the pre-adolescent child from the evidence of Bewley et al. (1975) concerning attitudes to, experimentation with and the prevalence of smoking, of Jahoda and Crammond (1972) concerning attitudes to and consumption of alcohol and from that of the Kreitlers (1966) concerning concepts of sexuality and birth.

> A common thread winds its way through each of these researches, a thread which emphasizes the importance of social experience as a background to the formation of attitudes in young children. There are many factors which play their part in the process of attitude formation in children, the most significant of which are thought to be the home, the peer group and the influence of the mass media.
> In many instances, however, there are very few opportunities for children to be exposed to influences which can act as a counter-weight to their informal social learning about health-related behaviour. Perhaps we ought to consider the influence of the school in this context.

One final point must be considered here; many teachers may well say 'If you provide young children with education on, for example, smoking, you will introduce them to the idea', or 'They're not all ready for such information.' It is important in such cases to try to stimulate discussion about the children's exposure to ideas outside the classroom as mentioned above. Young children, although neither smokers nor alcoholics, will through other means already be beginning to have clear notions about adolescent and adult smoking and drinking behaviour. I conclude this section therefore by quoting from the Hampshire Education Committee Working Party's Guidelines, *Health: Learning to care* (1972):

> There are stages of emotional development at which a pupil can accept and integrate information relating directly to himself, to his own development, and to his relationships with others. . . . These stages of development vary greatly between individuals, and information often requires repetition, and needs to be readily available at many levels. . . . It was felt that there is probably less danger in giving information to pupils too early than in being too late. (para. 4)

Some reasons why health education should not be left solely to parents
Desirable as it may be for many aspects of health education to be the responsibility of parents, only a proportion of parents seems both to acknowledge this and to provide the stimuli, discussion, information and support required. In addition, it must be stated that there are indeed some areas which might be difficult for parents to cover even if they wish to, perhaps because they do not know what they ought to be saying or are unsure how to raise and to handle sensitive issues in which they themselves are involved. They do not have easy access to group discussions or role-play exercises which might help to shed light on various factors of importance, and in addition they may not have the appropriate information or the necessary skills. It should also be said that, in certain cases, the transmission of ideas, attitudes and practices by parents may be most likely to lead to the long-term ill-health of children (e.g., smoking, drinking, dietary habits) – a vicious circle which may have to be broken at some stage by another person.

Some teachers may feel a little uneasy, however, about the possibility of undermining the role of parents by providing such education within schools. This fear can be allayed in some measure, first, by stressing that a school programme need not, indeed should not, be an alternative to parental responsibility. On the contrary, it is without doubt of infinitely greater value when conducted with the full knowledge, agreement and, where possible, active involvement of parents. Secondly, it can also be viewed in terms of helping young children in such a manner that they will, as parents themselves, be better informed and prepared so that they are perhaps better able then to carry out such education with their own children in due course. Any work carried out in school should complement and build on what parents have done. It should encourage their involvement and participation in as full a manner as possible and should be reviewed continuously in the light of the changing demands of children, their parents, the school staff and members of the local community.

The Plowden Report (1967, ch. 4) emphasizes the importance of this contact with parents, and suggests many ways of developing and improving it in primary schools. Reports from schools involved in the development, trial and dissemination stages of SCHEP would suggest that wherever schools do consult or involve parents concerning their health education work, they have a particularly good response. Local authority guidelines mainly concerned with the secondary school age-range nevertheless acknowledge the value of these early school-parent links, particularly if agreement is sought in more sensitive areas. This message is expressed very clearly in the Hampshire Education Committee's document (1972):

> In primary schools the need for a sense of partnership, understanding and shared responsibility is particularly important for not only should parents be acquainted with what is being attempted, but should be consulted, and invited to join in the programme of Health Education. (para. 5)

The aims of primary school teachers broadly support the aims of health education

Although we cannot assume that headteachers necessarily agree with health education appearing as such in the school curriculum, nor can we look to the easy adoption of such ideas because of current widespread demands for emphasis on aims such as raising basic 'standards', nevertheless Ashton's work (1975) clearly shows that in ranking their aims, primary school teachers place major emphasis, which is categorized as 'of utmost and major importance', first, on personal development, secondly, on social and moral development and, thirdly, on the basic skills. We must complete the picture by adding 'conspicuous by their absence among the priority aims were any references to the arts, music, physical education, religious education, sex education, science or a second language'. However, teachers did, nevertheless, 'accept aims in these areas as valid aims for the primary school'.

Health education can help children's school work in many ways

Through its concentration on self-awareness and relationships, on personal responsibility, on concern for the needs and feelings of others as well as on physical health, the work increasingly undertaken in the field of health education can be seen to have a valuable impact upon children's learning in other fields:

- by improving their attitudes towards school and learning generally;
- by providing an interesting vehicle for the teaching of 'the basics' or of another subject, such as history or areas such as environmental studies;
- by providing many ways of developing and enriching work in other areas of the curriculum to specifically recognizable and relevant, immediate and long-term purposes.

The general value of a broad curriculum to the development of basic skills was supported by the recent HM Inspectors' survey and has already been mentioned: 'The basic skills are more successfully learnt when applied to other subjects.' (Hampshire Education Committee, 1972). This tendency has been widely reported by many of the teachers involved in developing and using the SCHEP materials.

Health education is important in its own right and in relation to other aspects of the curriculum

The HM Inspectors' Report makes a statement which is of fundamental value in current curriculum debate, steeped as it always is in the history of subject specialism:

> Curricular content should be selected not only to suit the interests and abilities of the children and to provide for the progressive development of the basic skills, *but also because it is important in its own right.* (p. 113, author's emphasis)

Elsewhere in this book, the claims to the importance of health education for the present and future needs of the children themselves and of society as a whole have been adequately argued. Unfortunately, subjects such as health education normally have to argue defensively about 'taking' time from other aspects of the curriculum which themselves are all too rarely subjected to similar scrutiny in terms of their relative value and importance. Dearden (1976), writing on curricular aims and curricular integration in *Problems in Primary Education*, says:

> . . . we may ask of any suggested curricular proposal, from whatever direction or personal inspiration it may come, the following four questions: Does it provide a useful preparation for subsequent life? Does it provide a worthwhile contribution to achieving a balanced general education? Does it provide opportunities to cultivate educationally important attitudes towards one's learning, over and above the importance of the focal content of the learning? Does it merit a high enough priority to gain a place in that investment of the community's scarce resources called a 'school'?

I have every confidence in subjecting health education to a rigorous analysis on all these four questions. It would be interesting if certain other aspects of primary school curricula were at the same time forced to stand a test of re-introduction on similar terms! For all these reasons, and many more which could be mentioned, I would hope that primary school teachers will feel they can and should include aspects of health education within their curricula.

Concern is expressed in the HMI Report and elsewhere about the complexity and pressure of the jobs which teachers are being asked to do. If health education is viewed as just 'another responsibility' it will not be welcomed. Many teachers will suggest, as they have in the past, that it should be done by parents or others. Fulton and Fassbender (1972) talk of 'pedagogical buck-passing' and I conclude this section by quoting from the final paragraph of their introduction:

> It has been said that former President Harry S. Truman displayed a sign on his desk which read 'The buck stops here'. It is our hope that every elementary school teacher will adopt a similar philosophy concerning his health education obligations, for there are few areas of education that have the potential for such dramatic impact and lasting benefit.

I know that there are many of us working in the field of school health education who would wish to endorse such an expression of hope and to see it translated into actions as well as words by every primary school teacher.

Current Practice in Primary School Health Education

Content, definitions and patterns of occurrence

There is no doubt that an enormous amount of work which can be regarded as health education does go on in primary schools. For example, general projects about 'Me and my family' may well include aspects of physical growth and development or personal hygiene topics such as washing and cleaning teeth, particularly the latter since so much material is made available to teachers, mainly by the manufacturers of toothpaste. Another topic which seems to be covered fairly frequently is food. The history of medicines or the history of disease are other somewhat time-consuming topics which can be seen in many primary schools and could be identified as health education. Whether or not any of these actually reach the appropriate personal health messages, particularly if teachers are not including them for that reason, is a matter for conjecture.

The DES Handbook *Health Education in Schools* (1977) supports this rather fragmented picture:

> Health education is neither recognised, nor recognisable, in the school curriculum in the sense that mathematics is recognised and recognisable. But health education is unavoidable, even if its presence is denied. The infant teacher who instructs her charges in the appropriate times to wash their hands; the primary teacher who introduces boys and girls to the ways in which animals and human beings organise themselves to care for their young; . . . Their influence may be

greater than they suppose. If so ancient an educational aim as the development of a healthy mind in a healthy body is accepted, the contributions of teachers of all expressive and creative arts, and of gymnastics, games and sports are self-evident. Such teachers also help to maintain a healthy mind in a healthy body throughout life when they arouse interests which grow into absorbing leisure activities, which may include physical skills and exercise as well as the creativity of the craftsman. So in a fragmented way health education happens to boys and girls in all schools without anyone necessarily being aware of its totality. Nowadays, however, a growing number of schools adopt a more positive approach. (p. 29)

This more positive approach to planning is something we looked for in the early development and trial work involved in SCHEP, but even among those schools committed to the project and involved with the team for some time in developing ideas and materials, there was a lack of positive planning. Experience during the project's dissemination phase (1976–1980) confirms that a great deal of health education is still largely piecemeal, unco-ordinated, haphazard even, and that the coverage of topics is patchy and unlikely to be based on any developmental programme.

However, not to paint too gloomy a picture, there are, of course, some schools which do set out to provide a co-ordinated programme of health education based perhaps on a headteacher's or a specialist teacher's own ideas as to what is important, on LEA guidelines or checklists, a health education television series or the SCHEP materials.

There is generally felt to be a problem in planning programmes to meet the broad definition of health education, which often leads to the response of teachers, 'Well of course we do all that already!' or perhaps, 'Such things should be caught not taught'. In the section which follows I shall attempt to categorize some of the different ways in which health education may occur in schools, from those which rather grudgingly accept they must answer questions if they 'crop up' (but may not hear them!) to those which are implementing an internally developed, planned and co-ordinated school programme.

At one end of this continuum a great deal of health education may occur by chance, as a result of children's incidental questions or comments arising out of situations at school. It may occur as an additional health aspect of some other subject or topic or centre of interest, should teachers and children be prepared to follow that particular course. Alternatively, individual health topics – often the crisis areas to do with eating, drinking, smoking, safety and sex – may be covered from time to time, often in terms of 'lessons' in the final year 'before they go into the secondary school' or, perhaps, as school assemblies conducted by the head, teachers or groups of children. Again, it might be as a result of following a general interest 'miscellany', general studies course or television or radio series, such as BBC TV's *Merry Go Round*, where programmes on nutrition, safety and sex education form part of a very diverse output. Moving further towards planning for health education to occur, one could next mention those schools and teachers who choose to cover certain topics, often still the 'crisis' areas, but do not have a fully co-ordinated and planned programme. Next come those schools which do follow some externally devised programme of health education, possibly a local authority scheme, a scheme found in text books or children's books or a live broadcast-related scheme such as offered by the ATV *Good Health* series now seen in 25% of primary schools.

The penultimate category of schools would be those with 'written guidelines or schemes of work' (now 17% of all primary schools according to the HM Inspectors' survey), that is, where a headteacher or specialist has either worked out a school scheme or has adapted and developed LEA or SCHEP guidelines or others to suit the school.

I would, finally, like to add one more category, namely those schools which are implementing a health education programme developed through an internal process of curriculum development involving the majority of the school staff. I suspect that very few schools indeed can be placed in this category, although we are working hard to provide training materials and methods to facilitate this process.

These eight suggested categories of primary school health education provision can be summarized as follows:

1   Answer incidental questions if and when they occur (SCHEP estimate 75%).
2   Cover any health aspect additional to the main topic if time allows.
3   Cover occasional specific health topics if they fit in or if crises occur.
4   Cover health topics as selected and when presented by, for example, general studies courses or broadcasts.
5   Plan to cover specific but probably unrelated health topics.
6   Plan to use specific health education guidelines (e.g., LEA/AHA or health education TV series (ATV 25%).
7   Adopt written guidelines or schemes of work for the school (DES 17%).

8 Develop internally a planned and co-ordinated programme for the school (SCHEP estimate 5%).

Our experience would suggest that the majority of schools come within the first four categories if they do any health education at all; schools known locally to be in the forefront of progress in establishing health education programmes are often only at category 5. We know of very few schools as yet which have developed their programmes of work as a result of school-based curriculum development processes (category 8).

Aims and methods

Although we are doubtless seeing great changes in the field of health education, the many discussions with which I have been involved during the dissemination phase of SCHEP 5–13 confirm what the early research of the project discovered in terms of teachers' aims and methods in health education. While teachers tend to find it easy to discuss, debate and define health education in terms of content, they find it much more difficult to consider their aims and appropriate methodology. Most teachers still seem to be unaware that in many cases the way they discuss or present something may be more important in terms of the final messages the children receive, absorb and apply than the actual topic under discussion. Writing soon after the beginning of the project Williams (1975) stated:

> Our methodology in the recent past has certainly been concentrated heavily on prohibition and information giving – in our anxiety to protect children we often end up by telling them how to behave. In our eagerness to inform, acquiring information became an end in itself and what children did with it ceased to be our real concern. These approaches were in themselves not wrong but merely incomplete.

I would suggest that much current primary school health education is still primarily concerned with telling children about certain crises and how they should behave, normally in a negative manner such as 'don't drink, don't smoke, don't over-eat, don't touch members of the other sex, don't run across the road' and so on. More worrying is that such messages are still occasionally reinforced by shock-tactic films, pictures or stories which are designed to frighten children away from such behaviour. Such stimuli may heighten in some children the desire to gain status by 'getting away with it', may work totally against what is transmitted elsewhere in school and may understandably cause conflict with or anxiety about parents, relatives or close friends.

While there may indeed be a 'growing number of schools adopting a more positive approach', I summarize below some of the questions which they have doubtless had to answer and which many schools have yet to consider.

Planning and priority
1   Is our health education unrecognized, unrecognizable, or merely unplanned and unco-ordinated?
2   Is actual coverage patchy, left to chance, missing key areas?
3   If we have a programme, is it related to children's stages of growth and development?
4   Is it provided early enough to be of value (cf. early maturity of children; health careers; decisions children face)?
5   Is it given too little emphasis/too little time because of its low status?

Content and method
1   Do we concentrate too much on the physical growth and development to the exclusion of social/emotional factors?
2   Is what we do sufficiently practical and relevant to children's present decision-making situations and capabilities?
3   Is it information laden and is that what we intend?
4   Is what we do mainly based on the crisis topics?
5   Are most of our messages positive ones?

New Direction in Primary School Health Education

National bodies

Readers will doubtless be well aware already of the move towards a preventive role for the medical services as discussed in the DHSS Consultative Document *Prevention and Health, Everybody's business* (1976). In several contexts this document underlines the important role education might play in helping to meet today's health problems:

> . . . the key factor may be the need to educate the individual so that he can help himself.

It also recognizes the value of health education specifically:

> There is much potential for prevention in health education aimed at altering

people's attitudes towards such things as tobacco, alcohol and exercise – persuading them in effect to invest in their own health.

However, the DHSS document has little to say to schools directly. Schools are, of course, very much more the province of the DES, whose revised official handbook *Health Education in Schools* (1977) has a lot to say about general and specific aspects of health education, but little which is mainly aimed at or of interest to teachers in primary schools. It does describe the broad primary school approach as being favourable to health education, but seems to imply a somewhat 'passive recipient' role for young children:

> . . . the physical, emotional, social and intellectual development of each child is seen as a whole, a viewpoint which is highly favourable for the beginnings of health education. The health education of young children consists to a large extent in the acceptance of values by example and the learning of behaviour, including elements of training, from good practice. The influence depending on the attitudes of every teacher as well as the caretaker, members of the school meals staff and playground supervisors, is inescapable. (p. 30)

As mentioned earlier the recent survey by HM Inspectors, *Primary Education in England*, has little to say about primary school health education as such. Although its general statements about the value of a broadly based curriculum and mixed methods can be used to support the case for health education, certain of the listed aspects of scientific and social and moral learning can also be described as health education, if one wishes to classify them in that way.

However, a very small but significant memorandum (DES and Welsh Office, 1977) was circulated to all LEAs, teacher training colleges and departments of education in December 1977. This advertised the new handbook mentioned above; set health education in the context of the several recent specialist governmental reports on preventive medicine, violence in the family, child health services, the misuse of drugs, alcoholism, nutrition and smoking; and alerted members of the education profession to these and to *Prevention and Health* (DHSS, 1970). The memorandum emphasized the importance of these reports' recommendations for schools:

> . . . within education their common theme is that those responsible for the school curriculum should pay special attention to the health issues highlighted.

It also referred to the new curriculum development projects supported by the Schools Council and the Health Education Council, going so far as to name the SCHEP teachers' guides and to describe them as seeking to provide 'a balanced and co-ordinated programme of health education within the school curriculum'.

The amount of support which both the Schools Council (funded by the DES) and, more recently, the Health Education Council (funded by the DHSS) have provided for SCHEP 5–13 provides evidence enough that both bodies see curriculum development in primary school health education as important. The joint memorandum demonstrated that the DES then endorsed both the importance of health education in general and the current attempts at curriculum development in particular. It remains to be seen whether the more recent HM Inspectors' survey is merely evidence under-lining the fact that health education in primary schools is still 'unrecognised and unrecognisable', or is suggesting indirectly that it should remain so in the face of other priorities.

Local authorities

Until recently most LEAs which have drawn up guidelines for health education have concentrated mainly upon suggestions or checklists for content and lists of available resources. With one or two notable exceptions, in general there has been an absence of discussion on the major aims and rationale of health education programmes and in many cases the guidelines have been overwhelmingly concerned with secondary school programmes and with crisis issues, in particular sex education. In the past three or four years this situation has changed, however, and a few authorities now offer schools much broader guidance on the 'why' and 'how' of a wider health education programme as well as the 'what'. Some authorities are now relating their advice for primary and middle schools to aspects of the SCHEP materials. Others have involved members of the SCHEP team in the deliberations of their working parties and have actively supported dissemination conferences.

In its conclusions and recommendations the Devon LEA booklet *Health and the School* (1978) states:

1 Every school should develop a clearly expressed policy with regard to health education. . . .
2 All teachers as well as certain members of the non-teaching staff should be closely aware of the school's health education policy and of the contribution which they are expected to make towards its implementation. (p. 11)

The approval of parents, their active support and occasionally even their involvement in the school's health education programme are variations on another theme common to many LEA guidelines. The Hampshire LEA (1972), however, sounds a note of caution about making it too much of a special case:

> Many schools feel that it is necessary to involve parents specifically in Health Education. Others feel that, as part of the established school curriculum, there is no more need for the parents to be involved in Health Education than there is for them to be involved in any other subject.

The Bedfordshire LEA document (1978) sets the work of the school within the context of a key principle of continuity:

> The panel found the following principle crucial to their thinking:- Health education must be accepted as a continuing concern from infancy to old age, not merely for the personal welfare of the individual but also for the sake of society as a whole.

The same document also underlines personal choice as the basic aim for all school health education:

> The basic aim of health education in all schools, regardless of the age and ability of the pupils, is to ensure that boys and girls grow up knowing that, accident and misfortune apart, health is a matter of personal choice. (p. 4)

Some local authorities are clearly, therefore, offering more guidance than others on what is expected of schools. The Devon booklet (1978), indeed, gives clear direction through an extremely valuable and clear list of 'questions which schools have to answer', under the heading 'Action':

- What are the aims of the health education programme?
- What sort of attitudes towards health are being encouraged among children?
- Do the ethos of the school and the nature of the facilities provided enable children to put into practice the attitudes which are encouraged?
- Is the school working with other sources of pressure in the community and with parents to secure reinforcement of the attitudes encouraged in school?
- Are parents fully involved in the aims of the school in this area?

- How much preventive work is undertaken in the school in areas such as road safety, water safety, dental care and in the prevention of home accidents?
- What topics are being covered and what information is being given?

In summary, then, some local education authorities through their working parties or study groups are now giving a great deal more help, guidance and in some cases 'direction' to schools' health education curricula. Others, in fact the majority, have yet to formulate a specific policy or have deliberately left it to individual schools to decide how, if at all, they will carry out their health education. In many cases the LEA advisory staff have made it known at courses and conferences run as part of the dissemination programme for SCHEP 5-13 that the authority endorses the principles, aims and rationale implicit in the project materials and thereby encourages schools to plan suitable programmes based upon these. Some LEAs with written guidelines have also encouraged schools to use them in conjunction with the project's materials and vice versa.

SCHEP, its ideas and materials

For a brief introduction to the project and the way it developed, an outline of the two teachers' guides, *All About Me* and *Think Well* (Schools Council, 1977), and details of the associated video tapes and television series, readers are referred to the booklet *An Introduction to SCHEP*, which is available free of charge from the project, its regional co-ordinators, the Health Education Council or the Schools Council.

A superficial reading of these two teachers' guides may leave teachers with the impression that there is not much in them which is new. This is a reaction which we deliberately set out to engender through organization and design, hoping to reassure and attract many teachers who might easily have been put off by too radical an approach. The key ideas behind the project are outlined very briefly below.

Health education should be broader in aims, content and methodology

. . . our interpretation of the word 'health' is very wide, embracing as it does not only physical health and hygiene but also the emotional and social facets of human life. It follows that our interpretation of health education is also broadly based so as to include those planned experiences which we believe will benefit the physical, emotional and social lives of children. . . . Because we have defined health education so widely, its aims would seem to coincide exactly with the accepted aims of 'mainstream' education. Both seek to equip individuals with knowledge, skills, values and attitudes which will help them cope successfully with their present and future lives. (*All About Me*, p. 1)

Health education should start earlier than often currently accepted

Our concern is to ensure that children are able to consider alternative forms of behaviour at points early enough in their lives to be of value to the choices and decisions – concerning their health – with which they are faced. With this in mind many health questions which hitherto were considered appropriate only for older children have been covered in *All About Me*. (*Think Well*, p. 2)

Some of the ideas offered for consideration might appear to some teachers to be not very relevant to the lives of young children, but our reason for including them is based firmly upon two well established observations:

1   That children's out of school experiences are far wider and more varied than some teachers acknowledge.
2   That children's values and attitudes towards certain topics of health related behaviour (such as smoking) are already forming at an early age. Such values and attitudes are very important, in the long run, to the development of patterns of health behaviour later in life.

The importance of the infant and lower junior school in the formation of children's attitudes to themselves and other people, their habits and general social development is an established fact. This guide seeks to offer help and practical suggestions which teachers might find useful in encouraging positive attitudes and meaningful development. (*All About Me*, p. 2)

Health education should be planned and sequential

Often the term *incidental teaching* is used to describe a type of teaching in which the particular subject matter is only discussed if it crops up or if children ask questions about it. Health education is much too important an area of the curriculum to allow its teaching to depend upon such unplanned and haphazard treatment. (*Think Well*, pp. 2–3)

The guide can be used in many different ways, but our hope is that it will provide a framework for and a stimulus to staff discussions concerning the relevance and place of health education in the school curriculum. Experience has shown that the impact of this work is greater when considered as an integral part of the school curriculum and when a sequential pattern of work is planned to occur throughout the school life of children. Teachers will be aware of the importance of repeating work at different times to coincide with levels of development and interest of children. (*All about Me*, pp. 3–4)

Health education should adopt a more positive approach related very closely to children's self-concept and their social relationships

In terms of emotional and social health we believe that children who have a positive and wholesome image of themselves tend to be better balanced in their relationships and dealings with others than children with less positive images of themselves. An important element of health education should therefore be directed at helping children to explore what they know and feel about themselves and to help them appreciate their uniqueness in a way which will contribute to their feelings of self worth. (*Think Well*, p. 3)

Health education should be a process focusing upon relevant decisions and key situations within which these decisions may be made

Its major aim should be to help children make considered choices or decisions related to their health behaviour by increasing knowledge and clarifying the beliefs and values which they hold. Health education, in our view, should not only concern itself with the passing of information but should also involve children in the process of making choices or decisions. (*Think Well*, p. 3)

Ultimately our health is closely related to choices and decisions we ourselves make and the whole purpose of this book has been to help teachers clarify, for their children, some of the areas in which decisions and choices can indeed be made. (*All About Me*, p. 119)

Finally, and perhaps most important of all, health education should emphasize personal responsibility

The strategies to be found in each of the eight units of *Think Well* have been designed to emphasize the personal involvement and responsibility of children and call for investigation, judgement choices and decisions of various kinds. All the units contain material to be 'learned', but, equally important, they offer opportunities for children to put what they have learned to some use in a way which is relevant and meaningful to them. Such an interpretation of school health education reflects the growing awareness amongst teachers of the need to develop in children a sense of personal involvement and responsibility for their own health. (*Think Well*, p. 4)

Developing Primary School Health Education

Are schools missing the point?

Our experience in both the evaluation of the final SCHEP materials and during the dissemination of the published versions tends to suggest that many of these key messages are missed. Curricular materials such as these are unlikely, it would seem, to be used in the fullest way the project intended, except by a small percentage of schools and teachers. This percentage seems, not surprisingly, to be higher in those authorities which have appointed an adviser with responsibility for this part of the curriculum and/or where working parties and study groups have spent some time thinking through the issues. However, as I have suggested earlier, even these factors may mean no more than that authorities or schools have produced a rather more sophisticated topic list and list of resources. It does not necessarily mean that the fundamental questions about aims and approaches have been asked and answered in individual schools.

Indeed, the evaluation indications showed quite the contrary:

> . . . teachers working with the trial materials were generally very positive but they did express *reservations about those parts* dealing with the *social and emotional components* and particularly the *sensitive areas* such as sex education and smoking (with young children particularly).

> General concern was also expressed about the amount of *time* available for work such as this. It was apparent, too, that there was a lack of positive planning to make sure that the less secure or superficially attractive areas – areas felt to be of importance by the project team – were covered adequately. (Stephen, M.)

Despite the fact that the project materials were re-ordered, amended and emphasized in several respects to try to reinforce the points mentioned above, and despite attempts in dissemination conferences and courses to focus on these issues, our overall impression is that such questions still often remain largely unanswered in so far as they affect the whole school, even if individual keen teachers may be very clear about what they wish to do, and why, when and how they wish to do it. Their colleagues may not, indeed, accept the need for planning in this field at all. This is the fundamental issue which has to be debated before any further progress on those key project ideas can be achieved. No discussions on what the school is trying to do in this part of the curriculum are likely to be of any value unless it is in the context of planning for them to take place.

The need for planning

The case for curriculum planning in some form or other is an extremely strong one. The need to know what has been covered and will be covered in the future in order to develop knowledge and concepts sequentially, to avoid gaps and overlap, is supported even by those arguing for much more flexibility in the curriculum, a point made strongly by the Plowden Report (1967):

> There is little place for the type of scheme which sets down exactly what ground should be covered and what skill should be acquired by each class in the school. Yet to put nothing in its place may be to leave some teachers prisoners of tradition and to make difficulties for newcomers to a staff who are left to pick up, little by little, the ethos of a school. The best solution seems to be to provide brief schemes for the school as a whole: outlines of aims in various areas of the curriculum, the sequence of development which can be expected in children and the methods through which work can be soundly based and progress accelerated. (para. 539)

Razzell (1969) talks about the need for 'clear, precise thinking about what the school hopes to do, and how it hopes to set about achieving the plan', while Bennett (1976) suggests that 'careful and clear structuring of activities' is one of the 'keys to enhanced academic progress'.

It is often in the context of the more sensitive areas, such as sex education, that teachers question or reject the idea of planning the deliberate introduction of certain aspects at a time appropriate to the needs of most children, and in many cases are not even prepared to answer questions frankly. Yet the Plowden Report was fairly clear in stating the need for a 'definite policy':

> Every school must make the arrangements that seem best to it and should have a definite policy, which, in consultation with parents, covers all the children. It is not good enough to leave matters vague and open, hoping for the best. (para. 717)

The 1978 HM Inspectors' Report, in discussing the relationship between class and specialist teachers, stresses the importance of the role of class teachers but goes on to say:

> When a teacher is unable to deal satisfactorily with an important aspect of the curriculum, other ways of making this provision have to be found. If a teacher is only a little unsure, advice and guidance from a specialist, probably another member of staff, may be enough. . . . (p. 118)

What implications does this have for primary school health education?

Involvement in planning and planning for involvement

The work of Ashton et al. (1975), which was quoted extensively earlier, highlighted the way that patterns of opinion seem, not surprisingly, to be closely associated with the age, experience and length of service of teachers:

> Generally, school staffs are probably composed of teachers of different ages and different lengths of experience, who have served in the particular school for different lengths of time. This is likely to mean that different opinion patterns will exist among each staff group. (p. 88)

She and others have pointed to the link between the aims of teachers and the way they teach. For example, Bennett (1976) writes:

> A strong relationship was found between teacher aims and opinions and the way teachers actually teach. . . . Teachers aim to engender different outcomes in their pupils. (p. 151)

So are some children likely to be receiving different, even contradictory, messages from the same school?

We feel that it is of crucial importance that all members of a school staff should be consulted and where possible involved in the development of the school's programme of health education. At the very least this should ensure that colleagues become aware of their different stances and might help them to present a range of viewpoints in a more open manner, even if not to reach any common ground!

Planning – the role of headteachers and co-ordinators

Quite clearly, such involvement will not take place unless it is actively encouraged and supported by headteachers. In smaller schools, or where they are particularly interested in this aspect of the curriculum, headteachers may actually carry out the curriculum review and development process themselves. In larger schools heads may appoint a teacher to a post of special responsibility or give them the role of subject leader or co-ordinator.

The 1978 HM Inspectors' Report emphasizes the value of the work of such colleagues, and clarifies their functions as follows:

> . . . these teachers should learn how to lead groups of teachers and to help others to teach material which is appropriate to the abilities of the children. They should learn how to establish a programme of work in co-operation with other members of staff and how to judge whether it is being operated successfully. They should also learn how to make the best use of the strengths of the teachers of all ages and to help them to develop so that they may take on more responsibility. Particular care should be taken to foster the special qualities of intuitive and gifted teachers.

Heads need, in consultation with those concerned, to make quite clear the responsibilities of individual teachers. (para. 864)

It may be unrealistic to seek the appointment of specialist teachers for health education alone in primary schools, in the light of the financial problems associated with falling rolls in the late 1970s and early 1980s. There is no doubt whatsoever in my mind, however, that such skills and concerns require application to this particular field.

Towards school-based curriculum development in health education

The SCHEP team believes that all schools should review their curriculum in broad terms to establish whether or not there is a need for more work in the whole area of personal and social development. In particular, they should consider whether there are important aspects of children's health education, as defined by the project, which are missing, provided too late, inadequately set in context, inappropriately developed or presented, or left to the whim of individual teachers.

Key questions such as these and others mentioned at various stages above must be discussed by the whole school staff, since they are of vital importance to their general teaching role as well as to the overall philosophy of the school. Together these will determine many of the key messages taken away by the children.

Such a process is unlikely to occur merely as a result of purchasing curriculum materials or attending a one-day dissemination conference. In fact, in some ways, the adoption of a 'teaching pack' or adherence to externally produced guidelines may militate against questions of fundamental importance to the school being asked. A firm commitment is required for the school to consider such matters over a period of time, with the support of headteachers and often as a result of local authority guidance both written and through the work of LEA advisers.

Schools wishing to undertake this process need support and guidance. SCHEP have therefore developed a manual of workshop training materials and appropriate introductory courses designed to help heads or co-ordinators to review and develop their health education curriculum with their colleagues, normally back in the school setting. The manual focuses stage by stage upon some of those key questions which continue to be of concern to teachers, explaining some of the key ideas contained in the SCHEP materials, and using various instruments and tasks to bring the school's current curriculum provision and teachers' perspectives sharply into focus.

By relying heavily on teachers' own experience the manual ensures a practical and relevant starting point for every school, and by aiming at the production of a programme related to the needs of children and the skills and interests of staff, it should help to create a practical and relevant end product, that is a primary school health education programme implemented by the majority of the staff, known to all and preferably adopting at least some of the key ideas put forward by SCHEP.

In conclusion, I quote once again from the Plowden Report (1967):

> Habit is an immensely strong influence in schools and it is one that should be weakened though it is never likely to be removed. These words are particularly addressed to practising teachers and especially to head teachers, rather than to educational theorists who seldom fear innovation, but whose ideas may founder because of their ignorance of what schools (and sometimes teachers) are really like. (para. 503)

In this chapter I have attempted to describe what primary schools, teachers and their health education programmes are like and some of the new directions they are or are not taking. The success of the SCHEP teachers' guides to date demonstrates that they were not produced in ignorance of what schools want and can use in the way of curriculum materials. However, the fact that many of the key ideas are not being adopted indicates that we must look again at what schools and teachers are really like. We must then attempt to apply our own principles to the problem of transmitting ideas and emphases in curriculum innovation; we cannot just 'tell' teachers but must help them to go through a 'finding out process' for themselves. This is what our workshop materials attempt to do and we have yet to see whether or not they will be successful.

Summary

In this chapter apparent changes in the style of teaching in primary schools are questioned. The author expresses the view that change is much slower than it seems, and that curriculum and teaching styles are far from being child-centred. The increasing need to introduce more planned health education is stressed, and the difficulty in doing this is related to the slowness of real change in schools. The author explores the concept of health careers, and emphasizes that habits and attitudes (e.g., smoking) are formed at a young age. It is argued that health education clearly supports the aims of primary education, as well as being valuable in its own right as a curriculum area.

Current health education practices are discussed and the emphasis placed by teachers on health crises is questioned. The author explores a more positive approach to health education, discusses the SCHEP 5–13 and the help given to schools by LEAs. He makes a strong plea for better planning and the use of programmed materials to help schools review and develop their Health Education programmes.

References

Ashton, P., Kneen, P., Davies, F. and Holley, B. J. (1975) *The Aims of Primary Education: A study of teachers' opinions.* Schools Council Research Series. London, Macmillan.

Bassey, M. (1978) *Nine Hundred Primary School Teachers.* Slough, NFER Publishing Co.

Bedfordshire LEA (1978) Report of panel considering health education.

Bennett, N. (1976) *Teaching Styles and Pupil Progress.* London, Open Books, pp. 54 and 160.

Bewley, B. R., Halil, T. and Snaith, A. H. (1973) 'Smoking by primary schoolchildren. Prevalence and associated respiratory symptoms'. *Br. J. Prev. Soc. Med.*, vol. 27, no. 3, pp. 152–153.

Bewley, B. R., Bland, J. M. and Harris, R. (1975) 'Factors associated with the starting of cigarette smoking by primary school children'. *Br. J. Prev. Soc. Med.*, vol. 28, pp. 37–44.

Blackie, J. (1969) *Inside the Primary School.* London, HMSO, p. 9.

Board of Education (1931) *The Primary School* (The Hadow Report). London, HMSO, ch. 7, para. 83.

Central Advisory Council for Education (England) (1967) *Children and Their Primary Schools* (The Plowden Report). London, HMSO.

Clegg, A. B. (ed.) (1971) *The Changing Primary School, Its Problems and Priorities. A statement by teachers.* London, Chatto & Windus, p. 51.

Dearden, R. F. (1976) *Problems in Primary Education.* London, Routledge & Kegan Paul, p. 41.

Department of Education and Science (1977) *Health Education in Schools.* London, HMSO.

Department of Education and Science (1978) *Primary Education in England.* A survey by HM Inspectors of Schools. London, HMSO, pp. 27, 40 and 111.

Department of Education and Science and the Welsh Office (1977) Administrative Memorandum 15/77. London, HMSO.

Department of Health and Social Security (1976) *Prevention and Health, Everybody's business*. A consultative document. London, HMSO.

Devon LEA (1978) *Health and the School*. p. 6.

Froome, S. (1970) *Why Tommy Isn't Learning*. London, Tom Stacey Books, p. 113ff.

Fulton, G. B. and Fassbender, W. V. (eds) (1972) *Health Education in the Elementary School*. Santa Monica, Cal., Goodyear Publishing.

Hampshire Education Committee (1972) *Health: Learning to Care*. Working Party's Guidelines. Hampshire LEA.

Jahoda, G. and Crammond, J. (1972) *Children and Alcohol: A developmental Study in Glasgow, Vol. 1*. London, HMSO.

Kreitler. H. and Kreitler, S (1966) 'Children's concepts of sexuality and birth'. *Child Dev.*, vol. 37, pp. 363–378.

Razzell, A. (1969) *Juniors: A postscript to Plowden*. Harmondsworth, Penguin Education Special, pp. 27, 36 and 125.

Schools Council (1977) *All About Me*. Teachers' Guide. Schools Council Health Education Project 5–13. Walton-on-Thames, Surrey, Nelson.

Schools Council (1977) *Think Well*. Teachers' Guide. Schools Council Health Education Project 5–13. Walton-on-Thames, Surrey, Nelson.

Stephen, M. (1976) *Evaluation Indications* in Johnston, V. (ed.) *SCHEP Newsletter 5 Autumn 1976*.

Williams, T. (1975) 'Health education and children learning'. *R. Soc. Hlth J.*, August 1975, p. 214.

Williams, T. (1976) 'Health education and the school curriculum', in *Health Education in Secondary Schools*. Schools Council Working Paper 57. London, Evans/Methuen Educational, p. 55.

CHAPTER 5

HEALTH EDUCATION IN SECONDARY SCHOOLS

Trefor Williams

The difficulty of writing about health education for a wider audience lies very largely in the absence of any shared or common understanding of what it is or what its purpose might be. In attempting to set health education in the context of secondary schools, this difficulty is compounded by the fact that this subject area is not generally seen by them as a matter of priority concern. There are two reasons for this:

1 Health education is rarely accorded much status in initial teacher training courses and therefore has little tradition in the sense that subject areas like English, maths, geography and history have a traditional place in the school curriculum. It is therefore of second-rank importance in terms of the school curriculum.
2 The orientation of secondary schools is biased towards the academic and the needs of examinations, and this largely determines the availability of curriculum time and inevitably the status of subject areas in the curriculum.

There is, however, a growing awareness of the need for schools to pay more particular attention to the personal and social development of their pupils, an awareness sharpened not only by reports from the DES (1978, 1979) and DHSS (1976) but more pointedly by the experiences of teachers who are sensitive to the present and future needs of their pupils. There is little doubt that health education can satisfy part of this need; the difficulty lies in demonstrating to schools and teachers how this can be brought about. Convincing staff colleagues of the importance and relevance of health education depends heavily upon the support of respected, responsible or senior peers, and who is there on a school staff to stand as an advocate of health education?

The Function of the Co-ordinator

There is a need for such a person in all schools to act as a catalyst, to stimulate debate and discussion across the curriculum, to plan, to organize and to implement. It goes without question that such a person will need to have considered personally the many issues and concerns involved in the matter. The role which such a person, let us call him or her a school co-ordinator, can play in schools is elaborated in some detail in the Schools Council Working Paper 57 *Health Education in Secondary Schools* (1976), the broad outlines of which provide a useful background for this chapter.

1   To draw up, in association with colleagues (perhaps a staff working party with outside advisers), an overall, ideal programme for health education and personal relationships in the school.
2   To examine, again with the help of colleagues, the existing programme in the school in order to eliminate unnecessary duplication and to look for gaps in provision.
3   To devise ways of filling important gaps, perhaps by agreeing on changes in the curriculum within established subjects, and by introducing either a specialist, or a core course.
4   To take the leading role in organizing any major new initiatives, and to take a prominent part in the teaching programme.
5   To act as a source of expertise for the staff as a whole, both by attending relevant courses and by passing on key information to collegues.
6   To co-ordinate the evaluation of the course and to initiate any necessary revision.

The notion of the health education co-ordinator and the tasks associated with this role provided the starting point for the work of the Schools Council Health Education Project (SCHEP) 13–18. With the hindsight of experience it is possible to clarify, develop and perhaps re-arrange the many facets of the role as outlined in Paper 57 (Schools Council, 1976). Perhaps the most urgent of the tasks to be tackled by a school co-ordinator is to develop a distinctive school perspective of health education, without which it would be impossible to plan and implement a programme. Indeed in coming to grips with this first and vitally important task, a school is setting a context in which other important issues can be tackled, such as the when, the where and the how of health education teaching.

The Content Areas of Health Education

Inevitably a sampling of the views of staff colleagues about health education would reveal a range of opinions reflecting not only their perception of health education, but also of the nature of education itself. At one level of understanding health education might be considered to be a list of content areas ranging from, for example, smoking to sex education, and, with the exception of a few topics, there is little difficulty in establishing general agreement on them in a school. Such a content list is important in helping to define the extent of health education across the curriculum, and sets a visible agenda for its operation in schools. In this way a content list of health education provides an agreed and concrete starting point for discussion and negotiation between staff members. A content list, as shown in *Fig.* 5.1, was found to be a most useful tool by the SCHEP 13–18 team in its work with schools, although the experience of the project would emphasize the need to use it as a staging post for further clarification and development, rather than as an end in itself.

The content list only provides a map of the territories to be visited and explored and cannot of itself describe the kind or quality of experiences we expect to sample there. These can only be arrived at by asking ourselves what we expect the purpose of the journey to be. It is customary and useful, in exploring the purpose of educational activities and experiences, to express them as aims and objectives. Thinking about aims does provide an immense opportunity for sharpening one's perception of health education and getting to the heart of the matter which is a necessary, if at times a difficult and painful, exercise.

Differing Views of Health Education

It is possible to identify at least two general views of health education, each with radically different outlooks on what it is for, and they can provide the opposite poles of a continuum of health education practice. For convenience we can label them as the 'preventive model' and the 'educational model', respectively. The former is primarily concerned with the prevention of illness and disease (and is sometimes referred to as the medical model), and attempts to achieve this end by deliberately influencing or

Table 5.1 Health education in schools/colleges

Main content area	Examples of items for study within each main content area
A. Personal health, body management and human biology	1. The working of body systems. 2. Adaptation to environment, e.g., physical and mental stress. 3. Exercise – need for and effect of. 4. Health habits and personal hygiene. 5. Effects on body of alcohol, drugs and tobacco. 6. Common infectious diseases including sexually transmitted infections.
B. Food selection	1. Nutritional needs of the body. 2. Nutrition and health, e.g., slimming, obesity, stress and anxiety, etc. 3. Eating patterns of individuals and community.
C. Growth and development from childhood through adolescence to adulthood	1. Body changes at puberty including individual differences and sexual development. 2. Emotional and social development accompanying physical changes.
D. Relationships	1. Parents and adult authority. 2. Peers. 3. Sexual relationships – with other and same sex. 4. Marriages and/or other long-term relationships. 5. Learning to cope with loss and separation. 6. With mentally ill and physically handicapped. 7. As situations for smoking, alcohol and drug activities.
E. Education for parenthood	1. Growth, development and needs of young children. 2. Family roles and structures including one-parent families, etc. 3. Helping young children to cope with loss and separation.
F. Community health	1. The National Health Service and alternatives. 2. Roles and relationships with doctors and hospital staff. 3. National and community health issues such as contraception, abortion, immunization, fluoride, etc. 4. Attitudes to physical and mental illness and handicap. 5. Voluntary organizations and clinics, etc., e.g., Marriage Guidance Council, Samaritans, Brook Advisory Clinic.
G. The environment in which we live	1. Litter, pollution including noise. 2. Meeting the needs of the community, for living space, leisure and mobility. 3. Effect of the environment on physical and mental health. 4. Health issues such as sewage processing, refuse collection, etc.
H. Safety and first aid	1. Road-traffic education and driver education, etc. 2. Home. 3. School and work. 4. Leisure. 5. Principles of first aid.

changing the attitudes and behaviour of target groups in some defined way or to some predetermined end. The other model is more concerned with the development of personal autonomy than with specific behavioural outcomes. A clear and concise analysis of these models is provided by Tones (1977) who explores their application to specific situations and institutions; he also suggests the context in which these models and their derivatives are best employed. The major difference between the two perceptions of health education is that while the preventive model is primarily concerned with the *outcomes* of a process of health education, the educational model is concerned with the *quality* of the process, involving decision-making itself. The former view would emphasize the urgency of helping young people accept and adopt certain modes of behaviour in the interest of their good health, while the latter view would urge that individual behaviour should be based upon free choice and decision-making while reminding us that schools cannot ethically embark upon a process of decision-making if the outcomes of the process are very largely decided upon beforehand.

Teachers and schools need to be wary of compromises on this issue, for it is comforting to believe that we are indeed presenting young people with opportunities for decision-making while applying subtle pressure upon them to conform to behavioural goals which we consciously (or unconsciously) provide. Are we, for example, concerned with helping young people clarify their own position, knowledge and decisions about smoking or is our aim to help young people to decide not to smoke? There is a difference and one which affects not only the spirit of the process but also the confidence which young people might have in health education and in its teachers.

If we decide that health education is concerned with more than just the prevention of disease to include, for example, notions of emotional well-being, we are immediately concerning ourselves with value judgements about what makes human life attractive and worthwhile. Once we set considerations of health matters in the broad context of human values then our perception of health education is affected. Baelz (1979) develops this theme further, pointing out that when we deal with human values there are no professionals or experts, we are all ordinary men and women sharing our experiences and insights. In this context teachers are often troubled by the notion of changing pupils' attitudes to conform to some norm or other. Baelz's comments on this matter are worth noting:

It is sometimes said that changing people's attitudes is incompatible with respecting the individual's freedom of choice. There is a measure of truth in this especially if the methods of change are manipulative.

The difference between education and manipulation is not that the manipulator is all the time influencing his pupils while the educator is not influencing him at all. The difference, rather lies in their respective aims. The educator encourages his pupil to develop the capacity to think for himself, while the indoctrinator wishes to make it impossible for his pupil ever to question the doctrine that he has been taught.

There is the possibility then of ambiguity and misunderstanding in the way in which the term 'health education' is used; an ambiguity which needs to be picked over and clarified as thoroughly as is possible. As caring teachers we would all wish for young people to make decisions about their health so that they become and remain healthy in every sense of the word. In our eagerness and at times anxiety for the 'right' choice, however, we might be tempted to sacrifice our ethical qualms for the immediate gains of manipulation. Such immediate gains are very likely built upon the shifting sands of half-truths, rhetoric and false claims; the aims of health education, and indeed of education itself, rest more firmly upon individual autonomy resulting from decision-making skills and a democratic process. Unless schools develop a clear and shared view of what health education is about, further decisions concerning how it should be taught and evaluated become impossible to make. While not wishing to overtax this issue it is worth repeating and re-emphasizing the need to explore and discuss the purpose of health education fully as it will provide an essential baseline for future development.

The Health Education Team

Reference has already been made to the importance of discussion and debate about health education amongst staff, and the experience of recent curriculum developments in schools confirms the need for frank and open discussion if the developments are to take root and flourish. In a narrower sense, however, it is important for a school co-ordinator to have the support of a team of colleagues as it is wellnigh impossible for one person alone to think through and come successfully to grips with the many and varied tasks associated with this role. Experience and expediency dictate the desirability and indeed the advantage of forming a team of teachers, preferably from across the curriculum boundaries, who are chosen to provide a balance of experience, enthusiasm, skill and willingness to undertake the extra tasks associated with planning and implementing a programme of health education. It is important that members of the team be given the opportunity of thinking through issues and coming to decisions together, and for this purpose time for meetings has to be set aside either during or out of school hours. The cut and thrust of debate in a structured but common experience helps to provide a bonding and camaraderie which is essential to the continual well-being and health of a team. When discussing the tasks associated with the role of co-ordinator, therefore, it is necessary to see the team as an extension of the co-ordinator's role. The criteria which a school might employ to choose a team are discussed in more detail elsewhere (Schools Council, 1980), but generally speaking a co-ordinator needs to think not only of the experience, enthusiasm and skills which team members bring with them but also of the potential which the opportunity provides for the personal and professional development of the staff members themselves.

Co-ordination – What It Might Mean for a School

The term 'co-ordinator' implies the wish to co-ordinate some aspect of school-based work which is already in existence or which might be brought into existence by a conscious decision of the staff. Another early task associated with the role, therefore, would logically be to discover what health education teaching is actually being attempted in the school. In order to accomplish this task a team will need to have arrived at a consensus view of at least the content areas of health education. Using such a content list as a baseline it is possible to discover which of the content areas are already being taught in the various subjects across the curriculum. It is possible, for example, to construct a grid or checklist based upon the main content areas of health education and then to invite heads of departments and their colleagues to indicate whether or not they are included in the teaching of specific year groups. When the results of such an inquiry are assembled together on to a master grid for the whole school, they offer a picture of what is being taught by whom and to whom. It is for the co-ordinator and the team to decide upon the level of enquiry needed to give a clear picture of which health topics are covered and when. It is probable that two levels of investigation are needed; one at the initial and surface level to give a general picture of what is happening, and a second to provide a more detailed account and clarification of the depth of teaching and methods used.

When assembled with care, a master grid gives a reasonable picture of what health education is being taught in a school and provides an excellent baseline for further and future developments. It provides, for example, an opportunity for spotting gaps, weaknesses, overlaps and major omissions. From it a team will be able to see what particular health topics are covered in any one year-group and also in which particular subject area such teaching is concentrated. Further scrutiny will enable a team to see whether specific groups of pupils in any one year-group are missing out on health education. Many schools are surprised by the amount of health education being taught across the curriculum, but many are also disturbed by the haphazard and piecemeal approach to the subject. Health education is often scattered across the curriculum of any one year-group with little consideration of timing or co-ordination. Frequently certain topics, for example sex education, are repeated with, for the pupils at least, monotonous regularity within different subject areas and with no apparent reference to each other. At the very least co-ordination of the teaching could offer a more rational and coherent approach. Teachers are sometimes worried by the apparent duplication of health topics which an investigation such as this reveals. It is worth remembering, however, that individual subjects bring their own distinctive perspective to bear on a topic which undoubtedly complements and expands the pupils' understanding of it. Co-ordination should attempt to bring together these contributions in such a way as to be coherent, intelligible and relevant to the lives of the pupils and not just as unrelated bits from three or four subject syllabuses with no clear overall focus. Successful co-ordination should add up to much more than the sum of the individual parts from subject contributions.

When a particular topic has been or is being taught to a particular year-group, it can sometimes carry with it the force of tradition so that it continues year after year to be part of the curriculum. The fact that a health topic already exists in the curriculum for a particular year-group is no valid reason for it to continue to be there. The master grid provides a useful opportunity for questioning such existing health education teaching. Perhaps what is taught is there because it fits, in a subsidiary role, with other subject teaching or for other reasons not specifically related to health education or the personal and social development of young people. In this way some health-related teaching might be occurring with impressive frequency across the curriculum but with little regard to any order of priority associated with the needs of young people. The co-ordinator and team will need to satisfy themselves that what exists in the health education curriculum exists for the right reasons and not because of the machinations of the syllabuses of other subject areas. In order to satisfy themselves on this account, school teams will need to consider how best to plan a programme for young people ranging from ages eleven to sixteen or eighteen which successfully caters for their various needs.

Criteria for Planning a Health Education Programme

It is not uncommon for schools to plan their health education in response to what they see as health crises in the lives of their pupils. For example, teaching about drugs, smoking, alcohol, sex, sexually transmitted diseases and other matters is often made a focus of attention when the problems associated with these topics appear to manifest themselves in the behaviour of young people. Judgements about what needs to be taught can sometimes be based upon erroneous assumptions, eye-catching media reports, half-digested and not clearly understood reports or upon personal observations of a small number of young people. Clearly a planned programme of health education needs to rest upon far more substantial criteria than these. What then might such criteria be? There are four related points to be made here.

1   The social and cultural background

An inherent difficulty of many of our contemporary health problems lies in the fact that they are embedded in the social and cultural lives of people. The social experiences of children and young people in their families and in the wider community provide a background against which new ideas, concepts and knowledge are placed. With little learning in the formal sense young people develop many attitudes, values, beliefs and behaviours directly or indirectly associated with their health. Baric's (1979) notion of a health career line is important in understanding how children and young people are exposed to and often adopt the values and attitudes of individuals who are particularly significant to them, such as parents, older siblings and, later, peers. Generally the career line approach to health behaviour focuses attention upon the social and other factors which might influence the development of health-related behaviour.

Teachers who are doubtful about the effects of such influences are referred to the work of Jahoda and Crammond (1972) who show that by about the age of eight, groups of children in Glasgow have attained what is referred to as 'a mastery of the concepts of alcohol' to an exceptional degree. Their major conclusion is that attitudes towards alcohol and drinking are taking shape during the years from six to ten. Bewley et al. (1975), in a study associated with cigarette smoking amongst pre-adolescent children, confirm that permissiveness towards smoking by parents, the influence of older siblings who smoke and the desire to conform with peer group behaviour all combine to shape the attitudes of young children. In this way an early health knowledge is the product of a socialization within a specific family or community culture. Such experiences provide a distinct frame of reference in which new health knowledge can be received and interpreted.

The concept of the health career is then an important criterion to be considered in the planning of a programme of health education since it highlights the need to consider more carefully the scope and sequence of health education. It also exposes the 'response to crisis' approach which characterized school health education in the late 1960s and early 1970s and which still lingers on in some of our schools. The truth of the matter is that young people do not come to school *tabula rasa* but come possessing knowledge, values, attitudes and behaviours closely or directly associated with health education. It behoves the educator to find out what these might be and to take them into account when planning a school programme.

2   Developmental needs

A second criterion to be taken into account is that of the developmental needs of young people. One of the popular catch phrases of contemporary education is 'education for a changing world', and it has in it, for our purposes, a double-edged meaning. In one sense it poses further questions about the kind of world which our secondary school pupils of the 1980s will be facing in the 1990s and beyond. What kind of education will enable young people to cope successfully with the world of tomorrow? Do we know enough about the world of tomorrow to be able to plan the education of today? There are strong hints about the shape of tomorrow's world contained in debates about, for example, the effect of the silicon chip upon industry, upon the health and personal services, upon work opportunities, leisure, the economy and even upon democracy itself to cause even the most unthinking among us to pause for reflection. The need for reflection is obvious but the need for action is paramount; the aims of education and indeed of schools themselves need to be clarified in the light of whatever changes are upon us or are expected. Can schools and the education service adapt to the needs of the changing world in the same way that we hope to prepare young people for their adult years, or will the shadow of the 'saber-tooth curriculum' (Benjamin, 1971) re-emerge? In one very clear way there is a growing, rather than a decreasing need for personal and social education of young people, in terms of their making personal choices and decisions in an increasingly complex social and technological world.

In a second and different sense, however, 'education for a changing world' has a meaning of its own for young people passing through the physical and emotional changes associated with pubertal and post-pubertal growth. This meaning has more direct relevance to young people because they are experiencing their changes now, and there is nothing like the immediacy of the present to demonstrate how relevant to their lives health education is and can be.

Pubertal changes mark the beginning of a secondary phase of socialization which brings young people from childhood through to a mature adulthood. It is a time for learning and practising to be an adult, in the widest sense of the word, and, in a very direct and purposeful way, of working through important 'developmental tasks', the experience of which provides a basis for their very adulthood. Such developmental tasks are intimately inter-related with the physical, cognitive, moral and social growth of young people at this time and provide a context within which self-esteem and self-identity can re-emerge eventually into an adult figure and role.

The notion of 'developmental tasks of adolescence' will of course be familiar to many teachers, but Havighurst's (1972) original listing of them is still worthy of consideration, particularly within the context of planning a health education programme for young people.

Developmental tasks of adolescence

a   Achieving new and more mature relations with age mates of both sexes.

b   Achieving a masculine or feminine role.

c   Accepting one's physique and using the body effectively.

d   Achieving emotional independence of parents and other adults.

e   Preparing for marriage, for long-term relationships and for family life.

f   Preparing for an economic career.

g   Acquiring a set of values and an ethical system as a guide to behaviour – developing an ideology.

h   Desiring and achieving socially responsible behaviour.

Havighurst deals more fully with each of the developmental tasks, and interested readers are directed towards his work and that of Monaster (1977) for a more detailed consideration and development of these tasks. For our purposes the list provides a framework for discussion about the ways in which schools can best help young people to cope successfully with these developmental tasks. School is not the only voice in this matter of course, because young people have lives outside school in their families, amongst friends of different ages and sexes and amongst adult groups of many kinds. In planning a programme for school-based work, therefore, it is vitally important to take into account the developmental needs of young people which are made more explicit by the notion of 'developmental tasks'.

3   Adolescent health needs

A third criterion focuses more sharply upon the specific health needs of adolescents. This provides an extension and development of the adolescent tasks in providing a concrete 'health' basis for health education. For this purpose school teams will need to consult with medical colleagues and other sources of information concerning the patterns of health and illness of adolescents. Such information exists in national and international reports and the personnel of the school health service are important allies because they have access to more detailed local knowledge which will help shape a health education programme. The World Health Organization has also concerned itself with the health needs of adolescents and has published an excellent short report which provides much valuable and useful information (WHO, 1978).

Generally, reports concerning the health of a community show the incidence of death and morbidity (illness) related to age, sex and perhaps social class. For example, in the age-group ten–nineteen accidents of one kind or another are the main cause of death in all European countries including the United Kingdom. This fact should influence the shaping of a health education programme considerably, particularly if more detailed information relating the type of accident to sex and age-group were available. At sixteen young people are legally entitled to ride motorcyles and it is all too painfully obvious to the observer that the number of motorcycle accidents is appallingly high amongst adolescent boys. Similarly there is a fairly dramatic rise in the incidence of sexually transmitted diseases amongst older teenagers, a fact related to increased interest in the opposite sex and consequential sexual behaviour.

However, mortality and morbidity during adolescence should not be the only basis upon which to plan a health education programme. It is necessary to remind ourselves of the health career concept and what it implies for adolescent learning and behaviour. Adolescence is the period in which much health-related behaviour is initiated or where the continuation of already adopted behaviours are confirmed and hardened or rejected. The danger implicit in some of these behaviours becomes explicit only later in life during early, middle or late adulthood. Much heart disease amongst middle-aged and elderly adults, for example, is believed to be caused by an inappropriate life style characterized by a diet heavy in animal fats and sugar, lack of physical exercise and cigarette smoking. These are all patterns of behaviour which were learned and adopted much earlier in life. The huge number of deaths of both men and women, which are related to cigarette smoking – lung cancer, bronchitis, heart disease – is largely due to a habit begun during the adolescent years. If we were to concentrate upon those health problems which only manifest themselves during adolescence, our health education programme would be inadequate and educationally inept.

4   The expectation of society

A fourth influence upon the planning of a programme for schools is, in one sense, ever present through the expectations of society as a whole. Society demands much of education; its demands are wide and varied and some-times conflicting. There is, for example, an expectation that the chief aim of schools will be to turn out academically able pupils. There are also expecta-tions of the school to turn out citizens who subscribe to socially accepted norms of values, attitudes and behaviour. The difficulty is that the former expectations are largely focused on and measured by performance in public examinations to such an extent that they become almost an end in them-selves. The difficulty with the second expectation is that society itself is often deeply divided over social and moral issues. In emphasizing the political rights of individuals to decide for themselves within the law, a society cannot expect to have the tight grip of social control exhibited by a totalitarian state. There can also be a disassociation between the academic and pastoral life of the school, as if the one existed separately from the other. Success or failure in the academic sphere of school cannot but influence the way in which young people see themselves and will therefore influence their behaviour. The insights and reflections about self and relationships with others stemming from a broadly based personal and social education pro-gramme will help young people in their attitudes to work and life generally.

Education has become particularly vulnerable to the barbs of critics demanding more accountability; whether they are friendly barbs intended to stimulate thought or hostile barbs intended to wound and discredit, they all need to be taken seriously. Public accountability is particularly important in health education because its process is not easily understood by the public nor are its effects immediately measurable in the same way as academic subjects are. Whatever kind of programme of health education is developed by a school, it should be readily amenable to social justification and scrutiny. It is deserving of a rationale based upon the judgements and deliberations of a team of teachers and others who have given thought to the definition, place and purpose of health education in the curriculum.

The purpose of identifying criteria useful for course planning is to help provide a context and framework within which priorities can be established for year groupings in school. Priorities for each year-group, or indeed for lower, middle and upper school if preferred, depend largely upon the interpretation of the available information from each of the criteria thought to be useful. Thus the judgements of the co-ordinator, team and others involved in the planning are fundamental to the process. For example, for a first-year group of pupils in a secondary school the major considerations might be:

1 The change to a new school with new relationships and opportunities which it presents.
2 Around this time there is a peak of road accidents.
3 Pupils of this age (eleven–twelve) will have reached or be approaching puberty.

Course priorities derived from some of these considerations could be:

1 An emphasis on group work to establish methods of working in health and social education, for example discussion skills.
2 Work on body changes, physical growth and personal hygiene should begin. An emphasis on the normality of individual differences should be encouraged.
3 Some work on body systems linked with general science approach already in existence.
4 An introduction to the idea of choice/personal responsibility using the area of safety to exemplify the change from small primary to large secondary school.

(The above example is taken from *Programme Planning* in the Schools Council Health Education Project 13–18 trial material.)

Health Education and the Soft Area of the Curriculum

One of the important decisions of principle which a school planning team will need to make is what kind of programme is suitable for the school; indeed what kind of programme does the school want. In the preceding pages the terms 'health education' and 'personal and social education' have been used as if they are interchangeable with each other, and this has been deliberate. They are not, strictly speaking, interchangeable because the latter term embraces not only health education but other educational experience which contributes to the personal and social development of young people. This matter has been elaborated elsewhere (Williams and Williams, 1980), but it is worthwhile considering in more detail the implications for schools. What does 'personal and social development' mean and where does health education fit into it? The Assessment of Performance Unit (APU) established by the DES writes briefly of personal and social development as: '. . . the pupil's understanding of himself, his development as a responsible person and his moral response to his physical environment'.

Schools might be forgiven for identifying this description with the more general aims of their own school, or even of education itself. It is, however, an attempt to clarify what specific contributions help young people become socially and morally autonomous. It needs to be clearly understood that there is no attempt here to denigrate the contributions of the traditional subject areas to the personal and social development of students. It is accepted that the traditional areas of the curriculum can and do make significant contributions to such work but, nevertheless, the focus is most often upon the subject itself and not upon the pupil as a person. It can be argued that learning related to a particular subject does involve pupils in personal development, particularly so when in studying English literature, for example, understanding and insights of interpersonal relationships and of moral issues are broached and deepened.

Such instances are many and varied across the curriculum, but often occur incidentally to the ebb and flow of the lesson itself. It is obviously true that these experiences can be co-ordinated and thus made more effective, but there is clearly also a need for a focus of a different kind which pinpoints more clearly the personal and social needs of young people; a core or a 'home base' upon which contributions from across the curriculum can be directed. Such a core of experiences can be more specifically concerned with the personal and social development of pupils through a balance of social education, moral education, health education, political education, preparation for parenthood, careers education and other facets of human social experiences. Unfortunately these areas of work often compete with each other for curriculum time, chiefly because their respective supporters insist upon emphasizing the uniqueness and distinctive contribution to education of each. In emphasizing this it is easy to lose sight of the fact that they also have shared aims and common purposes. Each is essentially attempting to help pupils towards a personal autonomy, albeit in specific and slightly different areas of human experience, but in broad terms the word 'autonomy' is a suitable all-embracing word which describes the common ground between them. What is the common ground, and can it provide a contextual framework to house each of the contributions to personal and social education?

In his analysis of moral education, Wilson (1973) offers a perspective which can provide such a framework. The five points of his analysis are as follows:

To help students develop:

- the ability to reason and make rational judgements;
- understanding of the importance of objectives and factual knowledge to rational decision-making;
- understanding of the ideas and principles involved in concern for other people;
- awareness and understanding of emotions and their place in human experience and life;
- skills and determination to translate what they have come to know and understand into action.

This is not to deny that there are differences between health education, social education, political education and the others which together make up the 'soft spot' areas. There are, however, a great many issues in which there is a clear overlap between them, not the least being the teaching/learning methods by which each attempts to achieve its goals. This discussion is articulated with some force in the recent HMI survey (DES, 1979), but it is sufficient here to mention the growing feelings of many schools which have attempted to think through a programme of personal and social education for their pupils. It is possible, maybe even desirable, therefore, for schools to locate health education within the broader front of the personal and social development of young people.

Whether health education is carried out under the umbrella of personal and social education or on its own, there remains the problem of how a programme can be organized. There are two ways in which this might be accomplished:

1   As a course within the school in much the same way as the traditional subjects are organized and which is usually taught by a small group of two or three teachers. The content areas of the course are well defined, and the programme is timetabled and can be organized with the minimum of fuss and inconvenience to the rest of the curriculum or school.

2   As a cross-curricular activity, the strength of which lies in the utilization of the rich and varied skills, knowledge and talents of the staff as a whole. This model of organization is usually based upon a small core element in one or other of the subject areas or located in pastoral care or indeed in a health or social education course. It depends upon the involvement of a wider range of staff colleagues which brings the benefit of discussion and debate across subject divides. In this way health (or social and personal) education can become more closely associated with the ethos of a school and can succeed in influencing colleagues working in the more traditional subject areas.

The former method of organization is by far the most common but an increasing number of schools are giving careful thought to the advantages offered by the second. Indeed it would be wrong to view them as alternative ways of organizing a programme because the second can, and usually does, grow out of the first. Such growth has to be nurtured, however, through staff involvement and training of various kinds. Cross-curricular activities are notoriously difficult to initiate and sustain, and co-ordinators and their teams would be wise to move slowly by involving at first only one or two subject areas in such a collaborating venture. For example, assuming that a core of health education is located in science, teaching contributions might be forthcoming from the home economics and the humanities departments. Later other subject departments might be invited or would wish to become involved.

The complexities of organizing such contributory strands from an array of curriculum areas, some of which will be optional to most students, might seem so daunting as to discourage the most enthusiastic of teachers. It is true that such cross-curricular activities do challenge the organizational ingenuity of a school and are demanding of tolerance and goodwill amongst staff; such is the nature of school-based curriculum development. To facilitate a successful operation of this kind a school must be firmly resolved to carry it through. The resolve must stem from the headteacher and the senior staff of the school and needs to be sustained over very probably several terms of planning and implementation. Change, no matter how desirable, is rarely if ever brought about without conviction and commitment from senior staff and considerable skill in its management and execution. The *Co-ordinators' Guide* developed for staff training by the SCHEP 13–18 team offers considerable help here (Williams and Williams, 1980).

The Importance of Materials

The most carefully planned programme will be doomed to failure if adequate attention is not paid to the resources necessary for its operation. Co-ordinators and teams will need to acquaint themselves with the many and varied materials which are available from many sources. Excellent resource lists may be obtained from national organizations such as the Health Education Council, the Teachers' Advisory Council on Alcohol and Drug Education, the Family Planning Association and the Schools Council. Teachers will need to be discriminating in their choice of materials for use in their programmes, however, and to give careful thought once again to the aims which they have set themselves. Some materials, for example, employ the familiar factual format and are intended largely to impart information about a specific area, for example about tobacco or alcohol. Other kinds of material concern themselves with the social situation in which the health-related behaviour of young people occurs. There has been a tendency for pupil materials to reflect the 'topic' image of health education and to deal more with the hard subject matter than the social situation in which they are usually met by young people. There is a growing awareness of the need for material to be as much concerned with 'social facts' as with 'health facts', a recognition which owes much to the work of researchers such as Bewley (1975), Jahoda and Crammond (1972) and Dorn (1978). Experimentation with, for example, cigarettes occurs usually with friends or older brothers and sisters or when parents are permissive towards the habit. Motivation is a crucial consideration in such matters and the desire to experiment is located more in the social nature of the situation than in any intrinsic desire for the behaviour itself.

There is, of course, a need for materials which give objective factual information about specific health topics and also for materials which help individuals to reflect on the social motivation which surrounds them. Sometimes they are both embedded in the same material, but teachers need to give careful consideration to their use in the classroom.

The aspects of health and social education materials which concern themselves with setting the social scene within which young people operate and make choices about their behaviour do pose certain difficulties. Such materials require styles of classroom management different from those usually used in more didactic teaching/learning, and might well therefore require some additional thought and preparation. Generally materials of this kind – for example, trigger films, open-ended stories, case studies, group questionnaires, etc. – call for activities which require small groups and discussion experience of different kinds. Teachers not experienced in the ebb and flow of small group work often lack confidence in their own management and discussion skills and require reassurance and perhaps opportunities to regain their orientation to it. Help of different kinds is available through the work of Ruddock (1981), Button (1974) and SCHEP 13–18 (Schools Council, 1980), and any one of these could provide a focus for school-based in-service education for interested teachers.

Materials themselves can and do act as a stimulus to teachers and school activity in health education. Sometimes, however, the direction which a health education programme takes is dictated by the available materials themselves, for no other reason than that they are available and because they appear to have an 'authority' invested in them which teachers, largely untrained in health education, seek. Co-ordinators and their teams will need to view all material critically after assessing the needs of their own programme; existing materials can be changed, adapted and developed or indeed new material can be written and developed by the school itself to meet its individual needs. The writing of new materials or the adaptation of existing materials can provide teachers and schools with a most useful means of working through the many issues involved in school health education. Perhaps indeed it is one sure way in which the many issues surrounding health education can become personally relevant to participating teachers and meet the specific needs and aims of individual school programmes.

Materials and the methods employed in using them are inextricably linked to the aims which teachers themselves set. Whether such aims are educative or manipulative will depend upon their perception of health education itself and upon the direction which a school decides to follow. There is a wealth of material available, but the availability of certain materials should not in any way determine the content or the direction which a school programme takes. The programme, its general direction and its purposes need to be thought through and planned first.

Evaluation and Some Implications for a School Programme

The subject of evaluation is dealt with more thoroughly in Chapter 17, but its importance cannot be overstressed and merits some mention in this chapter. The matter of evaluation often gets lost during the planning and implementing of a school programme, despite its considerable importance. As a basic minimum it should provide a sharp monitoring edge to what schools are attempting to do. The type of evaluation should logically follow from the other policy decisions taken by a school; for example, if a school health education programme leans heavily towards cognitive input there is no real difficulty in evaluating the success of the programme. The more a school programme leans away from the purely cognitive to embrace the affective facets of health education, however, then the more difficult evaluation becomes.

A general view of the purpose of evaluation is that it should show whether or not an activity has been successful or to what degree it has failed to achieve some stated aims. In this particular sense it could be interpreted as the 'counting of heads'; a quantifying and interpretation of data followed by the presentation of results in some meaningful way. If, on the other hand, evaluation has to contend with matters of a more qualitative nature such as, for example, values and beliefs and their relationship to a range of behavioural options in response to a stimulus, then the collection of data and their interpretation and presentation become a profoundly more difficult evaluative task. More particularly, if the aims of the teaching/learning activity are concerned with the quality of the methodological process rather than their outcomes, traditional methods of evaluation might be severely challenged.

Some would argue that the evaluation of a programme which concerns itself with processes such as value clarification and decision-making as well as hard facts, is too difficult a task to contemplate because of the bewildering array of variables which would need to be considered. Another view would wish to emphasize the need for sound, longitudinal evaluative studies, spaning many years, as the only means by which to demonstrate whether the processes of decision-making or the acquisition of relevant knowledge make any difference in helping individuals choose healthier life styles.

I like to believe that whatever the aims or the style of teaching adopted, there are evaluative procedures to accommodate them. Perhaps we need to think of how evaluation could be brought nearer to the classroom as a useful tool for teacher and pupils. For example, it is generally accepted that a health education programme based on a decision-making model of teaching needs hard and accurate facts upon which the decisions can be made. It is not difficult to monitor the retention of facts but, I assume, it is very much more difficult to evaluate whether and how these facts are assimilated and become part of the repertoire of cognitive skills used to cope with personal and social decisions. In other words, how useful and relevant is the knowledge to the pupils? Do they use it? Will they use it? If so, how will they use it? I have a strong feeling that if we were able to design a simple process which could sensitize the teacher to the health education needs of individuals and groups of young people in the class or year-group, our health education teaching would become very much more effective. What is needed is a plain man's guide to Havighurst, Piaget, Bruner and Kohlberg turned into a readily usable and educational assessment tool. Maybe this is asking far too much.

One form of evaluation with which we are all familiar is the public examination, and there has been much serious talk about an examination in health education as the means by which it might be accorded status and therefore be given time on the curriculum. There is much to be said for such a scheme and equally there is much to be said against it. A variation of this theme which has a certain attraction would be to develop modules of health education within the context of several host subjects. I am sure that the host subjects might be enhanced as a consequence and the idea could be very supportive of health education co-ordination across the curriculum. If such a development were possible, one would, I think, need to look closely at the modes of examinations and to attempt to persuade examiners, if indeed they need persuading, to explore how public examinations might place greater store upon the judgements, arguments, value expression and rationality of discourse than upon clear-cut right and wrong answers. I do realize that subject areas other than health education also have such aspirations and maybe we could learn a few lessons from them.

The School Health Programme – A Postscript

No matter what kind of programme a school will finally decide upon, there are many school-based tasks and issues to be tackled. The lessons learned from a decade of curriculum development in the United Kingdom strongly suggest that curriculum development or curriculum innovation cannot succeed by being received 'gift wrapped' by a school. The ideas, concepts and issues which come in a packaged curriculum development have to be worked through and debated at first hand. They cannot successfully be put on like a second-hand suit of clothes, but have to be recut and stitched according to the specific needs of a school. Success will depend largely upon the skill and vision of the tailor and his assistants, as embodied in the co-ordinator and team, and this in turn will rest upon their perception of what a school needs and their creative response to that need. The work of the SCHEP has focused on a creative response to school-based curriculum development and has produced, as a result, in-service training modules of different kinds which are embodied in its *Co-ordinators' Guide* (Schools Council, 1980). It is difficult to see how, in the short term, programmes of health (or personal and social) education can thrive and develop without a purposeful and realistic in-service training programme for teachers.

The matters discussed in this chapter have hinted at the kind of tasks which need to be accomplished in order to discover and provide for the health education needs of a school. Essentially these tasks are as much concerned with school-based curriculum development as with health education, as much with the professional development of staff colleagues as with the development of the students. Such tasks are not, however, to be undertaken lightly because they do involve a major exercise of reviewing what a school already has, and building, shaping and implementing a school programme from that. They are nevertheless tasks which, if attempted in an atmosphere of sincerity, good humour and determination, will pay rich dividends in terms of the ethos and life of the school and, more importantly, the lives of the individual students themselves.

Summary

This chapter argues for the need in every school for a co-ordinator of health education who has considered in depth the many issues concerned with the development and implementation of a programme of health education. First and foremost is the need for each school to clarify what health education is, in terms of its aims, objectives and purposes. Alongside this task must go the investigation of what health education is already taking place across the curriculum subject areas. Together these tasks provide a platform for further planning and implementation. The chapter goes on to elaborate other important tasks which are essential to establish health education in the curriculum, including the possible location of health education within a broadly based programme of personal and social education, and the identification of priorities for such teaching. The need for materials and methods of teaching appropriate to health education teaching are also discussed, as is the difficult issue of evaluation.

References

Baelz, P. R. (1979) 'Philosophy of health education', in Sutherland, I. (ed.), *Health Education: Perspectives and choices*. London, Allen & Unwin.

Baric, L. (1979) *Primary Socialization and Smoking*. Health Education Council Monograph. London, Health Education Council.

Benjamin, H. (1971) 'The saber-tooth curriculum', in Hooper, R. (ed.), *The Curriculum: Context, design and development*. Edinburgh, Oliver & Boyd.

Bewley, B. R., Bland, J. M. and Harris, R. (1975) 'Factors associated with the starting of cigarette smoking by primary school children'. *Br. J. Prev. Soc. Med.*, vol. 28, pp. 37–44.

Button, L. (1974) *Developmental Group Work with Adolescents*. London, University of London Press.

Department of Education and Science (1978) *Curriculum 11–16: Health education in the secondary school curriculum*. Working paper by the Health Education Committee of HM Inspectorate. London, HMSO.

Department of Education and Science (1979) *Aspects of Secondary Education in England*. Survey by HM Inspectorate. London, HMSO, pp. 206–240.

Department of Health and Social Security (1976) *Prevention and Health: Everybody's business*. London, HMSO.

Dorn, N. (1978) *Teaching Decision Making Skills About Legal and Illegal Drugs*. London, Institute for the Study of Drug Dependence.

Havighurst, R. J. (1972) *Development Tasks and Education*. New York, McKay.

Jahoda, G. and Crammond, J. (1972) *Children and Alcohol: A developmental study in Glasgow*. London, HMSO.

Monaster, J. (1977) *Adolescent Development and the Life Tasks*. Boston, Mass., Allyn & Bacon.

Ruddock, J. (1981) *Making the Most of the Short In-Service Course*. To be published by the Schools Council.

Schools Council (1976) *Health Education in Secondary Schools*. Working Paper 57. London, Evans/Methuen Educational.

Schools Council (1980) *Co-ordinators' Guide*. Schools Council Health Education Project 13–18. Southampton University, Media Resource Centre.

Tones, K. (1977) *Effectiveness and Efficiency in Health Education. A review of theory and practice*. Edinburgh, Scottish Health Education Unit.

Williams, T. and Williams, N. (1980) 'Personal and social development in the school curriculum', in *Co-ordinators' Guide*. Schools Council Health Education Project 13–18.

Wilson, J. (1973) *A Teacher's Guide to Moral Education*. London, G. Chapman.

World Health Organization (1978) *The Health Needs of Adolescents*. Technical Report no. 609. Geneva, World Health Organization.

PART III

THE CONTRIBUTIONS OF SUBJECT DEPARTMENTS AND PASTORAL CARE

INTRODUCTION

In reviewing the development of health attitudes among young people it is, of course, immensely difficult to apportion influence. Most health attitudes of children are profoundly affected by parental and home influences, where health education takes place constantly, whether recognized or not. Influence is also exerted by, for example, the child's peer group and the media, and schools may come last on the list of those who shape a youngster's attitudes, skills and knowledge of health. However, while a child's life style may be largely shaped outside school, the influence of individual teachers and the cumulative influence of a well-run school may be profound. How profound that influence is depends on individual differences, and on many varied factors, but it is an underestimated truth that teachers influence children's lives more than teachers themselves acknowledge, and much of that influence lies through subject teaching and in pastoral care.

Although we are convinced that health education in its modern context requires a co-ordinated or integrated approach, as described by Vaughan Johnson and Trefor Williams, that co-ordinated approach is itself dependent upon the contribution of the traditional subject areas, which are unlikely to lose their authority in the near future. Most subject areas contribute aspects of health education, either intuitively or deliberately, and some subjects are traditionally guardians of various health messages.

The following six chapters illustrate the health education viewpoints of subject areas and of the pastoral care system of schools. From them we can again see how each subject department's contribution, particularly in secondary schools, could be integrated with others to produce a more effective school approach to health education. Health education overlaps most areas of the curriculum, yet each area may have its own distinctive contribution.

It must be emphasized that our selection of subject areas is not in any way definitive, and most other curriculum subjects could be dealt with in this way, if space permitted.

Science teaching has a traditional share in health education, especially in the teaching of biological science, and the science department has often been equated with the required element of sex education that schools have felt obliged to offer. This has given an unfortunate image at times, and one has memories of the dogfish as an important but confused part of sex knowledge. In Chapter 6 Tim Hull offers a modern view of how biology teaching can contribute to the teaching of health, and reminds us that emphasizing health education in biology teaching need not compromise the scientific balance of the subject, and that in human biology lessons the experimental material is there in the pupils, for interest in self and others is intense. After graduating from London University and obtaining an MSc from Southampton, Tim Hull taught biology in a variety of secondary schools. In 1975 he joined the staff of St Osyth College of Education as a lecturer in biology and environmental science. Between 1977 and 1980 he was deputy director of the Schools Council Health Education Project 13–18. He is currently a senior lecturer at Chelmer Institute of Higher Education, Essex and adviser for health education.

The home economics department has also been a traditional contributor to health education in schools, and Mrs Winifred Hart provides a personal view of the contribution of home economics teachers. In Chapter 7 she draws attention to the wide contribution that home economics departments can make for boys as well as girls in a subject area that has greatly widened its aims and objectives in recent years. Winifred Hart entered the teaching profession as a mature student, qualified as a teacher in home economics and taught for many years at both secondary and adult level, mostly with the Inner London Education Authority. She was then appointed as a teachers' centre warden and in 1972 joined the Home Economics Inspectorate in the ILEA. Since 1976 she has been inspector of health education.

Physical education should have always contributed to health education in schools, but it must be said that in some school settings such contributions have been very limited compared with physical activities, and at times have been limited to spasmodic wet-day sessions. Well-run physical education departments provide a major facility for health teaching, and the Physical Education Association, in Chapter 8, defines the contribution which physical education teachers can make. The chapter is provided by their kind permission and is from their Standing Study Group on Health and Recreation, summarized by John Wright as the group's chairman/ convenor. He is principal lecturer in movement studies at Nonington College, Dover.

In Chapter 9 Peter Farley comments on the contribution of English to health education, reminding us that 'the very use and existence of language implies relationships'. Peter Farley taught English and general studies in schools in Birmingham and Devon before joining the Schools Council Health Education Project 13–18. As a member of the SCHEP 13–18 dissemination team he is presently a research fellow in the Department of Education at Southampton University.

The place of religious education in the co-ordination of health education may seem debatable at first sight, but we have asked Ian Birnie to discuss this theme, and we are mindful of the way in which many other subject areas could review their part in the health message, as he does. After training at Cheltenham and Bristol, Ian Birnie worked as a head of department of religious education in Lancashire. Later as national secretary of the Christian Education Movement in London, he worked with teachers in secondary schools throughout the United Kingdom, both as an adviser and producer of curriculum materials. He is the author of a number of schoolbooks widely used in social, moral and health education courses, and since 1971 has been general adviser with special responsibility for religious education in Lancashire.

Chapter 11 argues the fundamental support that the pastoral system of a school can give to the personal and social education of pupils. Kenneth David points to the supportive nature of the tutorial system and suggests it could be more positive and planned, and could thus underpin the co-ordinated health education programme.

Kenneth David has recently finished a nine-year spell as a county adviser for schools in Lancashire, with special responsibility for pastoral care and personal relationships. Before that he was tutor-adviser in personal relationships in Gloucestershire, and played an important part in the development of the school and community personal relationships schemes there. He has taught in many types of schools and colleges, and describes himself as a kind of educational hobo. He is now a freelance lecturer.

CHAPTER 6

THE CONTRIBUTION OF BIOLOGY TO SCHOOL HEALTH EDUCATION

Tim Hull

Introduction

Biology in the school curriculum has long been seen as a vehicle for health education. For example, in 1918, the following appeared in *The School World*:

> The elementary biology course will form a natural introduction to that acquaintance with the working of the human body and the elementary laws of health which all young people should have towards the end of their school career. . . . If such a course were generally adopted in school education it would lead to the diffusion of sound biological thought on public health and other social questions.

Although the nature, purpose and place of both biology and health education in the school curriculum may have changed, one only has to look at current biology syllabuses to see that the links between biology and health education, at least in terms of content, remain strong. The following section, for example, comes from a CSE biology examination syllabus (EMEB, 1980): 'Biological aspects of such social problems as tobacco, drugs, obesity, birth control and venereal disease'.

The extent of the common ground has been illustrated by the work of the Schools Council Health Education Project 13–18 (1980). All the schools working with the project have used a grid for collecting information about where in the curriculum and to whom health education is taught. The grid listed the possible content of health education and heads of departments indicated which items were included in their subjects. In almost all project schools biology made a substantial contribution. Since biology is concerned with the study of living things this is perhaps not surprising, particularly now that the human animal is so often included among the living creatures studied. Readers might be interested to look into the contribution biology makes in their own school.

It would be misleading, however, to suggest that looking for aspects of health education in syllabuses is entirely satisfactory when trying to establish the contribution of school biology to health education. Labels, whether they refer to subjects or topics, tell us surprisingly little about the nature and purpose of what goes on within them, and it is quite possible to teach biology, even human biology, without including any health education. For example, work on teeth is likely to feature in most biology courses, but it may consist of drawing and labelling a tooth, learning the dental formulae of the dog, the sheep, the rabbit and man, etc., and allow no time for pupils to consider the importance of their own teeth and the extent to which they are responsible for the health of their teeth.

An understanding of health itself, as a dynamic interaction between a developing individual and his changing physical and social environment, is dependent on biological concepts. Dubos (1965) coined the term 'man adapting'; that is, the ability of man to respond to changes in himself, his physical and social environment and medical knowledge. Essentially 'adapting' is a biological concept which rests on further biological ideas. These include homeostasis both at the individual and community level, the co-ordinating roles of the nervous and hormone systems, individual variation, growth and development as a continuing process and ecological balance. An understanding and appreciation of such concepts seems fundamental to any school health education programme. Not only does it provide the background against which individuals make choices and decisions related to their health and well-being, but it also helps pupils adapt to changes in themselves and their environment. For example, by emphasizing the normality of individual differences and the nature of growth and development with changing individual needs, pupils may gain considerable reassurance about changes in themselves, particularly during puberty. The DES publication *Health Education in Schools* (1977b) considers in some detail the relationship between biological ideas and health education. However, knowing how biological concepts relate to health education and the way in which, for example, teaching about nutrition or the circulatory system in biology can be developed to include aspects of health behaviour, is not enough. It is also important to focus more closely on the nature and purpose of biology as part of the school curriculum. For many pupils, particularly those in secondary schools, it is a discrete subject and for others it may be included in an integrated science scheme. When schools come to review, plan and develop health education within their curriculum they will need to answer questions such as those listed below, which relate specifically to biology and integrated science as school subjects.

1 What are the aims of biology and integrated science teaching, and how far are these compatible with the aims of health education?
2 How does current biology or integrated science teaching in our school relate to health education?
3 How will health education be organized in school? (Schools Council, 1976).
   – as a specialist, subject approach;
   – as an integrated approach;
   – as an approach through the pastoral or guidance system;
   – as a combination of these?
4 What is the role of school biology or integrated science in the approach adopted?
5 To what extent is the co-ordination of biology with other areas of the curriculum, including health education or social education, practicable?

By looking specifically at the nature and purpose of school biology and integrated science I hope to consider issues which will help schools to answer such questions.

Since the primary school curriculum is not usually organized in terms of readily identified subjects, most of what follows will apply to secondary schools. However, it is interesting that both the HMI Working Paper *Curriculum 11–16* (DES, 1977a) and the Scottish Education Department publication *The Structure of the Curriculum in the Third and Fourth Years of the Scottish Secondary School* (1977) avoided subject labels when talking about the essential elements of the curriculum, and referred respectively to 'areas of experience' and 'modes of activity'. Both refer to the same eight areas as can be seen from the two lists on page 139 (the order of the lists has been changed for ease of comparison).

The HMI Working Paper *Curriculum 11–16* (DES, 1977a) emphasizes that any curriculum provided for pupils up to the age of sixteen should be capable of offering properly thought out and progressive experience in all these areas. This is possible through traditional subjects like biology, through various forms of interdisciplinary work, through special courses

Areas of Experience	*Modes of Activity*
The aesthetic and creative	Creative and aesthetic
The ethical	Concerned with morality
The linguistic	Linguistic and literary studies
The mathematical	Mathematical studies
The physical	Physical activities
The scientific	Scientific activities
The social and political	Social studies
The spiritual	Religious studies.

like the ones concerned with social and health education and through the pastoral and guidance organization of the school. In this context subjects like biology may need to make different contributions in different schools. Indeed we must pay particular attention not only to the relationship of biology to health education but also to the way in which both relate to education and the curriculum as a whole.

The Nature and Purpose of School Biology/Integrated Science

Biology syllabuses, as we have seen, often include topics or items which are also included in school health education courses. But while both biology and health education are frequently described in terms of their contents, this is far from a complete picture. The nature and purpose of health education is explored in some depth elsewhere in the book, but what about biology? Every school will interpret biology and its place in the curriculum in its own way, as reflected by the aims of the course and its content, organization and methods. However, while the question 'What is school biology?' will be answered in a number of ways, related to broader issues rather than merely the demands of an external examination, it is possible to consider general trends and developments in school biology and integrated science.

Prior to the Nuffield 'O' Level Biology Project (1966), school biology was very much concerned with presenting information about living things. One of the principal aims of this project, however, was to foster a critical approach to the subject with an emphasis on experimentation and enquiry rather than on mere factual assimilation. In other words process as well as content was considered important. Two of the curriculum projects in science which followed this, Nuffield Combined Science (1970) and the

Schools Council Science Project 5–13 (1972), maintained this emphasis on scientific thinking or method.

Primary school science

Primary school science does not have an agreed content and is seen very much as being integrated with other areas of the curriculum. Indeed the broad aims of the Science Project 5–13, which are outlined below, are clearly not unique to science.

Fig. 6.1   The aims of the Schools Council Science Project 5–13

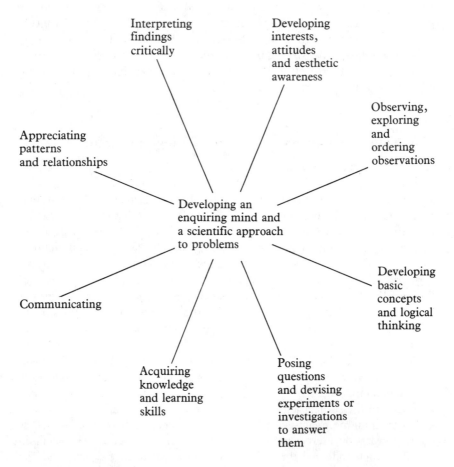

Interpreting findings critically

Developing interests, attitudes and aesthetic awareness

Observing, exploring and ordering observations

Appreciating patterns and relationships

Developing an enquiring mind and a scientific approach to problems

Communicating

Developing basic concepts and logical thinking

Acquiring knowledge and learning skills

Posing questions and devising experiments or investigations to answer them

It is only when specific objectives are identified that primary school science becomes more obviously scientific. While the importance of scientific method may be emphasized, we should also consider the content of primary school science and the criteria for choosing this content. The Schools Council Science Project 5–13 (1972) suggested the following:

> In general children work best when trying to find answers to problems which they have themselves chosen to investigate. These problems are best drawn from their own environment and tackled largely by practical investigations.

Many of the problems which meet these criteria will also be relevant to health education. For example, reaction times and stopping distances relate to road safety; the effects of exercise on heart and breathing rates relate to understanding oneself. Indeed, one of the units for teachers produced by the Science Project 5–13 is called *Ourselves* (Schools Council, 1975a) and gives suggestions about ways of helping children to find out about themselves and to gain an understanding of human variation.

In the process of finding answers to problems of their choice through practical investigation, pupils will inevitably accumulate factual information. However, the question is whether there are some items which all pupils should know by the age of thirteen. The Schools Council Project *Progress in Learning Science* (1975b) described a minimum set of ideas about the environment which children should build up whilst learning to explore and experiment scientifically. As well as enquiry skills and attitudes, a number of basic concepts, or generalizations, were included. Among these concepts were ones relevant to health education:

concept of life cycle,
concept of change,
concept of interdependence of living things,
concept of adaptation of living things.

Secondary school biology/integrated science

While the content details of secondary school biology syllabuses may differ, there is much agreement about the nature of the concepts or general principles which pupils should acquire. For example, the following are usually included:

maintenance of the organism/working of body systems
homeostasis
growth and development
reproduction
variation
ecology
evolution.

The Nuffield 'O' Level Biology Project emphasized the importance of pupils both developing a scientific way of thinking and working, and acquiring a fairly complex body of knowledge. It also tried to introduce the personal and social relevance of biological concepts. One of the aims of the project, for instance, is 'To develop an understanding of man as a living organism and his place in nature'. It is encouraging to note that more of the material in the second edition is concerned with 'the usefulness and social implications of biology to man's everyday needs, e.g. food and health'. For example, in Text 3 *Living Things and Their Environment* (Nuffield, 1975), there is a chapter specifically concerned with man and his environment. In Chapter 11 of the same text there is material for background reading under the title 'Natural selection in man today – survival in the urban environment', in which there is some attempt to relate the work to the lives of the pupils themselves. When an opportunity is provided, as in this case, for pupils to consider how a subject impinges on their own lives, their own behaviour or aspirations and how these may affect their health and that of others, then this is health education (DES, 1978).

In Nuffield Secondary Science (1971), the choice of content is based on the criterion of significance. It is suggested that in order to give significance to science each new aspect should develop from the pupil's immediate experience, and in this way pupils may be gradually introduced to fundamental issues which are likely to have considerable significance for them within a year or two. Using significance as a criterion for choosing the content of science clearly has importance when looking at the contribution of biology and integrated science to health education. Health education as we have seen is very much concerned with the individual and as such should have both intrinsic interest and long-term relevance for pupils. Indeed Nuffield Secondary Science, particularly Theme 2, *The Continuity of Life*, and Theme 3, *Biology of Man*, includes sections which relate very closely to health education. For example, while most school biology syllabuses for thirteen–sixteen-year-olds include something on variations and heredity,

Theme 2 has a section entitled 'Why I am like I am' in which 'The significance of the pupil's *own* variations is developed'. In making science more relevant to the lives of pupils, the problems of dealing with personal, social and moral implications will need to be faced when they arise. Social and moral issues can arise in the course of any scientific study, but they are likely to be particularly apparent in the work related to the human life cycle in Theme 3.

An orientation towards personal and social issues tends to mean more emphasis on human biology, and one of the criticisms that has been levelled at human biology is that it is not a very good 'science'. Indeed it was concern over the implications of the growing popularity of human biology as a school subject which led to a joint committee of the Royal Society and the Institute of Biology on 'The Teaching of Human Biology' (Biological Education Committee, 1978). Of particular concern was the suggestion that it was for some pupils the only science studied and that it was frequently taught in a non-experimental fashion. The opportunity for first-hand investigation is certainly more limited in human biology as is illustrated by 'Why I am like I am' from Nuffield Secondary Science, Theme 2. However, the main conclusion of the joint committee was:

> . . . that the study of human biology by pupils aged 13–16 can give a satisfactory introduction to biological science provided that it is experimentally and scientifically based.

It may well be that some human biology courses and also some social biology courses in schools are not experimentally and scientifically based. Although such courses cannot claim to be satisfactory as far as the scientific development of pupils is concerned, they may make a substantial contribution to the personal and social development of pupils. Where biology, human or otherwse, or integrated science is the only science which a pupil studies, a more balanced approach is necessary. Nuffield Secondary Science seems to have achieved a balance between basic principles related to an understanding of the physical world, scientific method (skills and attitudes) and aspects related to personal and social issues.

This is equally possible in human biology courses. The need for a balanced approach to science education has been emphasized in a number of publications (ASE, 1973; DES, 1977*b*; ASE, 1979). The HMI Working Paper *Curriculum 11–16* (DES, 1977*a*) has suggested that any science subject could have three components:

1 *Science for the enquiring mind* – underlying principles, the disciplines of the subject.
2 *Science for action* – use and application of those principles.
3 *Science for citizenship* – concerns the role of science in personal and collective decision-making.

Biology clearly has a wider educational role than simply contributing to the scientific development of pupils, in particular it has a legitimate part to play in the personal and social development of pupils. It is in this context that biology should make an important contribution to school health education.

Health Education in School Biology

Having argued that school biology does have a part to play in the personal and social development of pupils with which health education is concerned, to what extent can biology contribute to this development, bearing in mind the other demands on the subject? The major role which traditionally biology has had in health education has been one concerned with providing a basic health knowledge and an understanding of human development. This has been particularly the case for human and social biology courses where more emphasis is placed on man and the relevance of general biological concepts to health and social issues. However, the HMI Working Paper *Curriculum 11–16* science paper (DES, 1978) suggested that:

> No pupil should leave school without a usable understanding based on observation and experiment but not bounded by the limits of his own capacity for any of the following:
> 1 His own body and its functioning, with a reasonably clear notion of some of the many contributory causes of malfunctioning. . . .

The suggestion that the understanding should be usable has clear implications for the approach adopted in biology and integrated science teaching. Just as in health education, methods in biology must ensure that as far as possible the information and principles developed constitute, to use Barnes' (1976) terms, 'action knowledge' and not just 'school knowledge'.

Food selection provides an example of health education to which biology can contribute by helping pupils acquire an understanding of their own body and its functioning. Most biology courses in secondary schools include work on the composition of food, the importance of the various nutrients and the need for a balanced diet, the digestive process, feeding relationships and energy flow. It would not be difficult to relate such work to the eating behaviour of the pupils themselves, and in this way develop an understanding which they are more likely to apply to their own lives. An approach which attempts to increase the relevance of biology teaching, by relating biological concepts and understanding to the lives of pupils, is perfectly compatible with the more scientific aims of the subject. Indeed, experimental work involving, for example, food tests, the energy content of foods, and action of enzymes, etc., might have increased significance.

The multifactorial nature of diseases of the circulatory system illustrates the importance of understanding the relationship between body systems. Heredity, diet, smoking, exercise and stress may all play a part in diseases of both the arteries and the heart itself. Smoking may lead to lung damage which would impair the efficiency with which oxygen is absorbed into the blood. The oxygen transporting capacity is also reduced by the absorption of carbon monoxide from tobacco smoke. These effects mean that the heart has to pump more blood to ensure that sufficient oxygen is delivered to the muscles of the body. The increased work load that smoking tends to put on the heart seems to provide a reasonable explanation of the data which show that the risk of dying from heart disease in Britain is $1\frac{1}{2}$–$3\frac{1}{2}$ times greater for smokers than for non-smokers. However, one report showed that in some countries the differences between smokers and non-smokers is much less pronounced, and in some cases there appears to be no connection at all between smoking and coronary heart disease (Royal College of Physicians, 1977).

This apparently conflicting information may raise the question of whether smoking really is a factor in the occurrence of heart disease. Only when the interdependence of physiological processes is appreciated can we begin to understand the complex interaction of the various risk factors, for example smoking, diet or exercise. In those countries where there seems to be little or no connection between smoking and coronary heart disease, it may be because of such favourable factors as low levels of blood cholesterol or high levels of physical activity.

This discussion does not imply that there should be an emphasis on disease, indeed McKeown (1979) has suggested that a preoccupation with disease can develop when undue emphasis is placed on its precursors. He sees no disadvantage in suggesting, for example, that physical exercise and control of weight advance the quality as well as the duration of life. But he suggests that when people are also encouraged to monitor their weight, pulse and blood pressure, we are in some danger of crossing the delicate line which divides quiet confidence in health from a morbid preoccupation with its loss.

Biology is perhaps not usually considered to make an important contribution to those aspects of health education concerned with helping pupils explore and understand feelings, attitudes and values (the affective domain). However, biology teaching which aims to help pupils develop a 'usable understanding' of their body and its functioning should also contribute to the formation of responsible attitudes to the care and maintenance of the body. In most cases it is very difficult to separate knowledge and understanding from attitudes and values, and it is encouraging that Nuffield Secondary Science acknowledges that it has a role in this area. Any work concerned with the human body, for example a scientific investigation of the way the pulse rate varies with exertion, may contribute to an individual's body awareness or body image. However, it is more likely to do this if pupils are given the opportunity to relate the work to their own experience. Even courses which emphasize the factual content can make a contribution to the affective side of health education. For example, a caring teacher presenting the facts about human reproduction could create an atmosphere in which pupils might, through questioning, resolve some of their own worries and difficulties which could lead to a more open and less embarrassed attitude towards sex and sexuality.

Much has been said about the importance of decision-making in health education. Biology can contribute to present and future decision-making by providing relevant information, but it can also contribute to the decision-making process in a more general way. The Schools Council Integrated Science Project (1973) includes a section called *Science and Decision Making*, and the role of science in decision-making is also emphasized in the component *Science for Citizenship*. Health decisions in the future are likely to depend on the ability of pupils to interpret information, including epidemiological evidence, in a way which can be understood and related to personal life styles. Clearly biology can and does contribute here.

Fluoridation of the public water supplies, the effects on health of lead in petrol, and immunization, in particular immunization against whooping cough, could be issues considered within biology teaching, examination syllabuses permitting. Alternatively they could be part of a science or biology contribution to a sixth-form general studies programme.

I am not suggesting that health education can replace biology, nor that the issues relevant to health education should be a starting point for every aspect of a biology course. However, I think good teaching is relevant teaching, and where attempts are made to link the work to the lives of the pupils it not only makes a more substantial contribution to health education but can also enhance the other elements of the subject.

School Biology and a Co-ordinated Approach to Health Education

Whatever approach is adopted to secondary school health education, biology has a contribution to make. Even where schools decide to establish a specialist health education course, biology will still have a content and method which relates to a greater or lesser extent to health education, and co-ordination is therefore necessary. But co-ordination between biology and health education is not well developed in many instances (Scottish Education Department, 1979). Co-ordination is more than merely putting together elements of the existing curriculum, for it involves a synthesis of contributions in a way which has meaning and relevance to the present and as far as is possible to the future lives of pupils.

The extent to which biology can contribute to a co-ordinated programme of health education can be considered by first looking at the sorts of priorities a school might identify. Examples of such priorities are given below for year 1 of an eleven–sixteen or eleven–eighteen school. They are based on two considerations which seem particularly important in year 1: the change to a new school with the new relationships and opportunities which this presents, and the onset of puberty around this time. It should be remembered, however, that priorities for year-groups are likely to vary from one school to another, and that one year from a continuum does create a somewhat artificial picture.

Health education priorities for year 1

1   An emphasis on good group work and the opportunity to ask questions. The importance of a good pastoral care system.

2   Work on the change from the predominant influence of the family to the growing influence of peer groups.

3   Work on body change and physical growth should build on the work done in primary school. An emphasis on individual differences is to be encouraged.

4   Some work on body systems – to utilize the general interest pupils have in themselves to develop an understanding of body functions.

5   An introduction to the idea of choices using one or two areas that

exemplify the change from small primary to large secondary school; e.g., food choices and safety.

Biology and integrated science teaching, particularly in the first and second years, are increasingly emphasizing the importance of pupils working together in twos or threes, sharing ideas and suggesting things for themselves. Such teaching which also places some emphasis on helping pupils to relate the work to their own lives, has much in common with methods used in health education with its onus on good group work. Even when the content of biology courses cannot be co-ordinated with the health education priorities, it should be possible to ensure that the approach adopted in biology is supportive of the aims of health education without devaluing the other contributions which biology makes to the curriculum as a whole.

As far as the content of first-year biology integrated science courses is concerned, both Nuffield Combined Science (1970) and the Scottish Integrated Science Scheme (Mee et al., 1970) include work on body change and physical growth. There is considerable scope, however, for making stronger links with health education. Indeed the interest pupils have in themselves and in health issues could easily make more interesting starting points for some of the work in biology.

Nuffield Combined Science also includes material on human reproduction which introduces puberty and menstruation as well as providing information about the reproductive system. This could provide the focus for those aspects of health education related to growth and development, in particular the physical changes occurring at puberty. Social and emotional changes could be introduced here, but whether science is the place to develop them is more open to debate. Some schools, for example, might consider that a subject like English would be a better context for exploring with pupils the social and emotional changes occurring at and around puberty.

The reproductive system is the only body system to feature in Nuffield Combined Science. From a health education perspective, the first year seems to be an ideal time to introduce body systems in general. It could provide the vocabulary which pupils require to talk about their bodies without embarrassment, a balanced view of the body as a whole rather than the reproductive system alone, and could provide interest in learning more about the structure and function of their bodies. Although the Scottish Integrated Science Scheme, Nuffield 'O' Level Biology (1966) and Schools

Council Science Project 5–13 (1972) do include work related to other body systems, it does not form a major part of the biology work suggested for eleven–twelve-year-olds. It is unfortunate that human anatomy and physiology do not feature more strongly in lower school biology, since it is difficult to see from which other areas of the curriculum pupils will gain an understanding of body systems.

In years I, II (S1) and III (S2)* it is not, in theory, a difficult task to relate biology or integrated science teaching to health education and other areas of the curriculum. In other words, it is possible to approach health education through the co-ordination of traditional subjects of which biology or integrated science is one. However, there is a limit to the number of subject areas which can be closely co-ordinated, perhaps two or three, or at the most four. One of these subjects, maybe biology, will then need to be the focal point to which the others can relate in terms of content, methods and timing.

However, in years IV (S3) and V (S4) the option systems which operate in most schools make co-ordination a very different proposition. Biology is certainly not taken by all pupils, indeed some pupils will do no science at all beyond the third year. This means that the suggestion in the HMI Working Paper *Curriculum 11–16* Science Paper (DES, 1978), that no pupil should leave school without a usable understanding of his own body and its functioning, is not likely to be achieved. While a school will identify health education priorities for years IV and V, they cannot usually rely on all pupils doing work on some of them in biology or integrated science. However, we have already seen that many biology courses in years IV and V, as reflected by curriculum projects and examination syllabuses, include aspects which relate closely, at least in terms of content, to health education. Indeed the same is true of other subjects in the curriculum, for example home economics and religious education. One of the priorities for work on health education in years IV and V might be to look beyond the immediate health-related behaviour of pupils towards their future roles and responsibilities as citizens and parents. It would perhaps be appropriate to look at human needs, not just physical needs, within the context of growing and developing and the connection with 'good parenting'. The links this has with biology go beyond the fact that 'growing' and 'developing' are biological concepts, and this is reflected in Theme 3 of Nuffield Secondary Science where the introduction to the section on the human life cycle states:

---

* Transfer to secondary school occurs at the age of twelve in Scotland, and not at eleven which is more usual in England and Wales. Therefore year II in an English or Welsh secondary school would be the equivalent of year I (S1) in a Scottish secondary school.

. . . an attempt is made to present an outline of the whole human life cycle, including not only the physical and behavioural problems of adolescence but also those of child development, maturity, and ageing as well as the phenomena of human gestation and birth.

This raises the question of how far it is realistic to attempt to co-ordinate the various elements of the curriculum for fourth- and fifth-year pupils. The majority of secondary schools which have recognized that health education is an important part of the curriculum for all pupils in the fourth and fifth years, have established a separate course of health or social education. This core course may go under the name of social education, general studies, design for living, etc. There is often very little attempt to co-ordinate the work with that in other subjects because of the large number of optional subjects which only a small proportion of pupils study. Only when schools establish a policy for the curriculum as a whole and decide what all pupils should study up to the age of sixteen will the potential for co-ordination in years IV and V be realized.

In year VI (S5 and S6) health education is more likely than not to be part of general studies. However, within this context biology can make a contribution, for example to the community health issues mentioned earlier. There are a number of examination syllabuses at the sixth-year level which incorporate much of importance to health education, for example social biology 'AO' and 'A' level and human biology 'AO' and 'A' level. One of the drawbacks with these and other examination syllabuses is that only a small proportion of sixth-formers will be likely to take them.

Conclusion

Clearly biology makes an important contribution to school health education although the precise nature of this contribution will vary from school to school and will depend on what is going on elsewhere in the curriculum. Not only is an understanding and appreciation of biological concepts fundamental to health education, but an orientation towards health education when planning and teaching biology can give significance and relevance to school biology while not compromising its scientific and broader biological contributions to the curriculum.

Summary

Despite the traditional links that biology has had with health education it is possible to teach biology, even human biology, without making a major contribution to health education. The nature and purpose of school biology as reflected by recent publications and projects does, however, imply that biology has an important role to play in the personal and social development of pupils, with which health education is concerned. It is suggested that school biology can contribute to health education through:

- the development of biological concepts fundamental to an understanding of health and the scope for individual choice,
- the promotion of a positive self-image,
- the development of skills important in decision-making.

If biology is to make the most of its potential as a contributor to health education, it is also necessary to look at the way in which both relate to education and the curriculum as a whole.

References

Association for Science Education (1973) *Science for the 13–16 Age Group*. London, Association for Science Education.
Association for Science Education (1979) *Alternatives for Science Education*. London, Association for Science Education.
Barnes, D. (1976) *From Communication to Curriculum*. London, Penguin.
Biological Education Committee (1978) *The Teaching of Human Biology*. London, The Royal Society/Institute of Biology.
Department of Education and Science (1977a) *Curriculum 11–16*. HM Inspectorate Working Paper. London, HMSO.
Department of Education and Science (1977b) *Health Education in Schools*. London, HMSO.
Department of Education and Science (1978) *Curriculum 11–16: Health education in the secondary school curriculum*. HM Inspectorate Working Paper. London, HMSO.
Dubos, R. (1965) *Man Adapting*. New Haven, Conn., Yale University Press.
East Midlands Examination Board for CSE (1980) *Regulations and Syllabuses*.
McKeown, T. (1979) *The Role of Medicine*. Oxford, Blackwell.
Mee, A. J., Boyd, P. and Richie, D. (1970) *Science for the 70s*. London, Heinemann.

Nuffield (1966) O-Level Biology Project. 1st edition. London, Longman/ Penguin.

Nuffield (1970) Combined Science Series. London, Longman/Penguin.

Nuffield (1971) Secondary Science Series. London, Longman.

Nuffield (1975) O-Level Biology Project: Text 3, *Living Things and Their Environment*. London, Longman.

Royal College of Physicians (1977) *Smoking or Health*. London, Pitman Medical.

Schools Council (1972) Science Project 5–13. London, Macdonald Educational.

Schools Council (1973) Integrated Science Project. London, Longman/ Penguin.

Schools Council (1975a) Science Project 5–13: *Ourselves*. London, Macdonald Educational.

Schools Council (1976) *Health Education in Secondary Schools*. Working Paper 57. London, Evans/Methuen.

Schools Council (1977) *Progress in Learning Science: Match and mismatch*. Edinburgh, Oliver and Boyd.

Schools Council (1977–1980) Health Education Project 13–18. Unpublished.

Scottish Education Department (1977) *The Structure of the Curriculum in the Third and Fourth Years of the Scottish Secondary School*. London, HMSO.

Scottish Education Department (1979) *Health Education in Primary, Secondary and Special Schools in Scotland*. London, HMSO.

CHAPTER 7

HEALTH EDUCATION IN THE HOME ECONOMICS CURRICULUM

Winifred Hart

Introduction

Home economics entered the school curriculum during the latter years of the nineteenth century following concern for the health of the nation which had been prompted by various government reports. The intention was that girls, particularly working-class girls, were to be instructed in the management of their future homes so that standards of hygiene and safety would rise, and families would be better fed. Special emphasis was laid on economical budgeting and baby care. Moral undertones of wastefulness were to be eradicated, and acceptable standards of behaviour to be promoted. This curriculum was to be provided in the then elementary schools, although very soon domestic science found its place in the grammar schools. Historical attitudes and views of curriculum subjects remain long after they have ceased to exist, and both home economics and health education have to continue the fight to inform those both inside and outside education of the true nature of their work.

Both home economics and health education are concerned with areas of learning where incidental learning gained outside the formal system of education is often thought to be sufficient. The knowledge, concepts, attitudes, skills and competencies needed for optimal functioning on a personal and social level in the home and the wider social environment are neither recognized, nor thought to be of sufficient importance to be part of the basic curriculum of every pupil

Definitions of home economics and health education abound, and arguably this is to the detriment of both. It is difficult to define such subjects or areas of study because of their multidisciplinary eclectic nature. They draw on a range of other disciplines to make their own recognizable 'whole'. Both are academic and professional, and both contend that their essential aims are concerned with people in their social environment and with the relationships between people in that environment.

Statements on, or definitions of health education have been made in earlier chapters, but it is interesting to juxtapose two statements, one made by Professor Paolucci, a home economist, and the other by Miss Jean Arnold, a health educator. Paolucci (1976), talking about a group of men and women at the beginning of the twentieth century, said:

> (They) were aware of a simple but elegant idea, that if humans were to realise their potentialities they had to have a physical and a social setting which assured them of a continuous, reliable source of personal sustenance, and a setting which would help them to build, rebuild and nourish the health of the body, the mind and the emotions, a setting which would provide them with defensible standards that they themselves had evolved, that would give meaning to their lives as they coped with endless challenges of an increasingly complex and changing environment, and yes, many times a hostile environment.

Arnold (1977) said:

> Health is then both individually and socially a relative term, covering a wide range of standards which are complex to define and measure. Health cannot be regarded as absolute, it cannot be considered as a rigid and fixed concept; it is dynamic and flexible. . . . (It aims to) achieve optimal fitness or optimal functioning which will vary from person to person depending on the biological and genetic make-up, interacting and transacting with the context of their particular environment. . . . The key to health may be in the maintenance of homeostasis; health is seen as a condition of equilibrium and illness as a disruption of this balanced state . . ., giving a picture of health as man adapting to both his internal and external environments . . . . Health and disease are only meaningful when defined in terms of a given person functioning in a given physical and social environment. . . . Individuals have to find any proposed health practice acceptable in terms of their aspirations, beliefs and behaviour patterns of their daily living.

Paolucci continued: 'What is important at the everyday level is that we have some control, some possibility of managing our surroundings'; and to quote Arnold once again: 'Theoretically, health education is successful when it leads people to make decisions and to take action which for them are logical and sound, and which promise the greatest benefits and the least disadvantages whether or not *we* happen to agree with their conclusions.'

Both speakers were considering individuals in the social settings, and both wish to enable individuals to recognize the potential for change and the degree to which they may reasonably aspire to changing goals, and to which they may recognize and set goals. The speakers have a common thread of purpose and indicate the degree to which health education is an implicit part of home economics. Although many home economists and health educators may not necessarily share these views, they offer a useful basis for looking at the contribution of home economics to health education.

Home Economics and Health Education

Home economics is a practical, task-orientated subject offering learning experiences to pupils which enable them to acquire positive attitudes to themselves and others; to build concepts, through both knowledge and experience, some of which are specific to home economics and some which are of more general application; and to acquire certain competencies and skills necessary to operate successfully in this area of home and social environment. The morality of the choice made by teachers, of which attitudes and concepts, competencies and skills are to be fostered, particularly those relevant to health education, has been argued elsewhere. We shall concentrate here on those which are likely to be fostered and developed within the broad scope of home economics, child development and the family and textile courses, and thereby will be making a structurally recognized, or implicit but unrecognized, contribution to health education. The obvious danger is that implicit unrecognized attitudes and concepts may run counter to a structurally recognized, morally validated programme being undertaken elsewhere in the curriculum.

Home economics is concerned with satisfying the basic human needs for food, shelter, clothing and relationships of individuals living within an inter-related situation of family, home and community. At the present time, family, home and community embrace a multiplicity of various groupings within a pluralistic society, a fact that has strong implications for the approach to teaching the subject. Ultimately the degree to which these basic needs remain unsatisfied will have an influence on the health of any one individual. As with health educators, home economists may be unaware that they are teaching a variety of models of health education, and it may be that discrete areas of home economics fit better into one model than another. For example, teaching about the advantages of a medical immunization programme in child development courses may lean towards preventive medicine, whilst helping pupils to understand the growth of pressure groups for consumer legislation may tend towards a public health model.

Home Economics and Health Education

What then are the concepts encouraged and developed in home economics which make a contribution to the health education of the pupils? Central to home economics are the concepts of home and family. The concept of home has changed radically over the last three decades and home economists have had to reshape their ideas and values to maintain credibility in their teaching. Whatever the diverse nature of the homes in which our children find themselves in a multi-ethnic, pluralistic society, pupils can be encouraged to consider how home can be a secure base for action both within it and beyond. It is an environment where relationships encompassing both co-operation and conflict are experienced and utilized, where areas of co-operation and conflict can be examined and discussed. Pupils are guided to an understanding of socialization and security for the young and immature that is both positive and promotional rather than negative and deadening, and where cultural differences can be studied and appreciated. This work may be making a positive contribution to the health education notion that the creation of a secure self-image is linked to the sympathetic awareness of the needs of young children.

The concept of safety, or security, both physical and emotional, has always occupied a central place in home economics. Helping pupils to understand the idea of safety both in relation to themselves and others is no easy task. When teaching was instruction and unexplained rules were the order of the day, safe working was obtained in the controlled environment of the home economics and textile rooms. That this instruction did not, and perhaps still has not, become a working concept is demonstrated by the high rate of accidents in the home. Changes in educational thinking are bringing about changes in safety education. Pupils are being helped towards an understanding of the skills which need to be learnt before safety becomes an internalized concept. Questioning is encouraged on the value of habit; on who makes the rules, for young children, for adolescents, for adults; and if rules are necessary. Can security and risk-taking be balanced so that self-discovery, self-confidence and self-mastery are not thwarted, nor needless harm inflicted on the self or others? How can foresight and imagination be developed at each stage of development?

Home economics, as a practical task-orientated subject, offers opportunities for pupils to learn to cope with situations and problems of increasing complexity, and this is particularly true of pupils who pursue their home economics studies into the fourth and fifth years through to 'A' level studies. Within such problem-solving situations pupils gradually build up the concepts of choice and decisions. First, what is a problem? Can I recognize it? What is meant by a solution to a problem? Will it always be a compromise? How many others besides myself does it have to satisfy? What is evidence, what is judgement, do I know my judgement will be limited by knowledge and experience, do I know my values affect my judgement? The acquisition of the skills and competencies to define and solve problems, to evaluate and judge are implicit in home economics and are equally applicable when applied to health-related problems. There is a need to develop a concept of choice, which goes beyond a liking for one thing, or course of action, rather than another. It requires the ability to recognize and set criteria, to choose and justify the choice, to be able to recognize real and pseudo experts and evidence and to be stringent in assessing advice. Home economics and textiles encompass a wide area of consumer education where problem-solving, choices and decisions are constantly being encountered, not least in relation to health-related products and services. Also within consumer education is the notion of the consumer as an influence on future policies. With the knowledge and skills necessary to be a discerning consumer, discussion can take place as to how desired changes are or might be brought about.

Nutrition

Nutrition, as a concept, is probably one of the most difficult areas that home economists undertake. Consideration of diet is not new; in the *Syllabus of Instruction in Domestic Economy* (1912), teachers were exhorted, 'In planning meals due regard must be paid to instruction in the necessity for a varied diet', and the practical illustration given for a weekly budget of £1.18s was to plan, purchase, cook and serve a dinner for six for one shilling! The problems encountered in nutrition education are those endemic to health education. Attitudes to food are gained in early childhood; patterns of eating reflect family life styles and beliefs; advertising and public policy (or lack of it) exert strong pressures; likes and dislikes are well established and food and eating have a strong social value. All these influences are at work when food is chosen for eating. Home economists have too often concentrated on meal planning within a context which emphasized food functions, or nutrients, the seasons and the need for economy, without realizing the strength of the other factors. Consequently pupils plan ideal meals for stated people in particular situations, but do not alter their thinking or behaviour in relation to their own diet. The growth of both the pre-packaged and frozen-food industries has radically changed the contents of the weekly, or monthly shopping basket, changing work patterns and life styles have changed attitudes to meals, and a rising standard of living has extended the range of foods available to most families.

It is against this background that home economists can help children to an understanding of the concept of diet; towards the idea that whatever food is eaten it constitutes part of the total diet and that constant reviewing is necessary both to safeguard and promote health. The concept of a nutrient is difficult and requires a progressive approach leading to the knowledge that there are cheap and expensive sources of most nutrients. The choice of diet should be subject to the same criteria as other choices, but for many who may find some of the concepts too difficult, or who do not pursue the subject beyond the lower school, a simple workable meal-choosing scheme is vital. Such a scheme needs to be constantly used so that alternatives which cater for personal likes and dislikes and family and cultural differences can be considered. Home economists are faced with a dilemma when aiming to retain certain craft skills, allied to traditional dishes, which may be in conflict with modern nutritional thinking if they are overemphasized. Teachers and pupils need encouragement to redesign traditional recipes in line with modern nutritional knowledge, to look at diets in total – for example, being aware of 'hidden' sugars and fats – and to reconsider accepted portion sizes, whilst developing new attitudes and skills related to some of the more neglected but important foods which could find a place in the diet.

Care for Oneself and Others

The concept of care of oneself and others is an important aspect of much of the work undertaken in home economics. The needs of others are constantly considered in terms of food, clothing, shelter and relationships, but consideration extends beyond physical needs to emotional and social needs as indicated earlier in the chapter. Pupils work with a wide variety of people outside the classroom, including the young, the elderly and the handicapped.

Traditionally, concepts of growth and development were taught through the physical care of the young and the mothercraft element has a long history. But for many years now the emphasis has been on child development, promoting an understanding of all the needs of young children. This work is increasingly seen as having value for boys as well as girls. Pupils acquire the knowledge, skills and competencies to promote physical, mental and emotional growth. Through this work they are brought to a greater awareness of their own position in the growth cycle. They can begin to appreciate the range of normality and variation which exists at each stage, although the basic needs remain the same. This work enables pupils to study the relationships between parents and young children, between parents and adolescents, between the sexes in adult relationships and between adults and their parents. Concepts of gender roles and work roles are explored by encouraging pupils to study their own and others expectations.

Within the concept of growth and development is the further concept of learning as a continuous process beyond school. Through the study of young children adolescents begin to appreciate how learning can be promoted and encouraged, and child development courses are said, in fact, to provide good motivation for adolescent learning. The need for knowledge has relevance, is appreciated and makes a considerable contribution to self-development; the idea that learning can be a continuous, pleasurable experience might well enhance the future mental health of our pupils in a post-industrial society. One of the joint aims of home economics and health education is to enable pupils to attain a high level of autonomy and yet to care for and respect both themselves and others. Because of the task-orientated nature of home economics, and the fact that progressively more difficult tasks are undertaken through the years from eleven to eighteen, accompanied by the acceptance of increased levels of responsibility, pupils are given many opportunities to become aware of their own capabilities which are developed in relation to planning, completing and assessing their work. They become increasingly more self-confident and self-reliant, are more aware of their level of competency in a wide range of skills and develop the confidence to rely upon their own judgements. In terms of self-knowledge and its contribution to a secure self-image, home economics makes a positive contribution and offers many opportunities for pupils to experience success.

Classroom organization can provide a range of groups which promotes co-operation and sharing and encourages pupils to be supportive of each other. Whatever the ethnic, social or cultural mix within the classroom, home economics can be used to illustrate the diversities and similarities which exist in different groups, thus widening the pupils' understanding of life styles, family bondings and cultural influences which are different from their own. They can be encouraged to develop an open-minded curiosity, receptivity, and sympathy towards the differences between members of different groups in society.

Within the context of home economics, experiments in creative self-expression can take place. Clothing, self-adornment and the home environment continue to be the only areas where creativity is possible for many in our society, but these are also the areas where advertising pressure and fashion tend to dictate. Home economics should enable pupils to appreciate these pressures and leave them more free to create a home environment reflecting their own personalities, interests and values and chosen life style.

Conclusion

The emphasis throughout this chapter has been on attitudes, concepts, competencies and skills which can be acquired through home economics, particularly those which contribute to or coincide with aspects of health education. It has not dealt at length with content, but it should be clear that home economics and child development and the family courses, in addition to areas previously described, make a contribution to the pupils' medical knowledge and the responsible use and criticism of both the medical and social services, to the pupils' sex education and to their knowledge of themselves and others. From its inception home economics has been recognized as making a contribution to health education. The concepts of health and of home economics have expanded and altered since the beginning of the century, but the two still continue to be closely interwoven and are areas of study pertinent to both boys and girls.

I wish to express my gratitude to colleagues in the home economics and health education teams of the Inner London Education Authority with whom I have enjoyed a continuing debate, which has contributed in no small measure to the ideas expressed in this chapter. The views expressed here are those of the author and not necessarily those of the employing authority.

Summary

This chapter indicates how home economics and health education often subscribe to similar educational aims. It outlines those concepts, skills and attitudes which are likely to be fostered in home economics and which could also make a contribution to the wider health education of the pupils. Very little work has so far been undertaken which looks at these two subject areas in terms of concept formation.

References

Arnold, J. (1977) Lecture delivered at an ILEA health education residential course.

Paolucci, Professor (1976) Lecture delivered at the Conference of the International Federation of Home Economists, Canada, 1976.

CHAPTER 8

PHYSICAL EDUCATION AND HEALTH EDUCATION

John Wright for the Physical Education Association's Study Group on Health and Recreation

The Physical Education Association is mindful of the diversity and quality of the work already being done in schools by physical education teachers, and of the considerable and patient skill-building which forms a large part of their programmes. These guidelines are in no sense put forward to replace already valuable work, but rather to augment it and to underpin the planning and implementation of programmes providing central focuses for parts of some lessons and for the entirety of others. Some of the suggested material will be likely to be a recurring feature in lessons with different age-groups, for example those concerned with safety understanding and habits and with mechanically sound patterns of body use; others will be brought into central focus only at certain stages in the programme, for example certain aspects of the effects of exercise on the body would perhaps only be appropriate with older age-groups.

The guidelines have been formulated under headings closely related to the areas covered in the Schools Council Health Education Project *Think Well*. Thus the Physical Education Association's recommendations will be in accord with work already undertaken or being carried out by the Schools Council and the Health Education Council.

Self-Awareness – Awareness of Others

The nature of much of the routine of physical education, for example changing and showering, as well as of the work undertaken is such that young people are made more 'bodily aware' than in other subjects; this is particularly so in subjects like gymnastics and dance where concentration is focused upon muscular sensations in particular body areas in order to produce precise action responses and body forms. At appropriate times teachers can help pupils to appreciate the normality of differences in size, shape, growth rates and various bodily capacities, and this may involve discussion with individuals as well as groups. The use of a pupil demonstration in a gymnastics lesson to make a particular teaching point may sometimes provide an opportunity to highlight the relationship of certain individual differences to the effective performance of certain movements. Pupils should have ample opportunity to appraise their physical capacities, and the physical education programme should provide scope for them to test themselves, especially in non-competitive or self-competitive situations.

Tangible recognition and recording of skill attainments, such as are frequently done in the swimming and gymnastics programmes, can also be a means through which young people develop their body and self-images. In all these respects physical education teachers have a clear responsibility for the development of all pupils they teach; those whose physical and/or skill development is in any way inhibited or retarded are in particular need of the teacher's time, help and encouragement.

Mixed work

Some parts of the physical education programme in the lower school can sensibly be undertaken as mixed-sex work and can be used to foster sensitivity, awareness and respect for differences between the sexes. Depending upon a school's approach to sex education in the context of its total health education programme, it may be fitting for physical education teachers to discuss with older pupils the probable effects upon their performance in various physical activities of the changes in height, weight, strength : weight ratios and co-ordination which attend puberty. Ways in which programme content is adjusted in secondary schools to attempt to cater for developing manhood and womanhood could sensibly be discussed at this stage. The beginning of menstruation with older girls is likely to be a matter which involves women physical education teachers perhaps more obviously than other teachers; they may well be the most appropriate members of staff to provide the necessary education to both individuals and to groups of girls. At a suitable time boys, too, should be helped to understand the facts of menstruation and the more common effects on behaviour which it can cause.

Body Care

The reasons why high standards of cleanliness are insisted upon in working spaces, in physical education kit and in the body need to be explained to pupils; the special problems associated with cleanliness of feet, hair, nails and teeth should be discussed and the effects upon the feet of ill-fitting and poorly designed footwear should be highlighted. Thorough drying of the body after showers and swimming should be insisted upon and the reasons for this explained and discussed. Regular showering is only likely to become a pleasurable habit where lessons demand a high physical work rate from each pupil; insistence on showering when body temperatures have scarcely been raised is likely to be counterproductive. Appropriate understanding of the function of the skin during and after exercise would need to be developed in this context.

It is important, too, that pupils are helped to recognize that the body's functioning and general well-being benefits from the regular and moderate eating of salads and fresh fruits, and from the avoidance of excessive amounts of sugary and starchy foods. The benefits to be gained by avoiding such obvious internal pollutants as tobacco smoke need to be explained and discussed; similarly the importance of full breathing of clean, fresh air can be highlighted. The timing of such information exchange and discussion is a matter for sensible discrimination by teachers.

Safety

Pupils' safety awareness, understanding, attitudes and skills are likely to be fostered if the safety rules in the various aspects of the physical education programme are fully explained and justified. Pupils can themselves be encouraged to draw up appropriate codes of rules for particular working spaces and activities after suitable discussion. Safety in the swimming pool can be a starting point for developing awareness and understanding of the wider issues of open-water safety; indeed the whole wide area of safety out of doors can be opened up for discussion and instruction, particularly when pupils are taken camping and on field trips. Such discussion/instruction should pay due regard to regulations/guidelines concerning choices of clothing and equipment for different outdoor activities.

The whole area of accident prevention and the knowledge and skill needed to deal with emergencies can be taken to greater depth in secondary programmes. Blocks of work dealing with first aid and with life-saving techniques in swimming should be included (schools in coastal areas may well include lifeguard work for pupils with the requisite swimming skills). All pupils should master and understand expired air resuscitation techniques and opportunities should be given from time to time for recapitulation practice of those techniques. The particular safety issue of athletics and the various aspects of the outdoor pursuits should receive thorough treatment, both in terms of developing pupils' understanding and in making an impact on safety skills and habits. All pupils should be helped to acquire a healthy respect for the elements and a clear appreciation of the limitations of the human body in outdoor situations.

Body Use

Mechanically sound patterns of body use in standing, sitting and walking and in various lifting, carrying, pulling and pushing activities need to be taught to pupils and made a routine part of all physical education lessons, especially where the handling of all equipment and apparatus is concerned. Pupils should be taught, in appropriately simplified ways, why particular patterns of body use are sound and others are unsound, and this should be related to all skilled action learning in the programme. Well-poised standing, sitting and walking need to be patiently encouraged in every physical education lesson. A balanced, easy carriage in which pressure on joint surfaces is lessened rather than increased should be aimed for and pupils should be encouraged to identify in themselves areas of unnecessary and inappropriate muscular tension. All this should be a persistent feature of the physical education programme and pupils should be helped to understand the vulnerability to accidental injury of the lower back area if subjected to mechanically unsound use.

Effects of Body Activity on Key Elements of Physical Fitness

Physical education can make a valuable contribution in increasing pupils' awareness and understanding of the effects upon the body of different types of exercise and activity. It can also encourage involvement in balanced exercise habits, for example exercise with a predominantly muscular effect and that which has a chiefly cardio-respiratory effect.

Flexibility

The importance of maintaining an appropriately full range of movement at all joint complexes should be stressed, and pupils should be taught and should regularly engage in movement patterns which maintain and/or increase flexibility. They should be awakened to the possible excessive demands on flexibility made by certain activities, for example competitive swimming land conditioning, competitive gymnastics and aspects of certain forms of dancing. Pupils should be helped to recognize and understand the potential hazards in some of the methods currently used to achieve extreme flexibility, and simultaneously should be taught sound principles for building flexibility. In this work, as with other aspects of the physical education programme, they should be helped to appreciate the significance of individual differences in bodily make-up and to recognize that what is a normal range of movement for one person may be abnormal for another.

Strength

The significance of balanced strength to the pupils' all-round physical fitness needs to be stressed and they should be helped to understand which activities lead to strength in particular body areas. Teachers should also stress the importance of strength in critical body areas, such as low back and hip extensor strength and abdominal strength. Pupils should regularly engage in activities which make balanced demands upon their strength, and in this context upper-body strength, both flexor and extensor, should feature.

Endurance

The contrast between activities which make little and those which make great demand on the circulatory and respiratory systems needs to be highlighted, and pupils can learn to count their own and each other's pulse rates and breathing rates in various 'before and after' activity situations. The importance to total health of engaging in activities which make considerable demands on the heart, lungs and related mechanisms should be stressed, and short spells of discussion on the many features of modern life which make this difficult for many adults and some children to achieve should be encouraged. The pupils should be asked to suggest ways in which adults and children might adjust their habits to enable them to develop the efficiency of their heart and lungs. The school physical education programme needs to make regular and appropriate demands on pupils' circulo-respiratory capacities; for instance jogging and running on or off the school site could well be a regular feature of at least one term for each of the senior two years, but the emphasis should be on enjoyable participation for all rather than on the traditional cross-country racing pattern which tends only to be appropriate to a minority of pupils.

Relaxation

After bouts of intensive physical exertion the opportunity should be taken to let pupils experience short spells of total relaxation, and they should be taught to identify the appropriate muscular sensation in all areas of the body. At a suitable stage they could well be encouraged to discuss the value to bodily and mental well-being of relaxation, rest and sleep. They should also be helped to understand the different kinds of demands made upon the body and mind during a normal twenty-four hour cycle, and how a suitable balance of such demands might best be achieved. In this context the place and significance of physical education in the school week should be discussed and could well lead to a discussion of the enjoyment and benefit to be gained from both children and adults using part of their leisure time in suitable physical activities. The range and rationale of school physical education club activities should be such as to encourage maximum participation.

Where desirable, links with local sporting clubs should be fostered but great care should be exercised with the nine–thirteen age-range where youngsters with marked natural aptitudes can easily be drawn into club situations which make excessive and unbalanced demands upon their time and physical resources, thereby precluding a more catholic development of their leisure time activities.

Timing of physical fitness programmes

Although the attention and experiences of pupils will be suitably directed to ways of promoting flexibility, strength, endurance and relaxation as the need arises in relation to particular activities in the physical education programme, it is also necessary for particular blocks of work to be tackled which 'home in' on physical fitness, physique and figure control per se.

Such work is best undertaken when it has greatest relevance from the pupils' point of view. Thus boys in the fourteen-plus age-range not uncommonly become interested in the development of their physiques, and a block of work on physical fitness may well be apposite. During the course of such work they should develop a clear understanding of the overload principle and its application to physical fitness work, and should be educated to a stage where they can devise their own individual fitness programmes and keep their own record cards of attainments in, for example, circuit training. Fitness programmes like the Canadian Air Force BX systems could well form a useful basis for profitable discussion on the continued application of fitness knowledge in post-school years. Cross-country running and jogging has much to commend it as a winter activity, but distance and pace need careful adjustment to cater for all pupils. 'Minimum time' fitness routines which are also economical on space and equipment and could be suitable for home use should be practised in various forms.

The interest of girls of a similar age-group in figure and weight control can profitably be exploited and a variety of 'keep fit' activities should form the basis for developing understanding of the different functions of movement in relation to weight and figure control and to overall bodily efficiency. If properly organized and taught, with suitable music, such 'keep fit' programmes can be exhilarating and popular. At appropriate stages in the programme crucial information needs to be given concerning sensible eating habits. Schools with immigrant children should consider such basic nutrition guidance to be especially important.

Personal Responsibility Throughout Life

During the latter years of the secondary school it is strongly recommended that some discussion time should be included in physical education programmes to focus attention on the responsibilities which individuals should be prepared to accept for their own health once they have left school. The various aspects of the school programme should be referred to in terms of the understanding, attitudes and habits it was designed to equip pupils with, and the crucial need for life-long application of personal responsibility should be stressed. During such discussion periods some of the more common health-destructive factors of modern society might well be aired, such as, for example, smoking, alcohol, excessive and unbalanced eating habits (or insufficient eating with some young women) and lack of physical activity. The possibility of providing a school leavers' leaflet, which would succinctly summarize crucial issues of health responsibility and be made available along with the list of local sports and recreation groups, might well be investigated, and could provide a useful form of co-ordination with other subject areas in the school.

Teachers' Example

There is an important sense in which a physical education teacher's whole manner of approach to every aspect of every lesson can 'infect' pupils with constructive attitudes to their bodies and to participation in physical activity. The teacher's enthusiasm for his subject and, even more important, for the achievement and success of every pupil is clearly important here. So too is his example of caring concern for all individuals, regardless of their levels of competence in physical education. The teacher's personal example in grooming, poise, continuing delight in skilled movement and in maintaining a high level of personal fitness is also significant. By such consistency of example some of the more important attitudes to the body and to physical activity are likely to be 'caught' by some pupils.

The National Interest

The foregoing suggestions and recommendations reflect the concern of the Physical Education Association that physical education teachers should recognize and find increasingly effective ways of implementing their unique contribution to school health education programmes. This is held to be in the national interest at a time of economic constraint and when the limitations of high technology, medicine and a mechanistic approach to health are beginning to be recognized.

Summary

The chapter illustrates how the work of physical education teachers contributes to the aims of programmes of health education. It discusses the effect of skills, body care and safety, and adds self-awareness and awareness of others as elements of personal responsibility which can be developed in physical education.

CHAPTER 9

THE CONTRIBUTION OF ENGLISH TO HEALTH EDUCATION

Peter Farley

Introduction

This chapter offers a brief survey of the main concerns of current teaching in English and shows how these relate to health education. At the outset, however, is the problem of knowing what is meant by 'English'. The principal aim here is to consider English as a subject in the school curriculum, but there is a second and wider meaning which we should keep in mind. Language and learning are inextricably related, to the extent that educational success is often primarily a matter of linguistic success. In England, at any rate, the English language will be the vehicle for virtually all health education. Consideration of language for learning is not confined to that slot on the timetable generally called English. In this sense, English, like health education, crosses conventional curriculum boundaries with its concern for process and language/learning situations. There is a similar cross-curricular concern in that neither English nor health education have easily demarcated content boundaries. Indeed both could be described in the same way as John Dixon (1975) describes English: 'a quicksilver among metals – mobile, living and elusive'.

Models in English

In his book *Growth Through English*, Dixon suggests that historically there are three models of English: skills, the cultural heritage and personal growth. The skills model was ideally suited to the task of preparing a literate population, concentrating as it did on selected elements in the process of using language, such as correct spellings, vocabulary and punctuation habits. Its major drawback was that it confused, for example, 'menus' with 'meals', by leaving out vast areas of language use. The cultural heritage model offered a link between language and life by means of the study of literature. Beginning with Matthew Arnold's conception of literature as a 'criticism of life', this model derives much of its energy from the influence of the late F. R. Leavis. There is no doubt that this has charged English with much moral force and the need to relate English studies to life. Indeed 'criticism of life' has led to the development of social concerns on the part of English teachers by way of general cultural criticism. The third model, personal growth, implies a shift of emphasis towards the learner and his needs and experiences. These three models are not, of course, mutually exclusive and together they provide the framework on which the fabric of English in a particular school is stretched. Indeed the idea of personal growth may be best seen as informing current work generally, giving cohesion to the other two models rather than being distinct from them.

The concern with personal growth is, of course, shared by health education in schools, and it is not the only one with a direct bearing on English. If we compare a number of shared concerns we shall see that there is indeed a close match. Health education is concerned with fostering and developing an understanding of growth and development, with the idea of health as the ability to function actively in the world, with preparation for parenthood, with personal relationships and with the exploration and understanding of the feelings, attitudes and values of oneself and others. English is concerned with the acquisition of personal language and the development of language behaviour and skills without which it becomes impossible to function positively and with personal control in the world. Language cannot operate meaningfully in isolation and the very use and existence of language implies relationships of various sorts. Through language, and especially through the experience of literature, we are able to understand ourselves more fully and to extend that understanding in order to enter into the lives of others.

It will not be possible to pursue each of these connections in isolation, nor is it necessary. Instead I propose to concentrate on the broad areas of English already outlined; skills and the more general cultural/social concerns. As I have suggested, personal growth is seen to inform these for the most part. Normally our concern would be with the pupil's own growth and development in language competence, but there is no reason why that process itself should not be the subject of work in English as well as an aim. With preparation for parenthood in mind, some consideration of how people, especially young children, come to acquire language would be a valuable part of exploring language in English. After all it is the one school subject in which by far the greater part of learning occurs before school is even reached.

Skills

In considering skills in English, we should see that we are dealing with language skills generally. The basic skills are:

1 Adjusting intelligently to the great variety of communication situations one finds oneself in, each of which requires some different approach, there being no such thing as a correct English suitable for all occasions (and age-groups).
2 Working out meaning for utterances in such situations, whether one is the author or the audience of the utterance. This involves:
   a   understanding of content or subject matter,
   b   application of thought processes to it.
3 Generating wording to express that meaning
   a   with vocabulary indicating the content,
   b   and vocabulary and syntax indicating the thought processes.
4 Processing the wording in the complex acts of listening, speaking, reading and writing (CCAE, 1978).

From the perspective of skills, English can make a contribution to health education in three ways. The first is explicit: the teacher of English sets out to make a deliberate contribution to the health education of his or her pupils, whether in 'normal' lessons or as part of a team effort in curriculum time set aside for the purpose. The second contribution is implicit in that the normal concerns of English inevitably lead to the sharing of common ground with health, social and personal education. The third contribution is similarly implicit in that it relates to the fact that English is the language for learning, regardless of the subject, and is therefore not the monopoly of the English specialist. Much of the attention to language across the curriculum that followed in the wake of the Bullock Report (DES, 1975) is relevant here in that in this special sense all teachers are in some way teachers of English. The basic skills, then, inform all aspects of language in use, and we miss the point if we start from a conception of skills which places parts of the process in separate compartments. Nevertheless it will simplify matters considerably to proceed as if reading, listening and talking, and writing *can* be separated out.

Reading, Speaking and Writing

Reading is not simply a matter of decoding a text. Rather, the reader engages in critical and creative thinking in order to relate what he reads to what he already knows. Indeed the response to a text involves intellectual and affective processes, and it was once well said that we do not so much read a book as a book reads us. The development of reading brings a development in personal confidence, an increase in control over language and a decrease in the control of other people's language over us as we recognize how they operate. The potential gains for our self-knowledge and knowledge of others are obvious. This alone relates to health education by way of personal development, but within the context of the English teacher developing reading there are more pragmatic considerations for health education. There is no reason why, for example, health-related material should not be used when considering the language of advertising. Similarly, the development of skills in finding out information and assessing its value and effect can be health-related.

There seems to be general agreement that spoken language is the most neglected of English skills. This is ironic in that language is primarily a matter of speech and the most representative of all ways of using language is the situation in which two or three people talk to each other face to face. Language implies relationships, and spoken language implies the most immediate ones. The capacity to talk well in a variety of situations, to respond sensitively to other people and to understand what is really being said is necessary for social health, to make successful relationships and to learning as a whole. English has much to contribute to health education in this area, both within its own subject and in drama, and to the curriculum in general. It is difficult to organize exploratory talk and to provide experience of a variety of talk from the formal to the informal, but it is the case that group work provides the means of achieving a more effective situation for active language than the class discussion. Group work poses difficult questions of classroom management, teacher direction and intervention and this is not the place to resolve them. Indeed the whole question of talk in the classroom raises issues well beyond the reach of this chapter and some of the suggested further reading at the end may help to resolve them. Nevertheless the contribution of the English teacher can be a crucial one for health education. I am not only thinking now of a classroom contribution, but also that he or she could well act as a kind of consultant, whether for the staff as a whole or in the setting of a health education team.

With writing we again come up against the question of language use across the curriculum. By far the greatest number of writing tasks in schools (some estimates indicate 90%) relate to the recall of information and the representational use of language. A further problem is that of audience in that by and large the only person addressed in school writing is the teacher in her role as examiner. One hopes that the English teacher can provide a wider audience, both by carrying out his or her own role of sympathetic adult with concerns which are wider than those of simply examining for accuracy, and by fostering fellow pupils as a trusted audience. Beyond that, the values inherent in writing in English are ones which contribute to health education. Creative writing is much abused, but at its best is not about self-indulgence. Quite the reverse, in fact, since it represents the struggle for personal control and meaning. Further than that, I suggest that the values of personal space and privacy in writing have a part to play beyond the confines of the English lesson. The more personal modes of writing offer the means to relate knowledge to experience, attitudes, feelings and values – a central concern of the health education process.

Literature is the ground of the more social and cultural concerns of English. The range of possible connections with health education is vast and, of course, not unrelated to the way English teachers already make use of literature in their work. There are a number of possible starting points and these would include developing a health theme in a course of reading or simply being more alert to the health-related aspects of current work. I am not of course suggesting going to extremes about this; 'Keats as consumptive' or 'Coleridge as opium addict' would miss the point. Nevertheless, to fully explore those particular writers would inevitably lead to health issues without causing undue strain. Similarly the media, television and cinema in particular, which are legitimate concerns of the English teacher, have their part to play. But in the end the wider aspects of English in terms of content cannot be divorced from the value they have for the individual pupil. Personal experience is extended and access given to that of others from all ages and places in answer to the question 'What does it mean to be alive?'

Conclusion

The contribution of English to health education, then, can be viewed in a number of different ways. As a subject in schools it shares common concerns with health education. The normal range of English work complements health education and contributes to it in a number of respects. Equally the health education perspective can serve to sharpen and refine work in English. Last, but by no means least, English in the wider sense can offer support to health education across the curriculum, in terms of method and in terms of the relationship between language and learning. 'Language', according to William von Humboldt, 'intervenes between man and nature acting upon him internally and externally.' Health education attempts to do precisely that.

Summary

As a subject in schools English shares common concerns with health education, and the normal range of English work complements health education and contributes to it in a number of respects, particularly in the area of personal growth.

The health education perspective can serve to sharpen and refine work in English. English in the widest sense can offer support to health education in terms of methods and the relationship between language and learning.

References

Canberra College of Advanced Education (1978) *Material on Language.*

Department of Education and Science (1975) *A Language for Life* (The Bullock Report). London, HMSO.

Dixon, J. (1975) *Growth Through English: Set in the perspective of the Seventies.* Oxford, Oxford University Press.

Further Reading

Barnes, D., Britton, J. and Rosen, H. (1971) *Language, the Learner and the School.* Harmondsworth, Penguin.

Doughty, P., Pearce, J. and Thornton, G. (1972) *Exploring Language.* Schools Council Programme in Linguistics and English Teaching. London, Edward Arnold.

Doughty, P., Pearce, J. and Thornton, G. (1972) *Language in Use.* Schools Council Programme in Linguistics and English Teaching. London, Edward Arnold.

Postman, N. and Weingartner, C. (1971) *Teaching as a Subversive Activity.* Harmondsworth, Penguin.

CHAPTER 10

HEALTH EDUCATION THROUGH RELIGIOUS EDUCATION

Ian Birnie

As a preparation for writing this chapter I have read through the bulletins circulated by the Health Education Council during the last five years and have examined outline schemes and resource materials produced for teachers and pupils. It is interesting to note that while moral education receives fairly regular attention, religious education features almost not at all. One explanation for this might be the interest of the Schools Council in moral education. The same period has seen the publication of the Startline moral education materials for the middle school age-range (Schools Council, 1978), the Lifeline materials for older pupils having been issued some time before (McPhail, 1972).

However, the Schools Council has also recently published materials to support religious education in the primary and secondary schools, some parts of which might have been thought helpful by those concerned for health education. Also noticeable is the manner in which the frontiers of health education have stretched to encompass education in personal relationships (EPR), social education, moral education and some elements of environmental and community studies. A clear view has evidently developed which claims that health education is concerned with more than a transfer of information about such matters as smoking and drinking, the use of drugs, unwanted pregnancies and sexually transmitted diseases. If I have understood it correctly, those directly concerned with advancing the aims of health education recognize that if anything is to be achieved, teaching strategies will have to pay most serious attention to the individual pupil's assessment of how he is growing and developing as a person. Through introducing family life, boy-girl relationships, respect for other people, including those of a different race, respect for the environment, and community service into formal health education schemes, we observe a lassoing of human experience in order to provide the foundations of an approach to learning in this area. There can be little doubt that as pupils begin to explore and discuss in these territories, they will raise and encounter some of the most complex and controversial questions faced by people today. I refer to questions of value, meaning and purpose, sometimes termed 'ultimate questions', to which there are no answers in any absolute sense. It will not be misunderstood when I say that health education is not competent to answer such questions.

It is therefore both understandable and quite proper that a sound contribution to health education should be sought from the major human disciplines. Such contributions, if they are forthcoming, will give a depth to health education which will protect it from any accusation that it is, on the one hand, shallow when grappling with serious issues, and on the other, indoctrinatory in failing to acknowledge the controversiality of its subject matter. As a religious educator I welcome the direction which health education has taken and feel that this can only be helpful in ensuring fruitful links between these two areas. In continuing now to see how this relationship might prosper, perhaps we should also keep in mind some of the potential pitfalls hinted at above.

Education in Religion and Health

Let us consider the use of the word 'education' in association with religion and health. We do not normally see the terms english education, history education, science education, mathematics education used in schools, but have become accustomed to religious education, physical education, social and moral education, education in personal relationships and the like. The use of the word 'education' is in these cases quite significant, for it could be said that each of the afore-mentioned curriculum areas seeks to influence the personal development of the pupil in some way. The word 'education', as we know, derives from the Latin verb *educare*, meaning to lead out or to fulfil. For example, the usage of the verb could suggest the leading of an army out of a barracks to seek its destiny as a fighting force. An army does not fulfil its purpose by being confined to barracks! The context of the word 'education' is therefore that of helping someone or something to fulfil its true purpose. Such a view would probably be widely accepted in Western society, notwithstanding some disagreement concerning the 'purpose' of human existence.

At the heart of this view of education there is an assumption about the nature of man, and that is that the development, or future, of man, is not predetermined in an evolutionary manner in the biological sense, but is on the contrary an open-ended historic process. Teachers concerned with personal guidance and religious education will hardly need reminding that the education of a person takes place to a lesser extent in school and to a much greater extent in a world which is being transformed by social and technological revolutions. In such a world, events explode in the everyday life of people deeply influencing their attitudes, values and aspirations. Do we not have daily evidence of this in our classrooms? These movements in history have thrown up special problems for the teacher of religious education as they have for the great world faiths and their adherents. The recent history of the Christian denominations in our own culture illustrates the problem of the theologians struggling to restate the faith in the face of rapid change. In such times as these it becomes part of the general experience of all of us that we live in a runaway world. Feelings of helplessness in the face of change and of the meaninglessness at the centre of life, are not only intellectually known but emotionally grasped.

Those of us who risk attaching the word 'education' to our specialism are caught up in the history and the experience of our pupils. I would hope that the first co-operative act between health education and religious education would be an agreement on the part of the teachers that education is about equipping people for discovering what it means to be human, and how to live hopefully and humanly in a world which is largely denying human distinctiveness and human values. This understanding will certainly be decisive in determining how we approach the study of religion in school.

The Distinctive Concerns of Religious Education

In order to discuss the contribution which religious education might make to health education it is necessary to identify, for the benefit of those who do not have a specialism in the subject, just what are its key concerns. A number of different approaches to the study of religion could be proposed and justified on educational grounds as being worthy of the attention of pupils growing up in a world where manifestly religion is of great importance to the majority of men. But not all of these approaches would represent the distinctive concerns of the religious education teacher, for example the impact of a religion on the artistic expression of a culture, on its history, social life, literature, ethics, all these and more. But how curious it would be if, say, in the case of European culture, teachers of art, music, drama, literature, history, social studies and science were to avoid any mention of the Judeo-Christian heritage which so strongly influences our view of man and society. Any of these areas might feature in a religious education programme but they would not be central to it. If, however, pupils were involved in a study of certain important contemporary political problems, they might discover that some of the most intransigent of these have a religious source, for instance the problem of Arab and Jew in the Middle East, Christian and Muslim in central Africa, Marxist and Christian in eastern Europe, Hindu and Muslim in India and Pakistan.

If such problems are to be appreciated and some understanding inculcated as to why people take up the positions they do, then the religious dimension of individual and communal life will require careful study. This is an area where religious education has an important contribution to make to the whole education of the pupil. It is not necessarily the area which offers the best potential for links with health education but, as we shall see later, attempts to educate for multicultural or multiracial understanding will not get far without some rigorous study of this kind. Furthermore the consequences of taking up a faith position in life, another vital concern for exploration in religious education, will be important when health education turns to examine some of the moral dilemmas facing contemporary society.

Reference to a poster released by the Scottish Health Education Council entitled 'Children Learn What They Live', will most clearly indicate the central concerns of religious education. The poster presents eleven points about child development, each prefaced by the word 'if', thus:

If a child lives with criticism, she learns to condemn,
If a child lives with hostility, he learns to fight,
If a child lives with ridicule, she learns to be shy.

Towards the end of the list we read,

If a child lives with security, she learns to have faith,
If a child lives with acceptance and friendship, he or she learns to find love in the world.

This poster reminds us once again that in the planning of our teaching programmes and in the day-to-day relationships we have with children, it is important to have engaged in some deep personal thought about humanness and human fulfilment. All teachers/educators are inevitably brought face to face with questions about the meaning of human experience, whatever their subject specialism. The use of the words 'faith' and 'love' on the poster does pose a number of questions. Is there a purpose to life, if so what? Is there a meaning to be discerned at the heart of existence? Is there, as the poster suggests, something to find?

The Central Advisory Council for Education published in 1959 what came to be known as the Crowther Report (CACE, 1959). Although the report was concerned with post-compulsory education rather than religious education, we read in it the following:

> The teenagers with whom we are concerned need, perhaps above all else, to find a faith to live by. They will not find precisely the same faith and some will not find any. Education can and should play some part in the search. It can assure them that there is something to search for and it can show them where to look and what other men have found.

In 1963 the same body published the Newsom Report, *Half Our Future* (CACE, 1963), in which we read:

> Most boys and girls want to be what they call 'being good' and they want to know what this really implies in the personal situations which confront them. This is difficult enough but it is not sufficient. They want also to know what kind of animal a man is and whether ultimately each one of us matters and if so why and to whom.

I do not imagine that teachers of health education, especially those involved in education for personal relationships, would want to disassociate themselves from these statements. Similarly, teachers of religious education find such views very supportive. It should not be necessary to have to labour the point that religion is very much tied up with our understanding of what it means to be human and what interpretation we place on human experience. Here we touch on the central distinctive contribution of the subject, namely that of introducing the religious experience of mankind to persons who are becoming increasingly sensitive to the 'ultimate' on the boundaries of life.

What can we really know about ourselves and the world? Why is there a world supporting human life? Where does man come from and where does he go? Why is the world as it is? What meaning can be discovered at the heart of reality? What ought we to do? Why do we act as we do? Why and to whom are we finally responsible? What deserves our forthright contempt, and what our love? What is the meaning of suffering? What is the point of loyalty, friendship? What really matters for men? What can we hope for? Why are we here? What is life all about? How can I face death? What is there left for man after death? Does the fact of death render all talk of meaning and purpose meaningless? What will give us courage for life? What will give us courage for death?

Such questions, listed here largely as Kant formulated them, are vital in the process of developing self-understanding. They lie also at the heart of any mature programme of religious education for religions are concerned with what is true in human experience. Religious education aims to assist the maturing person in his quest for meaning and purpose. It can 'show that person where to look and what men have found'. An early discovery in this search will be that there is not 'the truth' in any universal or absolute sense. Different world religions and secular faiths, such as humanism, make opposing claims. They cannot all be right and they may all be wrong! The pupil will need to understand this if he is to begin to grasp what it might mean to take up a faith position in life.

When in 1970 the Church of England published a major report on religious education (SPCK, 1970), it echoed the Crowther Report when constructing an aim for the subject:

> The aim of religious education should be to explore the place and significance of religion in human life and so make a distinctive contribution to each pupil's search for faith by which to live. . . . The teacher is thus seeking rather to initiate his pupils into knowledge which he encourages them to explore and appreciate, than into a system of belief which he requires them to accept. . . . If the teacher is to press for any conversion, it is conversion from a shallow and unreflective attitude to life. If he is to press for commitment, it is commitment to the religious quest, to that search for meaning, purpose and value which is open to all men.

Health Education Through Religious Education

There is a lengthy tradition in religious education of devising schemes of work which contain just those themes which are now declared appropriate for health education. I refer to such themes as the concept of self, family life, caring relationships, personal responsibility and so on. In his book, *Teenage Religion* (Loukes, 1961), Harold Loukes, Reader in Education at Oxford University, recorded in transcriptions of conversations the issues which young people were most anxious to see tackled in religious education lessons. He went on to suggest a syllabus based on problems which were both intellectually and emotionally grasped by young people, for example friendship, sex and marriage, snobbery, money, work, leisure, prayer, suffering, death. The best teachers of the subject were already working in this way and a further stimulus to others has been given over the years by the publication of a number of new agreed syllabuses by such local education authorities as Lancashire, Inner London, Hampshire and Birmingham. In these syllabuses health education teachers will be gratified to see suggested such topics as population and family planning, drugs, racial discrimination, housing conditions, food, famine and world health, conservation, medicine and medical ethics. These and other topics are commonplace in religious education and through the consideration of them the teacher will hope to raise some of the fundamental human concerns we outlined earlier.

Teachers planning health education programmes should therefore take steps to familiarize themselves with the work of religious education in their own school for here they might find their strongest ally. There is a wealth of resource material in religious education and a long experience of dealing with highly controversial areas of human experience, both of which will be useful to teachers of health education. Religion, as we have said, is by its very nature concerned with 'hot topics', and teachers in both areas who are concerned to work with great sensitivity could, through close co-operation, strengthen the impact of the school strategies for health.

Work of this nature inevitably involves the teacher in discussion of ethical matters. The question, 'What ought I to do?' is central to many discussions. It is here that religious education has another important and distinctive contribution to make by focusing the attention of pupils on the ground of their decision-making. What dominant sentiment, what transforming principle concerning the nature of our humanity will be embraced by the student? We recall once again that phrase from the Crowther Report, '. . . finding a faith by which to live'. This can be a most difficult area within health education for the teacher may unwittingly pass on his own values as though they represent the agreed positions of the community. It is no more easy for the teacher of religious education who has to be careful to avoid suggesting that a particular religious view of an ethical problem is 'right', when there may be observable disagreement within the denomination. The debate in the Christian churches about contraception and abortion might serve as a good example here.

It is probably true to say that in the past religious education was expected to make the sole explicit contribution to the moral education programme of the school. Indeed, some headteachers of both primary and secondary schools have thought of religious education as moral education, which clearly it is not. Such an approach seems to suggest, on the one hand, that in order to be moral one has in some sense to be religious, and on the other, that a rejection of religion will encourage an immature approach to moral responsibility. It is of course true that one consequence of living with a religious faith will be an ethical outcome in daily life and this should be made clear in religious education teaching. However there are those who, acting on a different basis, will quite properly claim to be living a moral life.

Perhaps these brief remarks are sufficient to stress the need for careful thought and co-operation on the part of any teachers who find themselves naturally engaging in a particular kind of conversation with pupils. However, I am not suggesting that this area is so complex that teachers are better leaving it alone. It was stated earlier, when discussing the nature of education, that the process is directly related to, and thrives on, lively, controversial human experience. This is what makes it exciting to be a teacher privileged to be in close relationship with the growing mind of the young person. If teachers are aware of the danger of presenting controversial issues as though they were not controversial, and the school is open about its aims in teaching for personal growth, then accusations of indoctrination will be easily refuted. In such teaching programmes, as the Humanities Curriculum Project (Schools Council, 1970) demonstrated so well, far from not encountering clear views at all, pupils will meet them boldly presented in the material resources prepared to support work in the classroom. The whole question of the moral education task of the school as a whole could be strongly raised as a consequence of a lively relationship between religious education and health education. This discussion would be further supported by recourse to the handbooks for teachers produced by the two Schools Council Moral Education Projects and to the pupil materials of the Startline and Lifeline series.

It will be clear to the reader that I do see great profit in a close relationship between the teaching of health and religious education in schools. I am sure that health education is the weaker if it is not supported by the distinctive contribution of religious education, and it is inconceivable that teachers of the latter would choose to ignore the groundwork in developing self-understanding initiated in health education. This leads me to suggest that some formal link in teaching programmes would be most worthwhile. The term 'integrated course' has become commonplace in schools, sadly it is frequently used to describe doubtful liaisons between subjects not always happy to be blocked together for timetable convenience. A serious criticism of such courses is that they are sometimes constructed in relation to inadequate themes or topics, with the result that a given subject has to produce some part of its 'body of knowledge' which can be related, however artificially, to the object of the course. Here there is no integration of the central concerns of a discipline, only a curious demonstration of parallel studies. From what we have said about health and religious education it is clear that both focus on human beings, their nature and their development in such a way as to throw up overarching themes which would stand as excellent objects of an integrated study.

The Schools Council Health Education Project 5–13 takes a very broad view of 'health', ranging not only over hygiene, physical health and physical development, but also the emotions, social development and environmental questions. If religious education teachers need a demonstration of the splendid opportunity for a co-operative or integrated approach they should see it here. Likewise those explicitly concerned with health education might see in religious education, as I have attempted to describe it, a distinctive contribution to their programmes which will ensure that fundamental issues of human experience do not go unexplored, and that the faith responses of mankind are acknowledged as the way in which many people give shape and meaning to their existence.

Summary

Religious education is that area of the curriculum through which schools have traditionally explored values, attitudes and beliefs. The chief justification for this has been the central concern of all religions with the development and future of the human race.

While religious education will be fundamentally related to an exploration of this issue, Ian Birnie argues that the question of human potentiality is at the centre of curriculum theory and development. He draws attention to and welcomes those trends in health education which aim to broaden traditional content to encompass an investigation of what makes us human. The common use of the term 'education' by teachers of religion and health suggests both a view of the individual and the task of schooling which this article goes on to investigate.

Having identified the distinctive contribution to be made by the study of religion to this process, the author points to areas of common ground between health education and religious education and goes on to discuss how the teaching of health education will be strengthened where it establishes a good working relationship with religious education. Together, he suggests, these subjects can make a crucial contribution to the education of young people living in a world which is largely denying human values and human distinctiveness.

References

Central Advisory Council for Education (England) (1959) *15 to 18* (The Crowther Report). London, HMSO, p. 44.

Central Advisory Council for Education (England) (1963) *Half our Fortune* (The Newsom Report). London, HMSO, p. 52.

Loukes, H. (1961) *Teenage Religion*. London, SCM Press.

McPhail, P. (1972) *Moral Education in the Secondary School*. Schools Council Lifeline Series. London, Longman.

Schools Council (1970) Humanities Curriculum Project. London, Heinemann.

Schools Council (1978) *Moral Education in the Middle Years*. Startline Series. London, Longman.

Society for Promoting Christian Knowledge (1970) *The Fourth R*. London, National Society and the SPCK, p. 103.

CHAPTER 11

HEALTH EDUCATION AND THE PASTORAL SYSTEM

Kenneth David

A wide view of health education is more commonly accepted nowadays, and personal relationships and family life education are seen as parts of health education planning. This view of health has one disadvantage; it means that the subject area is diffuse and extends throughout a school's curriculum and activities. It is difficult, therefore, to encapsulate neatly in the timetable, and since health education co-ordination is demanding and frequently ignored, the subject area is very patchily dealt with in most secondary and primary schools.

In primary schools a co-ordinated approach through many subject areas is easier, for the class teacher controls all the planning, providing guidance and initiative are shown by the headteacher. In most primary schools there are easy personal relationships and a pleasing family atmosphere, and although there are strange prejudices and omissions, for example sex education and human biology are still widely ignored, the approach is likely to be managed well, especially with the impetus of excellent new curriculum materials for health education.

In secondary schools a director of studies may co-ordinate the personal and health education through academic subject departments, or a head of PE, home economics or science may have this responsibility. As schools put cognitive and examination matters into better perspective, so a managed, co-ordinated and professional approach to health may develop. In my experience a frequent lead for such co-ordination has come from the pastoral care staff. Co-ordinators are often pastoral heads, for the education in personal relationships courses, the welfare and counselling matters, and the constant attention on individual pupils are clearly appropriate links in a wide view of health. This pastoral co-ordinator, often a senior head of year, or a deputy head, will have certain questions to consider, and every school will have varying answers to suit their circumstances and staffing.

What system of meetings and consultations has to be set up, to ensure that there is efficient liaison with each academic department and pastoral head? Many schools are reducing the number of separate academic and pastoral team meetings held under different deputy heads, and are wisely attempting a more integrated approach.

How are health matters to be introduced into the teaching? This may be by occasional courses, in which departments join in teaching to a theme – perhaps third-year sessions on alcohol and drugs, a day on parentcraft during the fourth year, and so on. These sessions would be paralleled by arranged teaching on other themes in specified departments. An alternative would be to deal with major relationships themes at whatever residential courses the school organizes, though this may mean limiting valued work to those who pay for some residential experience. Some schools have a series of visiting speakers, or members of staff, who give extensive lead talks on major health themes, with discussion in tutorials during the following week. The best method of all will probably have a mixture of all these approaches, suiting the teachers' personalities and reinforcing their different methods in a flexible but carefully guided scheme. Then each academic department and all aspects of the guidance and pastoral care system will feel that they contribute equally and in a balanced and continuous pattern.

An increasingly popular way in which the pastoral staff can contribute to a school's efficiency is by having a timetabled weekly tutorial period, of the same length of time and with the same status as subject periods. This period, called 'guidance', 'tutorial', 'personal development' and various other titles, is then timetabled in such a way that a year-group of children, a group of staff responsible for the tutorial work of that year and a number of classrooms are available. The year head will then be responsible for a varied and flexible programme of work during the year. This can include large groups attending lectures on careers and health themes, small groups in discussion settings, an opportunity for regular interviewing and educational guidance of individuals and groups of pupils, and for personal counselling when needed. The school will need to plan carefully; staff will be invited to attend courses, so that the skills of counselling and group work are available in the team and those staff skilled in careers education will be allocated to each year team, perhaps after the first year. Someone in the team, not necessarily the year head, will have experience with health education themes and will be able to guide his colleagues. Headteachers may choose to ensure that selected and prepared staff are available in each tutorial team to lead discussions in more controversial areas such as sex education.

A number of schools have also linked some therapeutic group work with this tutorial period. Whilst one is properly suspicious of the word 'therapy' in a school setting, the average school does have a proportion of difficult or immature pupils who need specialist attention. Such attention from psychologists and others is often difficult to arrange, and a staff member skilled in developmental group work and counselling may lead a weekly supportive group, intended to help with problem personalities, perhaps under the general guidance of an educational psychologist. If there is a flexible system of groups in the tutorial period, varying needs of individuals and groups can be met in a very natural way; but care must be taken that group work of a therapeutic nature is not undertaken by enthusiastic volunteers of an emotional or sentimental nature who may see themselves as amateur psychiatrists, and who may do more harm than good.

Of particular value to all types of tutorial work is interviewing visitors. Through preparation of questions beforehand, practice in social care in meeting and looking after the visitor and discussing the occasion afterwards, pupils can learn a great deal. They can learn how different people, such as the head, a policeman, the caretaker, a clergyman, a health visitor, a young mother, view life, and they can learn many facts about society. If people are seen as individuals with their own feelings, cares and sensitivities, this usually has the valuable result of reducing stereotyping.

This tutorial cohort approach has many advantages. It is easily managed once the initial timetable and staff planning is done, it is comprehensible to pupils and it links health with a range of preparations for work and family life in a natural way. The major difficulty, of course, is the priority decision to allocate one of the week's teaching periods, in competition with the constant demands for more time in academic teaching departments. The demands of examinations appear so paramount, and the questionable feeling that health and guidance can be dealt with in normal teaching contacts is so easy to adopt, that we forget that good guidance tutorials make all the other work of a school more efficient and effective. We also forget that it is as important to be prepared for relationships in work and family, and to have a healthy life, in a satisfying job, as it is to be extremely well qualified in examinations. Unfortunately, success in examinations for some groups of pupils is easy to assess and publicize, and success in preparation for life for the majority can seldom be measured. Since learning and success in school are so closely linked with the motivation and happy personal development of a pupil, it seems very sad that more priority is not given to such well-planned guidance periods.

A demand more commonly met by pastoral co-ordinators is to incorporate elements of health and personal relationships work into a regular morning tutorial time taken by class tutors. Most schools have such morning tutorial time, with basic pastoral groups and a regular tutor. The planning of such groups will have been carefully done at the time of their entry to the school, based on various factors such as friendship groups, ability mix and personalities, and it is unusual to have many changes as the group moves through the school. One has regretfully seen schools in which tutor groups are reformed each year and based on ability in examinations, which seems a recipe for alienation and discipline troubles in the school. One also sees the very successful use of well-planned tutor groups as a firm and contented base from which different abilities will develop in sets and option groups, with several subjects taught in the basic mixed-ability groups. Games and social events can be based on such groups, and much learning and preparation for life can then develop with sensible tutorial leadership.

Such teacher-leaders may remain with a group throughout their time in the school, or there may be changes after lower school or middle school years. Some teachers manage younger or older children better, and some develop particular expertise in dealing with the affairs of entry or leaving classes so that they are best kept with a particular section of the school. It can be argued that pupils have to learn to deal with different adults at work, and that changes of tutors at least in the senior school help in this school preparation. The more timid and less confident pupils may need continuing contact with one adult.

Registration time is frequently a wasteful session. To take a register takes two or three minutes, and the remainder of the morning ten-minute tutorial time is frequently used then for an untidy package of tasks: dinner money, announcements, pupils finishing off homework, the teacher preparing for his next class. Confusion and lack of purpose are often the norm. Perhaps this is because many headteachers have not seen this time as anything other than a brief introduction to the day, and few demands have been made on staff.

There have been improvements recently in many schools, for a more purposeful content to the tutorial time is seen as setting the tone for the day's work in school, and is an opportunity for the tutor to get to know pupils and their work better. Many permutations of the time are possible:

sometimes an assembly time is added to registration time to give a twenty-
or even thirty-minute period, which gives an opportunity for more positive
work; there may be a case for reducing registration time on some mornings
to make a more worthwhile period of tutorial work on another day; pastoral
teams may meet to plan work while pupils are at an assembly; groups may
be put together to give one teacher a chance to take a discussion session,
while the other teacher deals with individuals and with administration. A
very satisfactory pattern in one high school is where each form group has
two twenty-five-minute morning tutorial periods in a week, with brief
five-minute registration times on the three other mornings when assemblies
are held. Forms are thus withdrawn from assembly time for their tutorial
period.

   We can now consider what the form tutor's task should be, and how this
is linked with health and education for personal relationships. The following aspects of the tutor's task have been discussed in detail at many school
in-service training sessions.

1   The tutorial period can represent the essence of the job of a good
    schoolmaster or schoolmistress, and represents the nature of good
    teaching. To know pupils well and to develop good relationships
    means that learning will flourish, with competent teaching.
2   These good relationships involve talking with and listening to chil-
    dren in a less formal setting and on a reasonably personal level.
3   She builds a family-type atmosphere in the group, using simple
    group work skills, as well as the effect of her personality.
4   The form tutor gathers and records relevant information about the
    pupils and ensures that administrative and welfare matters are dealt
    with properly. She will normally be the best informed member of the
    staff as far as knowledge of her group of pupils is concerned.
5   The tutor will learn to observe the pupils carefully, noting signs of ill
    health, of changing friendships, of hardship, attendance patterns and
    other matters.
6   She will support and enforce good order and discipline, for the two
    roles of counsellor and disciplinarian are compatible if a teacher is
    well respected.
7   Parents of the tutor's pupils will know that she is available to them,
    and she should endeavour to meet them on occasions.
8   She will monitor general standards of work, individual progress in
    different academic subjects and homework.

9   The tutorial period will be carefully planned and positively used.

In considering the last item one can now make certain assumptions:

a   there is co-ordination of health education in the school, including its social and moral implications;

b   the majority of this work is dealt with in subject teaching, or in special courses;

c   the tutorial groups have discussion time available to follow a planned series of themes, which link with and support the work done in subject classes;

d   this planned approach to tutorial time is flexible enough to allow themes of immediate interest to pupils to be raised, or for particular worries and anxieties to be ventilated by the pupils, even if planned work is postponed;

e   there is guidance, support and in-service training for staff in tutorial work.

The tutorial time should not be just another teaching period; it is a time for some factual teaching but mostly it is a time for discussion and an exchange of views. Pupils develop their attitudes to human behaviour and positive health largely from their home experience and partly from their environment, by observing, listening and talking about their feelings, and thus slowly forming their own style of living. Teachers in tutorial time can help by providing evidence and opportunity for discussion in a particularly acceptable and friendly setting.

Discussion is difficult with groups of thirty children, and too often the majority of pupils listen passively to an exchange between the teacher and a few articulate children. Such listening can, of course, be useful, if minds are busy comparing and reflecting. It is better, however, to have more children contributing, for to put thoughts and feelings into words is to clarify them. If the room allows it, a class can be broken up into groups of 4–6 pupils discussing, commenting and reporting back to the class later; a panel of pupils can be used to report to the class on what has been debated in groups; half a class can discuss themes, while half do other work, and there can be a sharing of teachers' tasks in this, with a year head taking some pupils to allow a tutor a smaller discussion group. Interviews are part of the pattern also. Each child in a tutor group should have a personal interview with their year head and class tutor at intervals, perhaps whilst the class is involved in small groups or while some are working with task cards on written work. The use of task cards can be helpful. The Health Education Council's project *Living Well* (Health Education Council, 1978) has cards on various health themes, with situations to discuss or write about (newspaper cuttings stuck on cards can be equally effective). Developing human relationships and health matters – smoking advertisements, car accidents caused by drink, household accidents, work incidents – all provide easy written and discussion themes. A well-trained class will regularly settle to small group work as a matter of routine, if some re-arrangement of desks is possible, or if pupils can 'clump' together somewhere. Such work needs consolidation, and there will normally be a teacher-controlled general session with the whole class before the tutorial period ends. All this can fit into a minimum of about twenty-five minutes, even allowing for registration. In addition to *Living Well*, Lancashire teachers have devised a co-ordinated course in health, personal development, careers education and study skills for secondary years 1–5, called *Active Tutorial Work* (Lancashire Curriculum Development Project, 1979).

So by general discussion in the class, by personal interviews and by small group work, the tutor will introduce a wide selection of themes, perhaps including some of the following examples:

Values and morals in our lives – family rules
Learning and motivation – study skills
Family life styles – parenthood
Adolescence and health – maturity difficulties and moods
Authority and responsibilities – rights and duties
Society and communities – vandalism
Sexuality – boy/girl friendships
Friends and acquaintances – peer group pressures
Personality and identity – emotions and individual differences
Communication and sociability – the language of feelings.

The tutorial discussion may offer an opportunity for pupils to discuss points heard in other lessons in a smaller group and with greater freedom, and it will be a time for further digestion of certain themes that the school deems important for living.

The following themes may be very testing for tutors in such discussion work and will need care, if indeed they are to be dealt with at all in tutorial time:

Bereavement
Aggression
Sexually transmitted diseases
Homosexuality
Deviance and abnormalities
Mental illness
Sex education (contraception, abortion, sensuality and other aspects)
Drugs and alcohol
Prejudice.

Some schools choose to have selected tutors dealing with these themes with different groups in turn, so that some greater experience and confidence with questions will be apparent. This destroys the point of the tutor's family group relationship, but may be necessary in some settings. The general knowledge of each tutor in a year team will almost certainly be limited where several of these themes are concerned, and pastoral heads and headteachers have to consider the quality and experience of their colleagues, and the need for more specialized work by prepared staff. This careful view of controversial subjects may inhibit the work of some staff, but may be more acceptable to parents, and to the local education authority who have to deal with unwelcome complaints and publicity at times.

The following more traditional health themes are often dealt with poorly, or not at all, and may need to be dealt with in small groups by one tutor from a team experienced in this area of work, or in occasional courses or subject teaching:

Smoking	Common ailments and illnesses
Home safety	Obesity and diet
Child development	The handicapped
Parentcraft	Community health
Suitable clothing	First aid.
Cancer	

Alternatively a lead talk can be given to all the year-group by one prepared member of the team, or by a teacher from a particular subject discipline, and followed up in tutorial discussion. Visiting experts may sometimes be asked to deal with a lead talk, or with visits to a series of tutorial groups or class lessons. Health visitors and health education officers are particularly helpful in this.

In such group work there will probably be questions by pupils and these must be considered with care, for mistakes can be made. A number of simple discussion techniques can be noted.

1   An informal setting is helpful, so that pupils can see each other as they speak. A group of fifteen or eighteen pupils is quite manageable, but a group of eight or ten often provides the best discussion opportunity.
2   Do not always interrupt when you disagree with a pupil's viewpoint, and do not attempt to answer every point raised. Members of the group will often do your answering for you.
3   Judge the right moment for intervening in discussion with your own experience, a question or a reminder of facts.
4   Do not be too provocative in order to liven up the discussion, and only give your own opinions at an appropriate moment, preferably when invited to do so by the group.
5   Help to clarify the discussion at intervals, by summarizing what has been said and what is being questioned.
6   Help shy members to contribute and restrain the over-talkative, by your interventions and by the way you look around the group.
7   Do not immediately present a group with a problem to discuss; ask them if there is a problem.
8   Keep good suggestions in the discussion by such questions as, 'How would that work out . . .?' Do not hasten your choice of answer by accepting the first good lead and emphasizing your agreement too quickly. Recognize all suggestions, and tolerate the irrelevant at times.
9   Fill awkward gaps by such phrases as, 'Someone was asking the other day . . .' and 'John, you were saying . . .'.
10 If response is slow, consider case studies, role play, question sheets and written work.
11 Sum up at the end of a discussion going over the main points and pointing out agreements and disagreements. Finish while interest is still lively, perhaps ending with a question.

In serious discussion work with pupils many moral issues will certainly be raised and ideally the main questions will be debated by the staff themselves before they start a discussion theme with their groups. Some year heads circulate handouts to their colleagues with a summary of views, for example on boy/girl friendship or family stress, and others invite colleagues to agree on general attitudes in response to testing questions from pupils. The school's aims and objectives may be the starting point for these discussions, and while there will inevitably be widely differing personal viewpoints, a general moral response can usually be agreed. Pupils know that life is controversial and some divergence in response from teachers is not too difficult a matter. Most teachers are, fortunately for society, 'on the side of the angels' in traditional moral matters.

The introduction of improved tutorial practices, co-ordinated health education and better discussion techniques with children needs very careful planning and preparation. It is better to postpone such plans than to set off too ambitiously with ill-prepared and reluctant staff, and cynical youngsters sensing an imposed innovation. Many schools start such improvements in the lower secondary classes, with voluntary teacher participation in a selected and keen team. This can then develop gradually through the school, involving more staff each year, and with a cohort of children accustomed to discussion work as they move up through the school. In other schools where there are few enthusiasts among the staff there can be some pilot schemes with keen voluntary teachers and selected groups of children. If the work is done well, and is seen to be useful, the idea will spread in time, if the school's leadership is positive and supportive. Critical attitudes by some staff may have to be faced, but one has seen many examples of the gradual reduction of criticism or even cynicism by a combination of careful development and preparation and accumulating evidence that such work is practical and effective.

A measure of what can be judged as effective may be the effect on learning and achievement. All pastoral care and tutorial work should contribute to an efficient school in which first-class classroom teaching is the prime factor, and in which examination successes are properly valued as a part of education. So in introducing such work we should lay emphasis on the fact that a school's efficiency and its learning should be safeguarded and improved. After that we can illustrate how the ideas of positive health, personal development and other concepts follow and permeate the work, gradually proving that positive attitudes to health have a productivity measure in pupils' traditional learning and qualifications. Staff can also be shown that life is more pleasant and teacher stress reduced by careful health education and pastoral care with pupils.

When the time is appropriate in a school's development of such work, an in-service session with all the staff is useful, and such a session may be held in school time. Various devices can be used to arrange such conferences.

Half the staff can be brought together for an afternoon with classes following a special timetable with the other teachers, and the process repeated on a further afternoon with a change of half the staff. Or the school may close earlier, and the staff invited to remain after the normal closing time as well. One has met many instances of both these methods being accepted and valued by staff. Teachers at the in-service session can then hear evidence from their colleagues, from visiting speakers, and even from pupils perhaps, can discuss plans, methods and materials, and develop support for and confidence in each other's work. In this way, by gradually involving more staff we can move from a simple tutorial system with few but clear demands on a few teachers to more purposeful group work by many staff, and from a tentative and simple co-ordination of health topics to a more inter-related and thematic approach, whilst still preserving academic rigour.

The final word should be on parents. They have brought up their children in their own style of life, and most parents are caring and responsible. They must be kept informed of all our tutorial work and health education. For the children of parents who are not caring and responsible the school has a clear duty to prepare them for life in positive health and with an understanding of human behaviour as well as on cognitive matters. Other children need teachers to complement the words and actions of their parents. At a time of adolescence the family normally needs teachers not only to teach facts but also to set adult examples and to provide evidence of how people live in a difficult society where health and relationships are vitally important matters. The staff of a school, whether as class teachers or form tutors, are models to their pupils, whether they like it or not, and our professional approach is infinitely more worthwhile and enjoyable if we acknowledge this.

Summary

This chapter emphasizes the wide-ranging nature of health education in schools, and relates responsibilities in this field to the pastoral system and tutorial work, this being seen as entirely complementary to the work done in classroom teaching. Appropriate methods and materials are reviewed, and particular attention is paid to the detailed work and responsibilities of the form tutor. Problem topics are discussed, and emphasis is laid on the total co-ordinated approach of a school to the personal development, both cognitive and affective, of young people.

References

Health Education Council (1978) *Living Well*. Health Education Council Project 12–18. London, Longman.

Lancashire Curriculum Development Project (1979) *Active Tutorial Work*. Oxford, Blackwell.

Further Reading

David, K. and Cowley, J. (1980) *Pastoral Care in Schools and Colleges*. London, Edward Arnold.

Manland, M. (1974) *Pastoral Care*. London, Heinemann.

PART IV

TEACHING METHODS IN HEALTH EDUCATION

INTRODUCTION

The three chapters in this section look at the methods and approaches used in teaching health education. All education has been under scrutiny in recent years in the search for more effective teaching methods to motivate pupils and to enhance real learning, thus reducing the boredom and disinterest which, it seems, form part of school life. Health education in particular needs fresh approaches in order to enable pupils to feel more involved; in some ways it can give a methodological lead to other areas of the curriculum.

As a classroom teacher and head of department, Tony Evans explains in Chapter 12 how he develops health education concepts through a variety of approaches. He emphasizes the experimental nature of health learning for pupil and teacher. After teaching biology and science, and gaining 'A' levels at evening classes, Tony Evans read sociology and social administration at Newcastle University, taught social studies and then set up a special unit for disruptive pupils at Thornes House School, Wakefield. In 1978 he was appointed head of the new personal and social education department at the school.

Bill Rice, senior assistant director of the Teachers' Advisory Council on Alcohol and Drug Education, is known to many teachers through his work with training conferences. He continues the theme of the previous writer and in Chapter 13 develops views on the part which skilled group discussion and other classroom teaching techniques play in developing health attitudes among young people. Bill Rice has worked with young people in various capacities since 1954; firstly as a youth leader, then as a school and college lecturer on alcohol and drug education and later as a counsellor to those with drug abuse problems. In recent years his work has included teacher in-service training and assisting in training youth and social services personnel. He is currently researching informal teaching methods.

The same theme of developing health attitudes through planned classroom techniques is taken up in Chapter 14 by Jeff Lee, a field officer with the Health Education Council. He argues that the basis of health education lies with the affective experience of young people, and with the skills they develop to make choices about their health career. After teaching in a secondary modern school Jeff Lee became head of year and head of social studies and religious education in a Hertfordshire comprehensive school. He co-ordinated health education which was taught through the pastoral system. In 1978 he was seconded to the Health Education Council with initial responsibility for the dissemination and training related to the *Living Well* Project. Since that time he has worked closely with curriculum development projects such as the Schools Council Health Education Projects 5–13 and 13–18 and the *Active Tutorial Work* scheme, which have all identified the need for in-service work to develop appropriate teaching methods in implementing their programmes of work.

CHAPTER 12

CLASSROOM APPROACHES

Tony Evans

Health education is a term which has altered in meaning over time. When I started to teach, as a biologist I was expected to teach the physiology of sex, contraception, general physical cleanliness and hygiene as part of a health education course to third-year pupils in a very large comprehensive school. It is significant that a shift of emphasis in my own career, which resulted in a move away from biological science to social science, did not involve any less teaching in the health education field but, in fact, distinctly more involvement in this area. This reflects the emergent philosophy that health education should not only be concerned with the physical aspect of the individual but should also include the social and psychological dimensions of the human being. This statement is all the more important because of its apparent simplicity and logic. This area of the curriculum is still dominated in many schools, however, by the illogical situation of appearing to remove the physical individual from his social and psychological context. My aim as head of department of personal and social education is to create a programme of work which will embrace all the interlocking facets of the nature of man, and attempt to synthetize them into a coherent whole.

The personal and social education department was originally charged with two broad objectives. These were to give 'educational and vocational guidance' and to teach 'the skills, knowledge and attitudes necessary for successful living'. The course focuses on a number of areas which are of concern or affect each pupil, and these include 'growing up', 'the family and marriage' and 'social problems'. Attention is also paid to political and economic literacy, multicultural studies and careers education. Personal and social education is compulsory for all the students in the third, fourth and fifth years with approximately three hundred and seventy pupils in each year; the department also makes a significant contribution to sixth-form studies. It would be easy but fatal to allow the work of the department to concentrate solely on factual material. Although the factual material which has been bought or produced by the teachers in the department is of a high standard, it is not an end in itself, and emphasis is placed on the need to develop the individual pupil's level of social skills, thus enabling him to make his own decisions on any matter which affects him.

Decision-making can be viewed as the process incorporating a logically ordered sequence from objective to goal. Realistic attempts can be made within the classroom to ensure that the pupils understand such a process. After formulating the objective it is necessary to find out all the possible information available to help towards the attainment of the goal. But within the health education field, when we are considering the social and psychological aspects of the individual as well as the physiological factors, the decision-making process must start with profound questions such as 'Who am I?', 'How do others see me?', and 'How do I see myself?' It is this area of self-image analysis which provides the distinctive teaching method which complements all other techniques of teaching and without which, I believe, the value of health education is relegated to a peripheral and unimportant place in the pupil's mind.

How can this statement be translated into practical terms in the class-room? I actively seek to create a group identity which demands participation on an active basis from both the pupils and myself. Of course it is true that all classes of pupils take on an identity. Normally teachers will refer to a class as good or bad, quiet or loud. I build from that base and, by means of simple exercises, encourage contact between all pupils. To achieve maximum contact I use ideas such as assembling all the class into a large circle and introducing the lesson as an exercise in getting to know each other. I ask them to write down six likes and six dislikes; the objective being to discuss their likes and dislikes with all the other pupils in the room. After they have completed this task they return to the circle and I manoeuvre the discussion towards pupils with whom they do not often make contact. 'How did you feel talking to strangers?', 'Were you embarrassed?', I ask. Another way to encourage communication is to instruct pupils to write down suitable questions which they could ask any stranger, for example 'What is your name?', 'Where do you live?'

Social contact can also be increased by distributing a worksheet instructing each pupil to grade various aspects of his character – for example, 'Are you sociable?', 'Do you get angry quickly?' – according to a very simple scale. Responses from pupils such as 'It's good because you start to find out about yourself' and 'I've never thought about myself like this before' suggest the effectiveness of this self-analysis. The pupils are then asked to obtain a score on all of these characteristics from all the members of the class. Communication is therefore encouraged, but also each pupil is building up his profile based on the perceptions of his contemporaries. Many parents see the value of this work and I recall the enthusiasm of the mother of a shy and retiring boy who acknowledged that this work could be the way to increase her son's self-confidence.

At times some members of the group, for a variety of reasons, will not participate nor be totally committed to the activities, but any negative reactions can be used as a learning aid. Thus refusal by an individual pupil to participate in a serious manner, reflected by cheating and trying to disguise the fact that they have not entered into the spirit of the exercise, is a useful point of departure to discuss different types of behaviour.

'Getting to know' themes are also a necessary part of developing self-awareness. I teach a group of fifth-year pupils who, in terms of academic ability, are likely to gain grades 4 and 5 in CSEs. Having been through the process of the 'initial knowing' exercises, they are now becoming increasingly sensitive to each other, and are stimulated to find out more about themselves and their relationships with each other and with me. Intuition is a necessary skill to be used at this point, because the pupils must feel ready to be able to cope with an exploration of themselves. An interesting exercise is 'space', where all the pupils move to a point in the room which they think represents in a physical manner their own perceptions of the degree of social contact they feel for me as a person. In this class a group of very dominant girls moved towards me whereas others showed indifference by keeping their distance. I chose to pick up this indifference as a teaching point, but what emerged was considerably different from what I expected. I expected a lack of contact which was acceptable, but in fact group discussion led to the conclusion that the dominant group of girls was actually frightening other pupils away, and so the issue of 'bossiness' was raised. One girl became very upset when they picked her out as the most bossy. I profoundly believe that this distressful situation for the girl was an essential prerequisite for her understanding of her own behaviour. We return to discuss the question of causing distress or anxiety later in this chapter.

The Schools Council Moral Education Project (McPhail, 1972) and Health Education Projects (Schools Council, 1976, 1977) and the Health Education Council's *Living Well* Project (Health Education Council, 1977) are among a large amount of material that helps social contact. For example, a work card may portray two young people talking behind the back of a third individual, who is presumably their friend. 'What would you do in this situation if you were the offender or the offended?', I ask. The class can be broken down into pairs or groups to talk about the problems presented to them. As McPhail (1972) says, the pupils '. . . are in other people's shoes'. The skill of the teacher is to try and create an atmosphere which will support the group and which allows the possibility of empathy or sensitive understanding between pupils. This climate can be used to initiate discussion of significant issues affecting individuals in the group, particularly when the pupils have the confidence and support of the group to express concern or anxiety about particular problems.

Confidence and trust in the group must be carefully nurtured and are vital to allow the possibility of changes in attitudes. For example, I teach a girl who is a heavy smoker. I introduced the issue of smoking and its associated health risks as a topic of a personal and social education lesson. The lesson included material such as nicely illustrated cartoons and a history of the subject. But although the class and indeed the girl enjoyed producing antismoking posters and developing all the available material into a worthwhile project, I would have been deluding myself if I thought a bombardment of this nature would have had any real effect upon her attitudes. The material did act as a stimulus however. The outcome was that the girl, with confidence and trust in the group, and given the group support, did at least make a commitment to give up the habit because of the health risk.

This example implicitly confirms the belief that in order to be an effective health educator and to influence a pupil to give up smoking or to reduce the amount of alcohol drinking, for example, attention must be directed towards the improvement of the self-image. Many of the social problems in society are in the last analysis related to an individual's low self-esteem. Group work has the potential to raise the self-image of each individual and to heighten the sense of worth and goodness which an individual should feel about himself.

This chapter has so far been concerned with the activities between teacher and pupils, but the introduction of a visitor into the group can provide the basis for an examination of social skills from a different perspective. I teach a fourth-year class, many of whom have additional English lessons because of their very limited linguistic ability. As part of a child development course I told them that my wife would visit the group to bath our baby if they considered the strategies necessary to make her visit worthwhile. For one lesson each week over a period of five weeks we talked about the various possibilities of meeting the visitor. Discussion centred upon meeting the physical needs in terms of arranging the classroom and bringing in the hot water for the bath. I asked probing questions such as, 'Who will meet my wife at the staff room?', 'What will you talk about?', 'Who will introduce my wife to the class?', 'What questions are you going to ask her?' Role play was used to allow the pupils to enter into situations which resembled as closely as possible the actual event. This encouraged the pupils to explore their own feelings and sensitivity about meeting strangers. All the teaching strategies employed in preparation for the visitor – discussion, role play and recording – were invaluable exercises in personal relationships. But the crucial point to be made is that although the visitor was important to the class, the decisions which they had to take created opportunities to learn more about themselves and others in the group.

I want now to return to the issue of causing distress or creating anxiety in a pupil, for it may seem a particularly insensitive act to initiate. The question is asked, 'Why do you want to create insecurity from apparent stability?' I justify this in terms not dissimilar to the rationale used in psychotherapy. Unhappiness about a facet of behaviour which has been brought to the attention of the individual by the group can be used as an important part of the learning process. All the caring professions tend to adopt and perpetuate the notion that the people who work in these professions are 'good guys', and therefore it is nasty to cause distress when distress is not present. However no social institution, indeed no concept of society, could exist if we tried to justify all the behaviour of everybody all the time. This point is illustrated in the following case. When I was in charge of a special unit for disruptive pupils I never at any stage justified any antisocial behaviour for whatever reason. After I had built up a relationship with each pupil based on mutual respect I would constantly confront them with their behaviour problems. I will always remember one girl who came to me as a frightened and aggressive person. For six months she would not allow me even to sit by her, so great was the hurt and anger. It took her two years to express to me that she understood and was aware of her antisocial behaviour. When I felt that the relationship was secure I constantly confronted her with the nature of her problem and encouraged the group to discuss her behaviour (and theirs). I think that it was a measure of success that she actually sat and listened to the criticism of her behaviour instead of running away from it and defending herself by aggressive behaviour.

In conclusion, there is a tendency in this field of health education, using the methodology which I have referred to, to create a mysterious aura about the work. There is nothing mysterious about it. The range of skills and techniques are all available to the good class teacher who, in my definition, is sensitive and articulate, and has achieved a relationship with the class based on mutual respect. He believes that the teaching should be a rewarding and satisfying experience, and knows that 'youngsters don't learn from teachers they don't like'. And so movement into this area of affective education requires confidence and belief in the method, and an understanding of the method not only in the theoretical sense (group dynamics), but also in an experiential sense. Any training programme for staff who want to move into this area has, I believe, to be carried out at an experiential level. After all it is very easy to ask pupils to talk to each other, but we can only understand their feelings if we have been placed in similar situations beforehand. As head of a faculty I have set up a faculty day to allow staff training in this field, and I also encourage my colleagues to apply for the appropriate courses. The next step in my school is to broaden the scope and include teachers from any discipline who are interested and concerned about the growth and development of the whole child. It is only by constant advertisement of this work that prejudices in the staff room will dissipate, ignorance will be erased and teachers will understand that these developments are grounded in thoroughly proven educational ideas.

Summary

The introduction to this chapter is concerned with trends in health education philosophy. This extends into a description of the broad aims and objectives of the personal and social education department, and the attempts to create conditions for social skill training. Decision-making is perceived as a vital aspect of social skill training and, as a starting point, exercises in social awareness are described in detail. Social skill training presupposes the need to work in groups, and the group is used to encourage and foster the development of social skills such as confidence, communication and sensitivity. The notion of group identity and support and the possibility of helping an individual with a health problem are explored. The chapter continues by acknowledging the inherent dangers present in group work but justifies its practice, and concludes with a personal statement about teachers and teaching.

References

Health Education Council (1977) *Living Well*. Health Education Council Project 12–18. Cambridge, Cambridge University Press.

McPhail, P. (1972) *Moral Education in the Secondary School*. Lifeline Series. London, Longman.

Schools Council (1976) Schools Council Health Education Project 5–13. London, Nelson.

Schools Council (1977) Schools Council Health Education Project 13–18. (Forthcoming).

CHAPTER 13

DISCUSSION, ROLE PLAY AND SIMULATION IN THE CLASSROOM

William Rice

Health and social education do not fit easily into a simple process of inputs and outcomes. Good health, like good citizenship, is more easily recognized when it happens to be absent. It is relatively easy to list the marks of ill health or to compile an index of social pathology, but to measure good health is another matter. Objectives, therefore, are difficult to state because we are all acutely aware of how problematic it is to know if objectives have been attained in those whom we are teaching.

In spite of these very real difficulties health education objectives have been postulated and most people will agree that in part at least health education should help the individual to deal with the changing circumstances of life, especially in a highly technological society with strong tendencies towards rapid social and other changes (Kime et al., 1977). In very brief outline that is what one hopes to achieve by engaging in health education; but what are the objectives of discussion and simulation exercises as parts of the total process?

Apart from the rather obvious fact that both approaches demand high levels of participation from those involved, and that they are associated with affective learning, there is the less recognized fact that both methods mimic aspects of behaviour found in everyday life. All of us engage in discussion, and all of us in some way and at various times enact or re-enact particular experiences and assume roles.

However, there is another and quite specific objective to be derived from discussion and simulation, and that is perhaps best described by the term 'fluency'. When one uses the expression, 'He or she is fluent', we usually mean fluent in language, where the flow of words is characterized by smoothness and confidence. We see a confident approach, a swift and accurate response to the demands of the moment. Similarly one can reasonably expect to see something of this same fluency in responses to the circumstances of life as a result of having had practice which has been founded on knowledge and appreciation of self, others and life situations (Coleman, 1972).

What Do We Talk About?

In planning discussion sessions we have to decide which topics to include, and in reaching our decisions all kinds of factors will influence our thinking. In a recent survey it was found that a high percentage of the teachers who formed the sample disapproved of the suggestion that they should teach about contraception, mental health, venereal disease and parenthood whilst 90% of the sample approved of dealing with smoking, alcohol, personal hygiene, road, water and home safety, first aid and conservation (McGuffin, 1978). It is striking to note that the former list includes some of the more sensitive topics whilst the latter consists of relatively open subjects about which a consensus exists. If one recalls that we are aiming at preparing people for later experiences as well as teaching for the present, our programme may be in danger of suffering from important omissions. As a guiding principle one must choose matters that are relevant to the pupils we are teaching. This principle clearly rests on the assumption that we *know* which are the relevant issues for our pupils. We *may* know, but it is likely that we shall have to undertake what has been called a 'social diagnosis' to be sure that we have got our impressions right and that our judgement can be relied upon (Skilbeck, 1971).

Social diagnosis consists of drawing up a picture of the overall characteristics of both pupils and environment. What are our pupils really like when out of school? What tone exists in their homes and the community? Such a process of putting substance on a rather bare skeleton may help us to avoid creating a mismatch between the aspirations of teachers and the needs of pupils. A number of studies have shown that both the setting and the *tone* of the setting are critical factors (Dick and Carey, 1978).

These searches take time and, if conducted without sensitivity and considerable tact, may be seen as plain and simple prying into the affairs of others; personally I never wish to know more than enough to prevent me from causing hurt or embarrassment to members of the group. This means that I need to constantly update my stock of facts about each member and also to be able to register the 'happy' news just as eagerly as we seize on the sadder bits of information that come our way.

It is clear that before people are able to pursue issues of central concern by means of discussion, there has to be a shared feeling of 'he/she knows and can understand my problems'. Without such a feeling it will be difficult for the person or group to relax and enter into a trustful exchange of views and ideas (Abercrombie and Terry, 1978).

What About the Environment?

We are usually aware of the human factors involved in creating a good atmosphere, for instance the warm friendly greeting and a minimal amount of formality. We are less conscious of the contribution made by the physical environment. Physical comfort and psychological relaxation are not necessarily related but one can say that discomfort, or the presence of intrusions such as desks and chairs acting as barriers, may make it more difficult to feel at ease and relaxed. Just think of the psychiatrist's proverbial couch and you will get the picture!

We might also give some thought to how much space we have in which to arrange ourselves. If the room is too crowded there may be an unpleasant 'fug' which is a fact of life when too many humans occupy too little space. But larger rooms also impose problems. On one well-remembered occasion I found myself trying to arrange a group of nine young people in a room which on Friday nights served as a disco hall; some of the group were so far from me that their faces were quite indistinct! And even when we had formed a tighter circle, the feeling of isolation in that large space was quite marked – and very disturbing.

How Much Time Is Needed?

'How long does all this take?', 'What about all the other demands on time?', 'Doesn't he know about the three Rs?' Of course there are severe limitations on time and resources. School life, like life itself, is a kind of competition where one legitimate need jostles with another for time and attention. But there are other constraining influences; research has indicated that more benefit to the learner occurs when the sessions are spread over time rather than closer together. Another point to consider is that during longer sessions a 'resistance to respond' might build up in those taking part (Borger and Seaborne, 1969). These comments serve as rough guidelines which can later be discarded in the light of experience with each group of pupils.

The Question of Numbers

How many should be in a group? We know that with four to ten persons in a group it is less easy to participate then when in groups of less than four. It is also more of a problem to influence others successfully within the larger group. Larger groups tend to display fairly wide extremes of interaction; most of the members will contribute little whilst a vocal minority can dominate the discussion (Bion, 1974).

On the other hand people will more readily express disagreement in a large group and there appears to be a less inhibited tone to the discussion. Most people seem to prefer to be in groups of five or six, and relaxed participants represent a potentially successful group session. However, we all recognize that it is more likely that teachers will be faced with classes of thirty-plus rather than units of four to ten pupils. Lancashire's *Active Tutorial Work* project (Lancashire Curriculum Development Project, 1979) is based on such larger group sizes.

One idea worth considering involves a kind of team teaching approach; two teachers are able to control informal discussion sessions even when the total class numbers exceed thirty, broken down into groups of five to six pupils. Another method is to make use of the services of an outsider, but clearly such a practice demands a full knowledge of the person, their background, training, contribution to be made and so forth. Outside helpers must be thoroughly briefed by the teacher in charge and must act under that teacher's guidance (Fantini, 1972). (Those interested in a fuller consideration of group size and its relationship to group dynamics are referred to the work of Barker (1968).)

Another and more difficult approach open to the teacher who must act alone on these occasions is to have one group of five or six in action while the remainder of the class act as observers noting down the flow of events on prepared sheets of paper. The group serving as models will at some point retire and be replaced by another group of five or six pupils. In this way every pupil will get the opportunity to contribute in two ways: as a direct participant in a group activity and with all that the exercise entails in the way of pressure to contribute, responding to challenges and recognizing cues, and by acting as a more detached analyst of the behaviour of others (Barker, 1968; Taba and Elkins, 1969). If such a method is adopted it is important to stress the value and importance of the observing exercise. Unless the pupils can appreciate the benefits to be derived from developing skills of observation they may well conclude that only the 'centre of the stage' episode is worthwhile.

Are There Objectives?

What is all this intended to achieve? Everything which has been proposed so far calls for considerable time and effort, but to what end? Broadly speaking we can take one of two stances: the *process* or the *product*. Under the former it is held that there are enough benefits to be derived from the exercising of one's mind and fostering creative thinking to justify the time spent in discussion and role play without worrying too much about grander objectives. The 'product' school does not deny the merits and benefits to be gained by the process of discussion and simulation, but stresses that there are end-products to be considered and planned for. An end-product might be that discussion skills will help to promote a more confident manner during social activities and better handling of formal interviews. One can argue that improved social skills contribute to the making of a more relaxed and competent individual.

The dichotomy is a very superficial one because both process and end-product are present in the exercises. Perhaps a more useful distinction may be drawn between discussion skills and the needs of the pupils in terms of effective social functioning. Many language theorists maintain that there is a need to be able to operate in a number of what might be rather weightily called 'language milieux'; social intercourse as between peers, a different variety when not with peers, the language of officialdom and so forth. These concepts may be valuable in directing a teacher's thoughts when he or she comes to try to see the place of discussion and, as I hope to show, simulation within the total context of a young person's learning experience.

It is quite likely that if Wackford Squeers of Dotheboys Hall could sit in on some lesson periods in a modern school he would find the entire proceedings enough to cause apoplexy. The involvement of pupils in a dialogue with the teacher is an important departure from the educational practices of the past, although the actual origins of the practice of teacher-pupil interchange have traditionally been ascribed to Socrates. The relaxed atmosphere and frank exchange of insights, the feelings of empathy and support all seem to indicate both enjoyment and a valuable learning experience for all concerned.

Planning and Preparation

This rosy picture bends reality for we all can recall occasions from our own experience when things fell flat! Some of us may have more worrying memories of times when matters got a bit out of hand. Can we find ways of preparing our sessions so that such failures are less likely to happen? As a starter one could say that useful, effective discussion needs to be planned in at least two senses. There is a need to place the discussion periods at suitable points within some broader programme of learning. It is obvious that in order to have interesting and informative discussion people must have something of value and interest to talk about. Therefore, looking ahead and planning well should enable a teacher to insert discussion 'units' at the most useful stages in the programme. But planning also refers to an ordering of each individual session. This does not necessarily mean that the vital spark of spontaneity must be lost. Rather, the suggestion is that the discussion is directed, or nudged gently here and there, exploring, rejecting, digging deeper when a particularly useful 'seam' of ideas is located. All the time one is trying to make use of the discussion as one uses a tool to effect some purpose. A brief example will help to make the plea for planning clearer.

A teacher, fresh from the summer vacation, invites the class to discuss bereavement as a starter to the term's discussion programme. What had gone unnoticed, because of the intervening break, was that one of the pupils had recently lost a parent. The child was unable to take part in the proposed class activity and was quite naturally greatly distressed by the subject matter and the very public handling of the painful topic.

Many people have found benefit in going to some trouble in planning discussion sessions, and what follows, by way of a personal checklist, has been tried and tested over a fairly lengthy period. There are, first of all, the two aspects of planning (as discussed above) plus the added matter of the choice of topic. It seems a sounder practice to dovetail the topics in such a way as to contribute to and build upon the syllabus as a whole. Remember that, in spite of the alleged language paucity of many pupils, comments elicited during informal and comfortable discussion will usually be 'rounder' than those conveyed in more formalized written work. It may be that some sensitive topics have to be kept for the privacy of written exercises, but it is worthwhile encouraging a preliminary exploration of such topics via the discussion medium and making the maximum use of the fuller picture obtained during the verbal exercises. Spoken adjectives can provide a crude but possible accurate measure of how a pupil feels towards issues of importance. And should we not strive for a balance between the all too real pathology of life and experiences which cheer? A diet of disaster is not only boring; it is probably damaging.

Do we require the pupils to review the discussion later by means of a written exercise? Such a practice may permit a pupil to withdraw, amend or otherwise qualify a view expressed in the discussion session. In my view this is a useful way of encouraging an active review of conclusions as well as allowing the individual to situate the experience within his personal moral framework, and to do so without undue and immediate pressure from peers or teachers. It also offers an acceptable escape route when a pupil has managed to get himself into an impasse situation brought about by trying to sustain conflicting public and private viewpoints.

In discussion and simulation exercises teachers should have gone over the ground very thoroughly *beforehand*. The intention should be that one is never completely surprised by a sudden change of direction, or an unexpected but erroneous conclusion which has escaped our previous notice. In short, the leader should be very familiar with the subject under review. In this way one can direct the discussion when necessary, and suggest avenues as yet unexplored by the group.

Another point concerns the way in which we organize the experience. Should we begin by posing a question to the entire group for a general response or should we first allow smaller groups to tackle the matter before joining in open discussion? Smaller, more intimate groups do not always discuss intimate subjects; embarrassment levels can be high when there is nowhere to 'hide' in a small group. A large group can offer the pupil a certain measure of anonymity, a chance to avoid making even a considered statement. We must always respect the privacy of the individual. Then there is the old problem of the 'know-all' pupil who has an answer for every question and never allows a lull in the conversation to pass without making some contribution. No one would wish to stifle such energy, so the task is to train and utilize it for the benefit of that person and the group as a whole.

We must also be alert to the possibility of discussion sessions providing leaders and pupils with a ready-made and apparently *approved* platform on which strongly held views may be aired, and indeed promulgated. There are no firm rules to guide one on this issue. If we really know our pupils we may be able to anticipate likely postures on certain matters and, without repressing the ardent contributor, seek to create a genuinely democratic discursive framework. One hopes that by employing relevant discussion structures of the kind dealt with later, the worst features of 'platforming' can be avoided whilst making use of the commitment and feeling which may underlie it.

The author sees the teacher or leader as occupying a very active role in discussion, but the word 'active' requires some additional comment. The teacher should be active in facilitating the discussion but not in dominating it (Abercrombie, 1979). The teacher is a guide who knows the terrain but does not insist on a particular route. He is aware of the answers (or some of them), but nonetheless encourages the questions to be asked whilst resisting the temptation to provide all the answers. He is a kind of nutritionist who is concerned to see that a balanced diet is placed before his pupils at all times.

Above all, the teacher should understand that he is not a therapist who feels obliged to sort out all of the tensions, worries and conflicts present in his charges and not infrequently brought to the surface as a result of discussing salient topics. Such treatment activities are properly the province of those trained in their use. This personal view needs to be qualified in the following way.

First, teachers can and do watch for the signs which can indicate serious needs and take action by referring the pupil to the appropriate agency. This is a general duty undertaken by all who have close contact with young people. Secondly, teachers *can* help pupils very directly by wise counsel and sensitive support, but teachers have differing views as to the kind of personal problems they can tackle. The point is that in successful group work confidences may be offered which give revealing insights into the pupil's home life and personal life style. Some of these pictures may cause teachers to be alarmed and to wish to take action, and in the desire to help we may take upon ourselves roles which we are simply unable to fulfil.

Simulations and Role Play

Simulations are segments of human behaviour or experiences and they are played according to rules and guidelines. These rules will usually refer to the number taking part, how long the enactment will last and, more importantly, outline the characteristics of those taking part and the circumstances in which the simulation takes place. Simulations have story lines usually called 'scenarios', and the players are provided with a set of personal identities (called 'role profiles'). An example from another sphere might help at this point. Pilots (and learner drivers) learn the rudiments of the required skills in machines called 'simulators'. If you crash whilst in a simulator you may be embarrassed but at least you will still be alive!

Role play differs from simulations in that there are fewer rules (sometimes none at all) and characterizations are left to the players. All of us during discussion have heard someone say, 'Can't you see my point of view?', or words to that effect. Although made earnestly, the cry has no meaning because the listeners cannot see the point of view in question without some real attempt to do so. There are some events in life which one must go through before one can gain the insights provided by those experiences. But there are other occasions when, by exercising our imaginative powers, we may perhaps very briefly and incompletely occupy another person's position and see as it were through their eyes. The insights to be gained from this experience can be very great and some may be deeply moving whilst others are transient and make no lasting impression on our way of thinking.

Perhaps it is the potential for lasting changes in thinking and possibly behaviour which may result from a relatively brief change of role that leads many practitioners to see role play and simulation as being a stage further than discussion (Argyle, 1968). The suggestion is that there is a continuum with, at one end, simple classroom chats followed by more exhaustive discussion brought about by planning and structure, followed in turn by simulations and role play which introduce greater levels of emotion and possibly provide deeper insights for those taking part.

Whilst discussion, simulation and role-play sessions cannot always produce clearer understanding and provoke deep insights, their potential for so doing is present. Conversely one can see that on occasions a brief end-of-period chat may get right to the heart of the matter whilst a carefully planned discussion and role-play session will grind to a stop, if it ever gets going at all!

There are levels of interaction to be enjoyed in all of the activities described, but it is my conviction that role play and simulation are most likely to offer a way into deeper insights, and of the two the latter is the most potent. More importantly simulations place greater emphasis on the structure of the experience than on personal roles (Taylor and Walford, 1974).

It is also significant that practically all simulation exercises are of a problem-solving kind. This does not mean that they must therefore of necessity be unexciting; much can be achieved by consideration of precisely how one will present an issue or problem to be solved so that the participants have a sense of confidence brought about by better understanding of the issues involved. In setting up a simulation exercise we might be tempted to introduce elements of theatre into the activity. It is true that many of the situations dealt with in role play and simulation are dramatic in themselves, and one may be justified in seeking to utilize that dramatic tone, but we should not confuse drama and theatre in this context. The author can recall one excellent simulation which was proceeding splendidly until the teacher in charge halted the entire class because one of the players had delivered a line rather badly! Role play and simulation can offer a way to a better understanding of the nature and function of relationships. Simulations, in particular, can permit us to explore various courses of action without having to actually bear the costs of a wrong or dangerous decision. We may also be able to get the 'feel' of the pressure and urgency present in some situations in which quite important decisions may have to be made.

One can say, to put it another way, that simulations and role play are examples of learning with knowledge of results – a kind of operant learning. Advocates of these methods believe that they help people to make more refined and skilled responses by virtue of having had prior exposure to social experiences in a setting which allowed for analysis and later correction of faulty behaviour (Argyle, 1968). When it is successful, role play may promote greater perception of and sensitivity towards the events of daily life.

More specifically, one can strongly suggest that the group structures inherent in simulations lend themselves to creating an awareness of the value of co-operation and of sharing tasks (and problems), and also go some way towards providing the skills needed in the many shared circumstances of life. Simulation is a way of accelerating the acquisition of social techniques by the processes of practice and analysis.

Some Constraints Considered

Classroom-bound simulations suffer from such things as immovable desks, cramped seating and a linear seating arrangement which does nothing to promote feelings of intimacy and closeness to the action. Of course one can recall many successful sessions which had of necessity to take place within the confines of a typical classroom, but many have failed because the essential atmosphere was missing. Ideally one needs some space and freedom to move, and certainly to feel and be physically relaxed. Observers need to be reasonably close to the events of the simulation so that subtle movements and changes may be detected and later discussed by those concerned. I have found a horseshoe-shape arrangement is the most useful in providing a feeling of distance for the players and yet can be close enough for the observers to see what is taking place.

In order to overcome the constraints imposed by time available, there must be planning at the level of the overall syllabus and also within the limits of the specific classroom session. It is so easy to run out of time and have to leave in the emotional middle of the exercise, even though it may be at the end of the classroom period. A useful way of gauging how long an exercise will require is to time, preferably with a stopwatch, how long it takes to open and close a door, put sugar into a cup of tea, shake hands and say goodbye and so forth. When one begins to form a picture of the relative amounts of time required for such everyday acts, we tend to become more sensitive to timing in general.

A brief word here about the role of the teacher. In a large measure the remarks made earlier with regard to discussion apply here as well. The teacher is a facilitator of the activity but if he decides to join in the game I think he should then be subject to the rules in the same way as every other participant. If the rules call for a reply to a direct question then the teacher should offer an answer as he would similarly expect a pupil to respond during the course of the simulation. This egalitarian approach must be maintained if a teacher decides to engage in the games situation. Having said that, one must again repeat a view expressed earlier; that at all times we must respect the privacy and intimacy of pupils and, we can now add, of teachers too.

Making the Most of Simulations and Role Play

It will be obvious from what has already been stated that careful planning and preparation bring real benefits. Both simulation and role play demand quite a lot from those taking part and anxiety levels, at the beginning at least, may be high. The situation will be improved if the group has had time to get to know one another and to build something like a group spirit. All this takes time and we need to give thought to ways in which the process may be fostered and even accelerated. One way is to see simulation and role play as parts of a three-phase process.

The preparatory stage makes use of formal teaching sessions, films, plays and readings. The basic objectives include acquisition of knowledge, 'getting to know you better' and, very importantly, orientating the group towards an awareness of the ways in which human beings handle their social experiences. Pupils then begin to learn the techniques of close observation and analysis.

In phase two we introduce the group to the experiences of simulation and role play. We offer explanations and frequent reassurances so that pupils feel as secure as possible. The early exercises are simple, brief and on fairly 'neutral' topics. As the players become more relaxed and interested we can increase the frequency of the sessions and begin to explore the more central issues of adolescent life.

An essential component of all simulation and role-play sessions is the follow-up 'talkdown' or debriefing. The importance of the debriefing is clear; we need to draw the lessons which emerge during the exercise and we may need to reassure pupils by restoring perspectives lost in a too close consideration of a particular situation. The purpose of these exercises is not to create emotional heat as an end in itself, but to learn from the experience as well as simply 'feeling' it (Taylor and Walford, 1974). One more point about debriefing is worth making: in order to exploit the potential of role play and simulations, participants need to become involved, 'immersed' as someone has put it; we cannot really benefit fully from these sessions if we remain on the fringes, we need to be right in the middle. However, debriefing calls for the exact opposite; we must assume a detached approach if we are to analyse and deduce. These are different skills and the transition from one to the other may be difficult for some people if we hurry the process. For that reason I always allow the players a little time to 'fade into the background' at the conclusion of an exercise and turn the heat off by drawing the observers into the debriefing. At a later stage, we must return to the players and ask for their impressions on what took place.

In phase three we should be able to get the group to plan and write their own scenarios and role profiles as well as playing them. This is not simply a division of labour, but a very active learning experience. In planning scenarios we act out in advance the likely permutations of behaviour, whilst in creating role profiles we search for expressions of behaviour which typify different kinds of people and, in so doing, live them ourselves for a brief time and in a limited way.

The Use of Structures in Discussion, Simulation and Role Play

In the case of simulations and role play some structures are already present in the form of scenarios, role profiles and rules, for structures are nothing more than the skeletons or frameworks on which the participants build their contributions. For example, a role-play session which seeks to explore parent-child relationships will almost certainly have a basic framework (or structure) of mother and/or father role and son and/or daughter role. The structure may be expanded to include particular elements of time and place so as to provide the players with a rough blueprint as to the way in which things might develop.

Discussion, especially in the context of the classroom or club, is usually without structure. There may be the minimum shape imposed by a teacher-pupil grouping, or the structure set by the male-female distribution of the group, but apart from such fairly obvious determinants most discussions are 'play it by ear' sessions. These can, of course, be entirely satisfying and valuable in their own right, but they are not the easiest experiences from which to draw conclusions or form systematic impressions.

Many practitioners make use of a series of structures by means of which those taking part may keep a closer watch on what is happening and be able in retrospect to assess more accurately the value and importance of what took place. The suggestions which follow can be applied to simulation and role-play sessions as well as to discussion.

The simplest form of structure involves giving participants some guiding rules. For example, certain players are asked not to express their own opinion but to spend their time supporting someone else's point of view. Another example asks selected members to observe their colleagues in action, recording by some unobtrusive means the gestures employed in putting forward opinions. It is worth stating at this point that what we have here called 'structures' are present in various forms in most, if not all, social exchanges. In talking seriously with people do we not ask for more information, offer advice, assert opinions, give support, provide information, persuade, pour oil on troubled waters? All these represent structures which one can introduce into discussion sessions and be confident that in so doing we are refining skills which we all need during our lives.

Argyle (1968) has provided a list of structures (or functions), and to this collection I have added others which I have found to be of some value in classroom discussion work.

Chairperson	– arbitrator
Salesperson	– persuader
Interviewer	– gathering information
Teacher	– passing on information
Counsellor	– offering advice
Leader	– assuming control
Follower	– taking directions
Negotiator	– reaching agreement
Supporter	– offering assistance
Facilitator	– making things easier
Analyst	– synthetizing arguments
Listener	– giving close attention.

A fairly cursory consideration of this list will surely bring to mind ways in which the functions may be employed in a learning context and still retain the enjoyableness of sharing ideas with other members of the group. The list contains two columns; one column is expressed in terms of functions, the other in terms of roles to be taken. The young person who dominates his group may benefit from being given a listener function or the role of a follower. Similarly, the pupil who is forever on the receiving end of directions could well enjoy being given the chance to be a leader in some suitable exercise, and perhaps thereby find unexpected personal qualities.

Structure can also be added by elaborating the process of discussion. This may best be explained by reference to the difficulties reported by many people in simply making sense out of the plethora of ideas, opinions, real and pseudo facts, statements and questions which are present in most serious discussions. We need some way of ordering the experience so that at least some of the wealth of discussion can be retained and used.

If one reflects for just a moment on this apparent unmanageability of some group discussion, we may begin to see that the breakdown occurs because we fail to list the contributions offered and we often do not explore the concepts which underlie our opinions even when we succeed in actually identifying concepts. For example, in a debriefing which followed a simulation dealing with personal autonomy in a peer group situation, members may draw attention to such diverse factors as loyalty to friends, being 'chicken', weak personality and the rights of individuals. Listing the ideas put forward by members will enable the group to form a picture of what is collectively known about personal autonomy and by the same token to begin to see how much the group needs to find out. By then identifying the concepts which are derived from a statement such as 'Everyone has a right to make up his own mind', the topic will be more comprehensively and systematically discussed. Listing the ideas and identifying the concepts are parts of a process of diagnosis which I believe to be at the very heart of discussion, simulation and role-play.

In terms of how one goes about listing, we may simply rely on the collective memory of the group, or we can write down the points which seem relevant to the topic. In a similar fashion we can repeat a number of statements and then ask the group what larger idea lies behind them. Alternatively we can note the ideas on a board or overhead transparency and draw from the collection all those items which seem to 'fit' together.

The latter exercise can be extended and become in itself a further elaboration which has been called *labelling*. In this exercise we attempt to categorize what has been said. For example, we might ask the group to decide if strongly held opinions are negative or positive attributes of those who hold them. Another use of labelling is that when we try to create categories in this way we frequently become aware of the relationships between the many statements put forward during a group discussion.

In all of this we must try to maintain a balance between an open and uninhibited exchange of ideas – an occasion marked by feelings of spontaneous enjoyment – and a thorough consideration of the matter under discussion. The purposes of the structures are to (1) facilitate understanding by means of improved powers of comprehension, (2) systematically exercise intellectual and verbal skills and (3) help individuals to enjoy the benefit from sharing thoughts with other people. When we undertake discussion, simulation and role-play activities we are placing certain aspects and issues of life under a kind of microscope. In order that our pupils may benefit from this detailed examination we need to provide some 'instruments' of an intellectual kind by means of which they can critically appraise what is taking place around them, and thereby manage their affairs more successfully, and with greater satisfaction (Coleman, 1972).

Summary

Three major aspects of informal teaching methods are dealt with in this chapter: planning and preparation, implementation and analysis. Attention is drawn to the size and composition of classroom groups and to the fact that individual and group characteristics assume a new importance in informal teaching. A special plea is made for choosing topics on the basis of prior investigation rather than on ad hoc grounds.

Simple techniques are suggested by means of which demanding and complex occasions can be made more manageable. One such technique, called structures, provides the pupils with clearly defined roles or functions within a group situation. As the skills of pupils increase, so their roles become more complex and their instructions less precise.

The author emphasizes the benefits to be gained from the various exercises of discussion, role play and simulation, and takes the view that not every participant can untangle for himself the many threads which are present in every form of social interaction. There are particular and unique insights to be gathered from group discussion, and these form a major raison d'être for informal teaching as an educational method.

The chapter includes some suggestions concerning ways in which the wealth of ideas generated by group activities may be systematically explored. Most people will agree that when there are decent levels of participation and adequate understanding of what has taken place, group work becomes a very satisfying experience.

References

Abercrombie, M. L. J. (1979) *The Anatomy of Judgement*. Harmondsworth, Penguin, p. 91.

Abercrombie, M. L. J. and Terry, P. M. (1978) *Talking to Learn*. Guildford, University of Surrey, Society for Research into Higher Education, p. 99.

Argyle, M. (1968) *The Psychology of Interpersonal Behaviour*. Harmondsworth, Penguin, pp. 12, 87, 188.

Barker, R. G. (1968) *Ecological Psychology*. Stanford, Cal., Stanford University Press.

Bion, W. R. (1974) *Experiences in Groups*. London, Tavistock, p. 26.

Borger, R. and Seaborne, A. E. M. (1969) *The Psychology of Learning*. Harmondsworth, Penguin, p. 142.

Coleman, J. (1972) In Raynor, J. and Harden, J. (eds) (1973) *Readings in Urban Education. Vol. 1, Cities, Communities and the Young*. London, Routledge & Kegan Paul, pp. 194–204.

Dick, W. and Carey, L. (1978) *The Systematic Design of Instruction*. Glenview, Ill., Scott, Foresman & Co, pp. 4 and 5.

Fantini, M. D. (1972) In Raynor, J. and Harden, J. (eds) (1973) *Readings in Urban Education. Vol. 2, Equality and City Schools*. London, Routledge & Kegan Paul, pp. 180–190.

Kime, R. E., Schlaadt, R. G. and Tritsch, L. E. (1977) *Health Instruction: An action approach*. Englewood Cliffs, N.J., Prentice-Hall, pp. 57 and 58.

Lancashire Curriculum Development Project (1979) *Active Tutorial Work*. Oxford, Blackwell.

McGuffin, S. (1978) *J. Inst. Hlth Educ.*, vol. 16, no. 1.

Skilbeck, J. (1971) In Raynor, J. and Harden, J. (eds) (1973) *Readings in Urban Education. Vol. 2, Equality and City Schools*. London, Routledge & Kegan Paul, p. 237.

Taba, H. and Elkins, D. (1969) In Raynor, J. and Harden, J. (eds) (1973) *Readings in Urban Education. Vol. 2, Equality and City Schools*. London, Routledge & Kegan Paul, pp. 269–270.

Taylor, J. and Walford, R. (1974) *Simulation in the Classroom*. Harmondsworth, Penguin, pp. 41 and 50.

CHAPTER 14

TEACHING SKILLS

Jeff Lee

The aim of this chapter is to consider recent work carried out in developing personal skills in young people. With reference to health education it assumes that the content area includes the physical, social and mental well-being of people. This means that health education is not only about the cognitive areas, and facts in isolation, but involves the affective area and people's feelings, emotions, attitudes and values. It is about translating the facts into a meaningful context which allows people to make decisions as to the appropriate course of action with regard to their health behaviour. Health education must be seen as a freeing exercise that gives the people the means to choose as a result of greater awareness and knowledge.

There is a strong case for beginning health education with the affective experience of people, for it is only by considering people's attitudes and feelings at the outset that one can expect to modify or confirm behaviour and attitudes to health issues. Obviously information and facts play an important part but if, as suggested above, health education is about encouraging people to make informed choices in their life styles, it has to take into consideration the current reasons for a particular aspect of behaviour.

Concern for the individual achieving his or her potential is one of the more common aims of school philosophy. However, whether schools achieve this admirable intention is another issue. The potential of individuals has to be considered beyond that of academic achievement, and has to encompass the social and personal potential of people in their relationships with others. The starting point for achieving or developing that potential is the person as she or he 'is', namely what the person says, thinks and does and the accompanying reasons for all that 'makes me what I am'. In other words health education has to start where the person is; it has to be child-centred. This, in turn, makes the role, attitude and approach of the teacher of paramount importance if health education is to be *effective*, particularly where teachers are involved in consideration of the *affective* areas of young people's behaviour. If one is attempting to promote the skills of making decisions and the ability to cope with incidents which young people experience, with a view to their making informed choices and decisions, it is vital that the training which is given to them to achieve this end is supportive of that objective and not opposed to it.

Having discussed and tried out various 'teacher approaches' with a large number of colleagues, one can propose a core of prerequisites for promoting students' skills in coping with the situations they encounter, and for making decisions about the appropriate behaviour. First, the teacher has to be a person, not an ogre, whose first aim is to teach children before subjects. Furthermore the teacher must be a facilitator of learning and not a law-giver or lecturer; 'teacher' is perhaps one of the more unfortunate misnomers in education. These comments may seem perfunctory and condescending, but experience indicates that many teachers in practice still tend towards being subject-based fact-givers. If a teacher wants to enable students to make informed choices about their health behaviour, the development of a relationship between the teacher and the students is vital. They have to know and trust one another. If people are to discuss their feelings, attitudes and behaviour there has to be interaction and communication between teacher and students.

The following comment of a teacher who had had a disagreement about whether a particular student should be allowed to attend his class because of a swearing incident indicates a barrier which cannot lead to positive health learning, nor to the development of students' potential. The teacher's view was, 'My job is to teach mathematics. I should not have to bother about kids' feelings.' This view is not uncommon; it may not always be voiced as such, but is seen perhaps in the way that teachers behave or treat their students – the message of the 'hidden curriculum'. I experienced a particularly good example of the hidden curriculum at work recently. I had visited a school and was just about to go out through the main door when a student walked across my path and bumped into me. One of the teachers saw this happen and bellowed angrily, 'Smith, lad, get out of the way. We talked about good manners and respect for others last lesson; now, get your grimy body off the floor and apologise!' How vital it is (and how easy) to detect the working of the hidden curriculum in a school – the ethos of a happy, caring community or an atmosphere of hostility and oppression.

So the teacher has to be a sensitive person, caring for the individual, concerned for the development of the whole student, and one who can communicate with others. Often this picture of a paragon teacher is said to be unrealistic. It would seem, however, that the majority of primary teachers and many secondary teachers seem to meet the demand, and certainly if schools are to achieve their aims in promoting sensitive, integrated, sociable, responsible and learned students, one is only seeking the sort of person that should be the product of the education system itself.

There are, of course, problems. One in particular is that of the amount of time spent with a particular group of students. The primary teacher has virtually the same students all week. The secondary teacher has *any* number – I once had to face something like 400 different students in a week, and being 'sensitive and caring' for each one was particularly difficult since learning their names was a big enough problem! Perhaps the solution to this predicament is that the teacher has first to limit herself to a particular group of students with the aim of getting to know one group very well. This, perhaps, indicates the vital role a form teacher can fill, though it does not have to be limited to the relation of the form teacher to the form group. It could equally be the decision of a French teacher to concentrate on knowing her first-year French group particularly well.

This may all seem an odd preamble to the role of health education and the affective areas in the development of skills. However, I think it is very important that any form of education, and that includes health education in particular, must be dependent on people – the teachers – to achieve its aims, and cannot rely on materials, or the authoritarian controller.

We must now ask what material props the teacher might use if she or he is to initiate child-centred learning which starts with the students and their feelings, leads into a consideration of connected factors and facts, and results in appropriate decisions being made or the students' ability to cope with life's situations? There have been a number of resources developed over the past few years which do have this starting point in mind. The ILEA have produced a wide range of materials. There has been growing development and use of 'Trigger' films as discussion starters. The Schools Council has produced two curriculum projects, *Lifeline* (McPhail, 1972) and, more recently, the 9–13 Moral Education Project *Startline* (Schools Council, 1978). *Living Well* (McPhail, 1977), sponsored by the Health Education Council, is a very good example of the type of resource that can be used flexibly in the classroom to promote and involve students and teachers with aspects of health education. Teachers do need a concrete material support, particularly until they become confident in their role and the aims and approaches for health education, and *Living Well* offers such material support.

Living Well is a curriculum development project sponsored by the Health Education Council and directed by Peter McPhail at the University of Cambridge. Begun in 1973, the project was published in 1977 and is divided into three parts.

'And How Are We Feeling Today?'

This is a set of 35 work cards presenting situations which are of direct concern to students and which arise from young people's experience at home, work and school. An entertaining cartoon on the front of each card introduces a topic, and practical straightforward questions and work on the back help to stimulate group discussion, role play, writing and other activities.

'Support Group'

This is a set of 35 work cards which illustrate, by means of photographs and drawings, situations which people might find difficult or complex. As with 'And How Are We Feeling Today?' there are questions on the reverse of each card which suggest possible directions for the development of discussion and group work. The material does not aim to provide many facts but rather gives experience and practice in identifying what is happening, recognizing what other people are feeling, deciding what to do, and taking responsibility for one's own actions, as well as developing the ability to communicate with others who are under emotional and mental stress.

The cards are intended to interest teachers and students in group activities which encourage the exploration of feelings, attitudes and possible courses of action in a variety of encounters with others.

'Who Cares?'

This is a collection of 43 dialogues involving teenagers and adults who are, in a sympathetic way, helping the youngsters to grow up and who reported the dialogue verbatim. The range of situations is wide, stretching from the major incident that rates a paragraph in the local paper to the minor challenges of everyday life with which every teenager has to cope.

Notes and linking passages set the scene, and every dialogue has the authentic flavour of reality, with its confusions and unanswered questions.

The student is invited to participate, to imagine taking the part of the adult or the young person and to answer the questions: 'What went wrong?' 'How could the handling of the situation have been improved?' 'What happened next?' 'What would you have done?' Through involvement with a situation which is not their own, students are helped to handle their own lives. The material will also help young people, as they grow in emotional maturity, to handle more confidently the feelings and difficulties of others.

The overall aim of the project is 'to promote healthy living by helping young people cope with and approach positively the challenges, complexities, difficulties and anxieties of everyday life'. It is the last two words of the statement that raise the project out of the realm of ordinary class materials to that of a relevant and useful class resource. However, rather than concentrate on the theory and description of the project, it would seem preferable to give just two examples of how use of this material can promote and develop young people's capacity to make decisions and cope with practical situations by reference to experience in the classroom.

The first example concerns a first-year class (11–12-year-olds), of mixed ability, in a co-educational comprehensive school. The lesson was humanities. Work in humanities was through a thematic approach and the class had been covering a theme on monsters. It was the end of the first term of the students' first year in secondary school. It was apparent to the teacher that John was not happy, nor was he integrated with the rest of the class. The rest of the class did not think too much of John for they saw that his ability to antagonize staff and be disruptive was affecting their work and reputation as a class. Indeed he had become the scapegoat for all trouble in the group, whether he was responsible or not. It must be added that he *was* frequently responsible for many of the problems which the teachers experienced with this group.

Something had to be done about this situation. The class attitude to John, articulated by the vociferous few, was that he should be punished, preferably caned, in order to 'make him behave'. The teacher in question decided things had come to a head, and as a varied approach, and because he wanted to confront the class with the problem of John, decided to use one of the 'And How Are We Feeling Today?' cards from *Living Well*.

He asked the class to move the desks and sit in a semicircle. He then started talking about the problem of bullying which he had encountered on break duty that day. He said he would like to consult the class for their views on how they would deal with bullying. He produced the *Living Well* card which shows a teacher wielding a cane and saying to a young student, 'I'll

teach you to hit boys smaller than yourself'. A number of students contributed to the discussion, raising various points about the value or otherwise
of corporal punishment, the problem of bullying and fear of teachers, and
once the topic had 'caught fire' the teacher suggested that the large group
should split into five groups of six and that each group produce a summary
of their response to the situation card. Ten minutes went by and the groups
discussed the issues, with more people making contributions than in the
large group. Many began to recount their own experiences of being
punished or being bullied and it was obviously a topic that had relevance for
the majority, if not all of the students.

After this time the teacher brought the whole group together in a semicircle and asked for the group reports. It was in one of the reports that a group
mentioned that the issue of how to treat an 'offender' was similar to the way
John's misbehaviour was being viewed by the class – 'when one of us
misbehaves, John, for example, the rest of us say he should be punished or
we all get at him'. The reporter continued by saying that the group did not
think corporal punishment or bullying had a good effect and 'so we think we
don't handle John properly'.

The discussion had now moved to a real problem which the class had
identified and personalized. Other contributors came in and suggested that
people only behave badly for a reason, giving examples from their own
experience, or noting that the more one shouts at a person the more likely he
or she is to cause trouble.

The next stages, to be very brief, consisted of the teacher initiating more
small group work on what makes people behave antisocially and how *they*
would go about dealing with someone who was a behaviour problem. He
encouraged some role play to try out situations and ended up with the full
group together asking for final comments. The most articulate lad stood up
and said, 'Our group thinks we have been wrong in the way we treat John;
it's no wonder his behaviour does not get better.' There was general
agreement. The lesson ended with a promise of follow-up of how the
treatment of John or any other person who has problems might be handled
in a better way than the one suggested by the teacher on the card. The class
had already, in their groups, made some decisions on how to cope with their
own behaviour and John's, but obviously needed time to structure their
ideas with reference to particular cases.

Obviously the teacher had been keeping a close eye on John all this time.
He had kept quiet during the large group discussion, beaming when his
name was first mentioned for he was getting the attention which his whole

behaviour pattern indicated he craved for. In the small groups he contributed quite freely and when his group asked him why he behaved as he did he was inclined to be defensive and put the blame on 'you lot' (i.e., the class). As the lesson continued John became more subdued and it was obvious to the teacher that he had to have a personal chat before the lesson finished and John disappeared. In this chat John became tearful at first, and then, obviously puzzled by the concern of the class, started to talk about some of the things that he felt made him behave in a way that led him into trouble. The chat ended with John (not the teacher) deciding he would 'try and make more effort to be good' and that he was glad that the class had been able to talk openly about the situation.

What happened next? Well, it is not the happy ending one might have hoped for; at least, not entirely. However, it was obvious to the teacher, and from the comments of other teachers who took that class, that John was making efforts not to be so disruptive. The class, in particular certain individuals, were at one extreme supportive and keen to be friendly towards John, and at the other extreme ignored the behaviour which they previously might have become indignant about. The development since then has been somewhat varied. John's problems are deep-rooted and need more specialized effort than the school is able to offer, and even if the class are more sensitive and supportive of John than they used to be, the same cannot be said for some of the staff whose attitudes have an effect on both John and the class.

I have gone to some lengths to tell this story because I think it indicates certain features that are vital to positive health education. This is not to say that because *Living Well* was used problems were solved. It does say that teachers need to be sensitive of the interaction among the individuals in a group, and when problems exist to try and do something positive rather than ignore them and continue with the subject teaching. It does infer that material support such as the *Living Well* material is a useful stepping stone into the area of personal relationships, of understanding and trying to cope with human behaviour. It does indicate that the way the class is organized in terms of physical environment and the use of small groups is an important key to encouraging students to discuss and understand different points of view on human behaviour and how to cope with the variety of behaviour. It suggests that the chance to try out certain ways of behaving through role play, drama or other activities, gives individuals an opportunity to work out various ways of coping with other people; this can then be carried over into the realities of everyday interaction and behaviour. And, perhaps most importantly, it would seem to indicate that allowing the above things to happen does have an effect on the way groups and individuals behave, support, understand or cope with one another.

My initial stress on the role of the teacher is borne out by the above example. The teacher has the important function of allowing things to happen. She or he needs to be aware of the undercurrents of the particular situation, and to be sensitive to the individuals whose behaviour may come under discussion. The teacher needs to see such work not only as crisis-based, as in the example, but as a general pattern of allowing students to make decisions and have a chance to see the outcomes of such decisions. This means a willingness to move into the affective areas, the everyday behaviour and experiences relevant to people's interaction and communication. It means providing opportunities by the teacher's attitude and the choice of resources and different approaches and methods (group work, role play, drama, creative work, audiovisual material, tape, etc.) for students to explore their behaviour and learn what behaviour is appropriate. Passive acceptance, rote learning, note-taking or copying, isolation, anxiety, irrelevance, the notion of 'filling an empty vessel' are common features of some teachers' methods, and can hardly be promoted as inducements to self-discipline, autonomy, or to decision-making skills or the ability to cope with people or situations. Action, participation, collaboration, discussion, involvement, relevance must become apparent if the teacher hopes to reach the stage where young people can decide and act responsibly for themselves.

The second example is shorter but re-iterates all that has been said above and indicates that the development of coping strategies and decision-making skills is not confined to the more abstract areas of inerpersonal relationships, but can promote an input of knowledge which previously had been seen as the only requirement for health education lessons. If one can marry the knowledge with the behaviour and attitudes, then such knowledge can be transferred from 'head knowledge' to 'action knowledge'.

A fourth-year group was working on the theme 'My body'. Within this theme there was a section on drugs, and the teacher began this session by producing the 'Support Group' card about smoking, which bore the statement 'I know all the facts but I can't give up'. He then initiated various activities. Those who had a sympathetic response to the statement formed one group, those who did not smoke formed another group and those who said they really did not know the facts formed a third group. Each group had to present their case to the others. Obviously some interesting views were put forward, but perhaps most interesting were the two issues which led to the work of the next three weeks. First, the majority decided that they did not know the facts even though they thought they did. Secondly, there was a desire to try and influence those who smoked, or did not smoke. The youngsters sought to consider the nature and operation of 'feelings' and their relation to 'knowledge'; which should have priority or how could they be allowed to interact? The activities that ensued involved all manner of research into people's smoking habits, reasons for and against smoking, interviewing a doctor, display work on the effects of smoking, graphs and charts on smoking habits of various age-groups, antismoking posters, a chart of the case in favour of smoking, discussions on why people start or stop smoking and so on. Not only were those students involved in an issue which they felt to be relevant to themselves, their parents and friends, but they were also learning why people behave in certain ways, a tolerance of different views and the facts on smoking. Furthermore they were employing all the skills that society stresses ought to be acquired at school: reading, writing, research, comprehension, factual information, social, numerical, technical and creative skills.

Finally, the pupils met together again in their original three groups, and each person in the group presented the work they had done individually or with others and gave their case for or against smoking once more. A notable change had occurred in the group that had smoked even though they knew the facts. Not only did the majority of the group decide to try and give up smoking, or had already done so, but those who continued to smoke were at least able to give account of their feelings as to why they smoked and would continue to do so.

So, once again, with the teacher as the initiator and guide, young people had been able to start from the area of human experience and go out into the cognitive domain, to consider other views and attitudes, and then to return to their own behaviour in relation to an informed decision or an ability to cope with the issue of smoking.

Surely this is where health and education come together. They are concerned with understanding and, as a result of this, with a self-imposed modification or continuation of behaviour. The use of such materials as *Living Well* allows the teacher to start with the all-important affective area, and from this base one can move into the knowledge or cognitive areas, and then back to pupils' attitudes and behaviour. The effects of equipping young people with the skills of being able to cope, make decisions, and make aware and informed choices about behaviour can be far-reaching, as in the experience of a Nottingham school. Beginning with a discussion on student attitudes to the elderly there followed a survey of amenities, involvement with the old people in their community and a document to County Hall about the need for more to be done for the elderly in their community. The report was in fact acted upon by the Council. In this instance the experience of the pupils had developed from an initial sharing of feelings and experiences, through a process of finding out and acquiring knowledge, to action and involvement, and finally out into the community. Is this what we mean by health education?

Summary

This chapter examines recent developments in health education resources which allow consideration of the affective areas. It centres in particular on the Health Education Council Project *Living Well*, and attempts to illustrate that the approach and attitude of the teacher is all-important if such resources are to be effective in allowing students to develop their own attitudes and strategies of behaviour. Any development in the resources needs to be supported by a consideration of the most appropriate methods if their implementation is to achieve the desired objectives.

References

McPhail, P. (1972) *Moral Education in the Secondary School*. Schools Council Lifeline Series. London, Longman.

McPhail, P. (1977) *Living Well*. Health Education Council Project 12–18. Cambridge, Cambridge University Press.

Schools Council (1978) *Moral Education in the Middle Years*. Startline Series. London, Longman.

PART V

DEVELOPING AND EVALUATING HEALTH EDUCATION

INTRODUCTION

Visitors to be interviewed by pupils, visiting speakers and outside resources are of continual benefit to teachers in numerous subjects. In health education there exist extensive resources and manpower in the paramedic services, and we therefore need to look at responsible ways to use them. Liaison between education and health authorities in health education in schools appears to us to have been improving considerably in recent years. This is associated with increasing professionalism among health staff concerned with health education, and with a growing understanding of health education and confidence in its practice among teachers. The role of the Health Education Council in supporting projects and schemes of school health education has been increasingly important in the improvement of liaison. Whilst the major work of health education in schools must inevitably lie with teachers, the development of extensive co-operation with other professional workers is essential. In the past too much responsibility for health education has been given by teachers to health staff; now the balance is becoming more sensible and more professional in our opinion.

Ian McCafferty taught for ten years in a comprehensive school and a college of technology. He then worked as deputy director of the Schools Council Health Education Project 5–13 for three years before becoming area health education officer for Nottinghamshire. He is now extensively involved in local dissemination and training related to various school health education curriculum projects at primary and secondary level. He is also currently engaged in the development of training materials designed to improve the teaching techniques of health service personnel, particularly community nurses. He is in an extremely good position to review the use of visitors and other resources from a wide range of perspectives, having worked both inside and outside schools.

Increasingly teachers ask for in-service training. In our current economic situation a heavy responsibility therefore falls upon providers to ensure that courses and other facilities are as effective as possible. James Cowley reviews the field of such training in Chapter 16, and his concluding remarks crystallize important thoughts in the quality versus quantity argument.

James Cowley was originally a secondary school teacher. For five years he was the national director of TACADE, a national organization specializing in health and social education generally, and in drug and alcohol education specifically, leading a full-time staff concerned with in-service training, resource publication, resource services and consultancies and research. He then moved to the Open University with responsibility for developments in personal and social education in the section concerned with the in-service education of teachers. He is now Director of Health Promotion for the Government of South Australia Health Commission. His studies, all of which have been part-time, are mainly in psychology.

Continuing the theme of Chapter 16, Marilyn Stephens explores the necessity for evaluation in Chapter 17 and suggests various methods and ideas which teachers can use as they think about evaluating their work in health education. Increasingly health education is being asked to prove itself useful, and Marilyn Stephens has seen the need for this as a teacher, as a health education officer and then in the role of evaluator to the two Schools Council Health Education Projects. She has also acted as consultant to a number of research projects.

CHAPTER 15

THE ROLE OF VISITORS AND AREA HEALTH EDUCATION TEAMS

Ian McCafferty

Health education holds a curious and in many ways unique position in the school curriculum today. A historical view of health is that over a period of time it has become the province of what we now call the medical profession. This profession has by force of circumstance mainly performed a curative role, and the word 'health' therefore has now become synonymous in people's minds with the cure of disease. As the patterns of disease have changed, however, it is evident that the majority of diseases now causing serious illness or death are largely the result of man's own health behaviours. Obvious examples of this would be lung cancer brought about by smoking, heart disease due to smoking, diet or the absence of exercise, accidents and the increase of venereal diseases. A logical progression of the argument is, therefore, that if these diseases are the result of particular health behaviours, then we should be able to prevent them by altering those behaviours. How these health behaviours can be changed or whether they should be changed is not the province of this particular chapter, but in the context of the present discussion we may observe that one thread of the argument suggests that if people were better educated about their health then they might make better health decisions.

Health education, therefore, should form an integral part of the attempt to prevent ill health. Thus a variety of recent reports, such as those dealing with nutrition, alcoholism, child health and violence in the family, to name but a few, have all pressed the demand for schools to provide more health and social education which may lead to greater understanding of these and other areas. Education is therefore being encouraged to take a major role in the field of prevention, and to develop the partnership between health and education to a degree never attempted before. Health education is at present lying uneasily balanced between the two professions.

The medical professions see clear health trends as the result of activities such as smoking, drinking, eating particular types of food and failing to exercise. Their demand is that information regarding these activities and their likely outcomes should be placed before people in an attempt to alter their behaviours. On the education side of health education there is a recognition of these basic health trends, but a recognition also of the great complexity of effective educational processes. Health education can be seen as a fusion of health, which describes the content, and of education which should provide the process.

Given that the cause and effect of a majority of health issues are relatively clear – accidents, smoking and venereal diseases for example – and that only a minority such as heart and circulatory disease are not so straightforward, it would seem logical that the major effort in health education should be the exploration and development of the complex issues of changing attitudes, values and health behaviours. In other words it is important now to make serious attempts to improve the process of health education rather than to argue about its content. It is curious then that the greatest commitment to health education remains with the health service at both national and local level, for the majority of work on health education is either carried out by the DHSS through the Health Education Council, or locally by area health authorities through their health education departments. Though the DES has made clear its support of health education in schools through its own publications and through the Schools Council, it remains true that the greater level of finance and initiatives remain with the health service side of health education.

The purpose of these opening paragraphs has been to outline the context from which a teacher often has to begin when attempting to develop health education in the classroom. He may well have been subjected over a period of time to the view that health and its attendant issues are the province of the medical profession, and may therefore feel unsure as to his role in educating children about their own health. It is unlikely that he will have received any initial training which will have equipped him to teach health education as a subject in schools. It is by no means certain that there will be anyone in the local education authority team of inspectors or advisers who will be providing support or training. It is not altogether surprising, therefore, that many teachers, faced with their own increasing conviction that something needs to be done to educate the children in their care about the health and social issues which they will face, turn to the health profession whose province this appears to be. Many schools with health education programmes have begun in precisely this way, with teachers seeking the active teaching support of doctors, health visitors, nurses, dentists and so forth. Some schools developed complete programmes around visiting speakers, and thus treated this area of the curriculum in a way which they would not contemplate for any other area.

The situation is of course changing rapidly. Many schools have now incorporated health education as part of their own curriculum and are increasingly supported by new curriculum development and other health education materials which are now reaching the market in profusion. There is, however, no clear pattern or policy for training in health education either at initial or in-service levels, and it is still quite possible for teachers to feel that they lack support to take the initiatives in this area. The purpose of this chapter, therefore, is to look at the nature of the support teachers might receive from health and other professions, and at the ways in which schools may profitably use them, but this will always be in the context of the belief that health education in schools is basically the province of teachers.

There are a very large number of people outside schools whose job either normally requires that they should be prepared to contribute to health education in schools, or who feel themselves, that as a result of experiences in their own field, they would like to contribute in some way to health education. Most schools refer to them as outside speakers. An obvious but not exhaustive list would include such people as health visitors, school nurses, school medical officers, general practitioners, hospital staff, dentists, chiropodists, pharmacists, dieticians, and from the non-health fields people such as education welfare officers, environmental health officers, the police, social workers, workers from voluntary agencies and so forth. In a recent exercise in Nottinghamshire a secondary school found nearly thirty actual or potential local visitors to the school who could possibly have something to contribute to a health education programme. Health education officers were not included in the list because they form rather a different category. As distinct from visitors who may wish to contribute in specific areas related to their own qualifications or experience, health education officers have a responsibility to promote and support health education in the schools within their area and it is obvious that this is a far more onerous and complex task. The two groups are clearly different in terms of both their character and roles, and it is important to establish at an early stage the background and training of both groups and how they are at present used by schools. We will then examine ways in which current curriculum development and organization might change the setting in which these groups may work in the future, and conclude with a discussion as to what realistic future role the two different teams may have in schools.

Training and Backgrounds

The problem with any general discussion of the background of visitors is the obvious one that there is no uniform pattern. A major criterion which may be used to judge their suitability for health education in schools must be the question, 'Are they capable of talking to groups of children?' Within the health professions, for example, only health visitors will have had any formal instruction in talking to groups of children, but much will again depend on where and when the health visitor was trained, on the amount and type of school work that her field-work teacher was involved in and so forth. Health visitors are the only members of the visitors' group, as outlined above, who have a professional responsibility to contribute to health education in schools within their own areas. One has to be realistic, however, about what can be expected, for within the ranks of health visitors there will be those who can talk to children and enjoy doing so, and equally there will be many who cannot and who do not enjoy teaching.

For the rest, doctors, nurses, pharmacists and dieticians may well be expert in their own fields but there is no guarantee that this expertise will be translated into dynamic and interesting teaching, for at the present time no part of their training includes formal teaching techniques and many do not receive help in group discussion techniques either. Much will depend on their own personality and teaching ability as to whether they relate well to children, and it is a risky business to base any health education programme on the contribution of expert outsiders until they have been tried and tested. One point to be borne in mind, however, is that those who work regularly in schools, on medical inspections or dental inspections for example, are perhaps more likely to pitch things at the right level than those who do not. There is also the point that many outsiders still fear the unfamiliar school situation and are thus less likely to wish to contribute than those who are familiar with it on a day-to-day basis. We shall consider later how outside visitors may be selected and used.

Health education teams, however, should be in a different position, for part of their professional requirements should be the ability to communicate well. In 1971 the Health Education Council carried out a survey of the backgrounds of health education officers (Tones, 1977). Of the 80% who responded over 50% were from nursing, 16% were from teaching and the remainder from administration or some other background. Health education officers therefore may come from a number of disciplines but may also have completed either one of the health education diploma courses or one of the higher degrees now being offered in health education and allied subjects (see Appendix II). It is quite possible that an area health authority may have a team of health education officers who are able to offer both insight in their own particular disciplines and a good level of overall knowledge as to content and method in the delivery of health education.

The Present Role of Visitors

The ways in which visitors and health education officers are used in schools vary widely. The Schools Council (1976) describes the ways in which a number of outside speakers felt themselves misused. Some were left with very large groups of children, of 200 or more, some complained of being given very little information as to the background or progress of the children. Other visitors felt that they were brought in to deal with the topics which teachers did not wish to get involved in, and were only asked to talk about venereal disease, contraception and abortion, for example. Some of the more educationally aware speakers complained that theirs was the only input on a particular topic, and rightly wondered just how much was likely to be retained by the children in these 'one-off' lessons.

It would be wrong, however, to suggest that misuse is the most common practice with visitors. Many schools have developed a regular liaison with a number of outside speakers, and many of the speakers see contact with a school as being important to their own knowledge of future generations of local citizens. Health visitors, for example, may well see the opportunity to regularly visit a school within their area as an admirable way to develop the confidence of future parents who may be their responsibility. One could see a case for the police, dentists or general practitioners to feel the same. Such development, however, requires the use of the same people over a period of time to develop this confidence, but in many cases staff turnover or reorganization unfortunately may well make long-term development and confidence difficult. It requires also that the school has established health education as part of the curriculum which will continue, despite staff changes. Too often established liaison declines or ceases because one committed member of staff moves elsewhere.

It is interesting to look at exactly what some visitors are asked to do by schools. Perkins (1978) sought to establish what health visitors in one large health authority taught in schools and how this teaching was planned. Counselling pupils on health matters, and advising schools on health problems as a precursor to the planning of health education programmes were comparatively rare occurrences. It is not really surprising that the advisory role remains limited, for comparatively few schools have an established structure for health education which would facilitate the use of outsiders as curriculum advisers. A health visitor cannot be expected to fully understand the organization and curriculum problems of a large comprehensive school, for example. It is the school's responsibility to nominate one person, a co-ordinator, who can liaise with and learn how to use the expertise of outsiders like health visitors. By contrast with the advisory role, the greater part of the health visitors' time was spent in teaching groups of children. Half the teaching was done in secondary schools and one-third in junior schools. The principle findings of the survey indicated that the majority of health visitors were teaching courses which mainly comprised the body systems and hygiene with the younger age-groups, or a general course on health including some basic physiology and such areas as smoking, alcohol and sex education with the older groups. The third highest utilization of health visitors' time was in teaching child development or child-care courses.

A number of questions need to be asked about these findings. Is it really necessary to have a trained person of this calibre to teach simple physiology and hygiene to younger children? These are subjects which any competent teacher could learn enough about for the needs of primary school children. In the secondary schools is it realistic to ask health visitors to teach about the dangers of alcohol, smoking, venereal diseases, accident prevention and so forth? Most health visitors, though informed on these topics, would not describe them as being their first concern or one requiring their particular expertise. Again there is a great deal of resource material and information available which a competent and interested teacher can use, and which can be fitted in many cases into existing subject areas. In addition, the contribution of the outsider is limited in most cases to factual input, by time and availability if nothing else. When one considers that the affective side of most health topics is at least as important as the factual input, it is difficult to see how any visitor can take on the major contribution in any subject area.

In the case of child development and child care however, there is a very obvious case for using the health visitors' expertise, but it would seem that on the strength of this study such work did not occupy the majority of the health visitors' teaching time. This point, I think, brings to light some of the difficulties which health education faces in its initial stages of development in schools. Many teachers feel that they are not competent to handle what they consider to be a specialist subject with some potentially difficult or embarrassing areas. They may therefore rely on outside experts to carry the responsibility for this in the school. For their part many health visitors are loath to refuse to help in a school, particularly if they are aware that the children there are in real need of this type of education and that if the health visitor does not carry out this function then nobody will. Some openly hope that by taking on the responsibility in the first instance they may encourage the teachers themselves to take over as time progresses. To some degree this hope has been justified by a subsequent growth of health education in schools, but this does not happen in all cases and there are still too many instances where the withdrawal of a health visitor who has been teaching in a school has been followed by an end to any health education activity. It is certainly the case that guidance and advice for such visitors should be available from health education teams, but the central point remains that health education must be the responsibility of the school itself. The contribution of visitors should be an outside stimulus and support, and not the major part of any programme.

The very positive value of outside speakers is often emphasized by the schools themselves. In the secondary age-range particularly, some children show a reluctance to question or confide in members of staff about personal or health matters, even sometimes where a pastoral system exists. However, after the teaching session has ended, many speakers such as nurses, health visitors and doctors find themselves talking to individual children who are happier to discuss things with an uninvolved outsider than they would be with a teacher who is part of the school establishment. Sessions such as these are often valuable and perhaps point to the need for greater accessibility of such people to children. Though this may throw a justifiably unfortunate light on the pastoral system in some schools, it would be unfair to suggest that this is automatically the case. However good the pastoral or counselling staff in a school may be, children, just like adults, might prefer to choose their own sounding boards and sources of information rather than the official channels.

This would be an opportune time to mention the possible contribution of school nurses, particularly those who are based in an institution such as a comprehensive school. Apart from their statutory medical duties, many who are based in a school find that they will often be seen as a person who can be confided in on health and personal matters, and will over a period of time develop what amounts to an alternative counselling role. They are thus well aware of the real needs and problems of children in this age-group, and apart from any formal teaching which the school may ask of them, they will certainly be in an excellent position to advise on the need for teaching in certain subject areas within the health education curriculum. Many head-teachers who are in the fortunate position of having good school nurses, prize the contribution they can make.

When we come to examine what schools may at present expect of an outside speaker, more fundamental questions arise. Let us use one situation which is not uncommon. Some schools like to invite outside speakers to talk to children about some particular aspect of health education, for example drugs. The school may see drugs as having connections with legal problems and may therefore consider a policeman to be the right person to invite to talk. The policeman in turn may see his duty as being to warn children of the dangers as he sees them, perhaps in terms of health or social problems, or more particularly regarding the law. The children, depending on their individual ages, backgrounds and experiences, may be at a variety of stages in their knowledge, they may have different attitudes and different behaviours with regard to drugs.

The potential problems here are clear. The school itself may well not have a clear picture as to what the session is supposed to achieve. Is it to inform the children about drugs or about using drugs? Is it to help them clarify their own views about drugs or to alter their views, or to attempt to bring about direct behavioural change? We might ask if the session is supposed to do any of these things, for one disturbing element in much secondary education is the assumption that by having a topic 'covered', something intrinsically satisfactory is happening. The clearest answer to this would be if the visitor's session was only one part of a process where all these cognitive, affective or behavioural issues had been clarified. This is not always the case; were it so, the need for a visitor and the clarification of his role would be evident.

When we consider the session from the visitor's viewpoint, further considerations need to be made. Apart from the person's ability to com-municate, one would ask whether he has been made aware of the role which the school expects him to play in this process. He will need to know the level and background of the children, the preparatory work which has led up to his visit and how the school proposes to use his work afterwards. He would also need help with any audiovisual presentation he wanted to make. It is not the duty of a visitor to do this preparatory thinking; it is the responsibility of the school to make him aware of what part in the process he is to take, of the most valuable contribution he could make and to assist him to deliver just that. Not all schools are prepared at present to take this sort of trouble with their visitors. The fundamental questions to be asked then are these: does this topic require a level of expertise which cannot be provided by the teachers? Has the school thought through the precise requirements to be made of this visitor? Is the visitor aware of and capable of fulfilling these requirements?

The Present Use of Health Education Teams

The role of health education teams is rather more clearly defined. Following the reorganization of the National Health Service and local government (DHSS, 1974), their function as regards schools was outlined as follows: 'AHA's should be prepared to co-operate with local education authorities, education establishments, teachers and parents' associations in assisting in identifying health education needs, and by providing speakers, materials, information and advice on health education matters. They should also be prepared to help local education authorities on the in-service training of teachers in health education.' It is as well to point out, however, that school health education is only one of their functions, since they are required to provide health education for the whole community. Apart from working through schools they would also be expected to provide health education assistance for community nurses, hospitals, general practitioners, the social services, voluntary organizations, environmental health officers, occupational health services, the media and all the many other agencies who may carry out some health education function and require support from the health education department. When one recognizes that in an area of say 250,000 people the total number of health education officers in a department might be no more than two, with some clerical assistance, the enormity of the task becomes clearer, and sympathy with what may have seemed inadequate support becomes rather easier to give. In their support for education, however, they have three major functions: to define needs, to provide resources and to provide or assist with training.

The resources aspect is clearly the most straightforward of these. Most health education teams would see one of their traditional functions as being the running of a resources centre. These will not be uniform in the quantity and quality of their contents, and will depend to some extent on the level of financial support which the department receives from the area health authority. The resources will probably include a wide variety of films, slides, tapes, models and possibly video cassettes. There will also be a large quantity of printed materials in the form of leaflets and posters. Some health education departments will have a library of appropriate books and journals and may also be able to provide specific information and statistics on health matters. Many centres now have technicians who are skilled in the use of audiovisual aids and who are able to assist schools and give them the benefit of their expertise.

The character and type of many of the resources are to some extent determined by what is commercially available at the time, films being an obvious example. Some schools rely heavily on outside resources to support a programme of health education, and will build a year's work around either what is available on film or whatever television series are running at the time. A certain similarity of pattern may therefore be deduced in many schools, which develop their work around what is available from health education resource centres, which have in turn gathered their materials from available commercial and other sources. One ought not to under-emphasize the amount of influence which resources have on what is taught. In an area where many teachers are uncertain, they will rely on what is available to support their programme, particularly in the initial stages. Many visitors to schools will also rely on some sort of aid, such as a film, to help them through if they are uncertain as to their own capacity to teach. It is by no means unheard of for a teacher to visit a resources centre and plan a term's health education programme around what is available on the date and time when the class is to be taken, or for a visitor who has to teach in a school to book the resource being used solely to fill in the amount of time allocated. The function of the health education department may therefore be to provide both a breadth of resources and some clear guidance as to their worth and use.

The fact that what is actually done in schools is often overshadowed by the resources available may well be only a temporary situation, for as schools develop their own programmes and resources they will often tend to regard health education resource centres as a means by which they may be kept informed about new materials and ideas, and not as the definers of what they may do. In some ways this leads on to one of the other stated functions of health education teams, that of helping to define the health needs of children. This is an exceedingly complex matter, and not one where some glib definitions could be suggested. The observation that might be made in this context is that many schools new to the planning of health education will make the conventional assumptions that a programme, for example in the secondary sphere, should comprise work on smoking, alcohol, drugs, sex and so forth. These assumptions are often reinforced by the type of resources which are available to them, a large proportion of which fit exactly into the above pattern. Clearly schools have to have some recognizable framework to begin with, and this will often be topic-based. One of the functions of the health education team may be to encourage schools constantly to redefine their perceptions of the needs of the children they are teaching. Certainly where schools have been invited to reconsider what they teach, either by the use of teaching grids or questionnaires, even some established ones tend to find areas which are not taught or areas where there is a fundamental lack of purpose to that which is taught.

Many health education departments will also translate national concern into local action, through localized campaigns, etc. Through the provision of resources, information sessions, displays and so forth, they may bring to the notice of teachers some aspect of health education which is deemed worthy of national action, the eradication of the head louse or the reduction of adolescent drinking being examples. Not all departments work to support national campaigns in this way, but they will be aware of the relevant information and will be able to help in some respect.

A third function, that of in-service training for teachers, is of growing importance. The word 'training' in this context can have many meanings. Some work described as training is in fact information-giving. A particular topic is chosen, speakers assembled and the teachers are lectured to. In some cases there will be discussion groups, and if these predominate the training is then sometimes described as a 'workshop'. The giving of information is certainly one vital and viable aspect of the work of the health education department, and most teachers would recognize this as being valuable. Certainly where health education is in its initial stages, then an adequate level of knowledge about particular topics is essential for the teachers, in order to give them the confidence to work in these areas. The implication is that if teachers are given such information then it is up to them to use their basic expertise to translate this into work in the classroom.

However, if this approach goes no further than upgrading knowledge on particular topics, it ignores what is now happening to health education in schools; by far the most significant movements are those which are taking teaching away from a simple information-giving process, and looking more closely at, for example, the distinction between behaviour modification and education. Method in health education is becoming as important as content, and the school's organization in its delivery of health education is as significant as the topics which are taught. If health education officers are to fulfil their functions as partners with the local authorities in the provision of in-service training for teachers, there must be some clear recognition that these rather more sophisticated processes deserve at least as much attention as traditional information-giving.

Health education departments work for the health service and are seen as important arms of preventive medicine. The guidance and pressure which form and influence the work of such departments is primarily medically orientated, with a strong epidemiological impetus. Smoking, for example, is seen as an activity with known health implications, reductions in smoking would bring about known effects on chest and heart disease; therefore, the argument continues, one of the functions of health education should be to dissuade people from smoking, and let it be said that one of the methods approved of is the creation of anxiety as to the consequence of smoking. This is rather a long way from McPhail's aim (1977) in the *Living Well* material of supporting 'the growth of happy and creative involvement in which, as far as humanly possible an individual's needs, feelings and interests are recognised and met, and to combat children's slide into a lifestyle which is unhappy, sick and destructive of self or others'. Health education by this definition has radical overtones which attack social and political assumptions, and it contrasts sharply with what may be expected from those who take a behaviourist standpoint on specific health hazards. Tones (1977) has pointed to this problem within the ranks of community health education specialists, as he describes them. Are they by virtue of their links with the education system to propose and support educative materials with these radical overtones and the emphasis on free choice, or should they accept and support a behaviourist role which may more accurately reflect the views of a number of their medical colleagues? It is probably too early in the development of health education services to give any clear picture of what the likely responses would be to such a question. One has to accept that at this moment the response is more likely to be governed by the numbers and calibre of the staff involved and perhaps more significantly by the background of the officers themselves.

The Future Role of Health Education Teams in Schools

Tones (1977) brings us to the final consideration of the future role of health education teams in relation to health education in schools. It would clearly be erroneous to suggest that centrally developed curriculum materials will be accepted in their totality into any school curriculum. One might argue in fact that the fate of most Schools Council projects indicates precisely the opposite. Many have been received with interest upon their launching and have largely been forgotten after the passage of a comparatively short period of time. It would be equally erroneous to suggest that only centrally developed curriculum materials have any worth, for there is a case for suggesting that locally developed materials have a far greater chance of acceptance in their own area than those which may be imposed from without and may often be regarded as lacking relevance to major local problems. Considerable interest has, however, been shown in recent centrally developed materials by both schools themselves and by people responsible for stimulating this interest at a local level. Health education is in fact unique in having two possible agencies who may have an interest in stimulating, supporting and developing the quality of work done in schools, namely the education department's advisory team, and the area health authority's health education team. The words 'possible agencies' are used advisedly for one of the immediate difficulties is the lack of any standard pattern in the provision of specialist health education advisers in education authorities, or of education specialists within health education teams. Where both exist and are able to work in partnership then it is to the advantage of schools.

There are, however, potential pitfalls in the relationships. There is a considerable difference between an education authority giving a health education team carte blanche to work in its schools, and an education authority taking on its responsibilities in conjunction with the health education team. The former shrugs off responsibility, the latter recognizes that to be effective the partnership has to be seen to exist and initiatives have to be seen to come from the education authority. For example, a statement on health education from a director of education, or a questionnaire in his name asking about the organization of health education in his schools is likely to produce a more fundamental reaction than anything that a health education department can do on its own, no matter how good it may be. Regular queries from local advisers or inspectors on health education matters in their schools are more likely to produce results than persuasive publicity and handouts from health education officers, however good and well prepared these may be. Courses run by the local inspectorate are more likely to draw substantial numbers, whatever the topic, for it is natural that many good and ambitious teachers would wish to be seen by the inspectorate who may influence their later prospects. Such views are not, I think, cynical, but may represent a realistic view of what avenues of approach are more likely to have long-term effects in schools rather than short-term success.

Without responsibility for health education being shouldered equally by the education authority and the health education team, the latter is essentially in the position of an outsider without authority or access to decision- and policy-making and this is a less viable position in the promotion of this area of the curriculum. The fostering of this partnership is therefore of key importance in the long-term development of a health education service. As regards the functioning of health education officers in schools, the study by Tones (1977) of the role of health education officers points to some possible dichotomy in the ways in which they think they should work. Nearly half the officers in 1974 considered that direct teaching in schools was a continuing and important part of their function. It will be evident from the descriptions elsewhere of new curriculum materials that the emphasis now is totally on the ways in which the schools should involve the children themselves in the process of discovery, or discussion or decision-making, looking at the roots of health education, attitudes and health behaviour, rather than treating or attacking the results. One of the most common manifestations of this different approach is the emphasis on group work and discussion, demanding small groups and high levels of staffing. It becomes less clear how direct teaching by outsiders on a regular basis can be justified, either in terms of their own time or in terms of the overall aims of the health education programme. It will take time for many schools to become confident in their total responsibility for all aspects of health education teaching, notably in the more controversial areas of contraception, abortion, venereal disease and so forth. Some areas do indeed benefit by the inclusion of some first-hand professional experience, for example child-care courses where the health visitor has so much to offer, but the ultimate aim should remain the same: teachers themselves should be encouraged and enabled to teach health education.

What then is the future contribution of health education teams? Many officers in Tones' survey included training as a major part of their function. The meaning of training in this context has already been examined, but an immediate determinant of what can be attempted will be the background of the officers involved. It has to be accepted that there are many levels of training, from straight information-giving to highly structured workshop techniques such as those used by TACADE, which have taken years to develop. Many points on that spectrum are within the compass of a health education team, with the right background and training, but I think that it is significant that new projects such as the Schools Council Health Education Projects 5–13 and 13–18 (1977) have invested a great deal of time in devising highly developed workshop training techniques and are suggesting long-term training programmes for teachers, leading possibly in the future to diplomas in health education. No health education department has the time, resources or even techniques to develop this level of training, but certainly the team should be aware of training organizations in the field and should be willing and able to support such work in their own areas, in addition to more straightforward dissemination or information-giving work of their own.

As mentioned earlier, the function of the health education department as an advice and resources centre is vital. Many teachers will be interested in new curriculum developments, but they may well require assistance in the early stages of use and information as to how other schools are using the materials. The team should therefore familiarize itself with how such materials may be used, and of the results of work done in the schools. Many areas have run pilot trials of materials in selected and interested schools as a means of creating interest and a pool of expertise in the use of the materials. If this type of work is carried out in conjunction with the advisory staff, maximum advantage will be taken of the possible cross-fertilization of ideas into other schools. Many of the projects suggest specific resources which have been used in the trial stages and have been recommended by teachers. If a health education resources centre carries quantities of these materials this will be of considerable help to teachers embarking on the work for the first time, for there is nothing more frustrating to teachers than to see recommended materials and have no local centre where they can be obtained. This is particularly true of course with items like films, slides or video tapes which are too expensive for the schools to procure themselves.

It might be suggested also that much curriculum development material has failed simply because interest has never been sustained after the initial impetus. It has been the experience of the author that even in schools where a great deal of early work has been done, it is possible to find that after two or three years little knowledge remains, staff may have changed, other subjects may have made demands and so forth. However salutary this may be to the initiator the case remains that many teachers know nothing of health education and one should not assume that because materials and ideas have been introduced once into a school, this means that the process will not have to be repeated many times. It may be necessary for health education teams to continue to reintroduce materials which, although familiar to them, may well not be to many of the teachers in their areas.

Increasingly in the secondary sphere the idea of planned and co-ordinated health education programmes is becoming accepted, but not all schools will have the personnel to begin these tasks. The assistance of a knowledgeable health education officer who is aware of the school structure, and of methods and styles of organization which would fit its particular circumstances, is often welcome, particularly in an area where there are no specialist advisers in health education to carry out this function. The current curriculum activity has certainly created considerable new interest in health education at both primary and secondary level, and it is all the more distressing therefore to hear of a minority of health education officers who see such development as a threat to their own situation, rather than as an opportunity to work in a different way with considerably more schools.

Conclusion

We conclude by summarizing the arguments so far presented in this chapter. It is indefensible to misuse outside visitors' time in teaching subjects which could easily be within the domain of the teacher. Some who have contributed for a long time to health education programmes in schools, for example health visitors, are concerned that what they have considered to be a vital and rewarding part of their work should be taken away from them. They consider that their presence in the school has a value over and above the teaching which they carry out, and many teachers would support this by pointing out the value of a new face talking about familiar subjects, and an authoritative and experienced viewpoint on matters where this is of value. None of these points are to be discounted, but it would seem that there is still an over-use of such people by some schools in teaching very general subjects. The criteria should be whether or not the visitor brings in some attribute which is vital to the health education process and which cannot be supplied by the school itself. Ironically the problem may in time solve itself, for increased demands made on fewer and fewer professional staff in the public sector have reduced their availability to a considerable degree.

What may a teacher reasonably expect from a health education team? Many teachers are unaware of the existence or location of the health education services for their area. Those wishing to locate them would be best advised to contact the area health authority headquarters direct, and ask for the whereabouts of the health education department. What level of support they may then expect from the department will depend very much on the personnel involved and the investment which the area health authority has made in the service. At the very least they should find quantities of printed materials such as leaflets and posters, together with a selection of films and slides which they may borrow without cost. If they are fortunate they will also find knowledgeable and experienced staff who have up-to-date information on all aspects of health education in schools and good advice to give on current curriculum developments. They will in this case probably already know of the existence of the health education service because they will have received information and publicity about the resources and services available, and will have been invited to courses and meetings on aspects of health education. In the best of all possible worlds they will also have been recommended to visit the department by the adviser with responsibility for their school, who is helping to implement a joint policy on health education devised by both the local education authority and the area health authority.

Summary

The position is taken that visitors can only have a subsidiary role in a school's health education programme, and that it is the school's responsibility to develop and structure this area of the curriculum. Reference is made to the benefits and shortcomings of visiting speakers and to the evidence that there is substantial misapplication of their skills and knowledge.

The role of health education teams is extensively discussed. The background of health education officers is considered and their traditional role as resource providers is seen as a vital but severely limiting factor. The development of health education as a curriculum issue by a number of national projects has demanded very different understanding and skills which have to be incorporated into the training role of health education officers.

It is suggested that benevolent but uninterested patronage by the LEA of the health education team's work leaves it in a fundamentally weak position. Without the active support and co-operation of the LEA such work lacks any real foundation in terms of lasting curriculum development. Genuine partnership with the LEA on in-service training, advice in schools and the development of policies is seen as essential.

References

Department of Health and Social Security (1974) Reorganization of National Health Service and of Local Government: Operation and development of services. *Health Education*, Circular HRC (74)5. HMSO, 1974.

Health Education Council (1977) *Living Well*. Health Education Council Project 12–18. Cambridge, Cambridge University Press.

McPhail, P. (1977) *Monitor*, vol. 46, p. 4.

Perkins, E. P. (1978) *Is Your Journey Really Necessary? The Role of the Health Visitor in Schools*. Leverhulme Health Education Project, Occasional Paper no. 8.

Schools Council (1976) *Health Education in Secondary Schools*. Working Paper 57. London, Evans/Methuen.

Schools Council (1977) Schools Council Health Education Project 5–13. London, Nelson.

Schools Council. Schools Council Health Education Project 13–18. (Forthcoming).

Tones, B. K. (1977) *Hlth Educ. J.*, vol. 36, p. 106.

CHAPTER 16

THE IN-SERVICE EDUCATION OF TEACHERS IN HEALTH EDUCATION

James Cowley

Early Influences upon the In-Service Education of Teachers

In the nineteenth and early twentieth centuries a large number of people who were developing the in-service education of teachers concentrated upon the social and physical health and well-being of the child and the role of the teachers. For instance, John Ruskin, to whom we are told we owe such developments as art teaching in schools, interest in nature study and the extension of playgrounds and playing fields, also has ascribed to him the responsibility for the major increase of interest amongst teachers in the medical and physical care of children. In the late nineteenth century we find Arnold, the well-known inspector at the Department of Education, travelling on the Continent. He brought back to this country the realization that schools were not solely concerned with academic learning but also with preparing children for a society which they would soon have to enter (Arnold, 1894).

Arnold recognized from his visits to the Continent that the outside world was increasingly moving into a philosophical turmoil. The traditional views that had been relatively unchallenged in England for several centuries were now being challenged by the influence of Darwinism and the new developments in teleology outside the Church, and the influence of the Oxford movement within the Church. He saw that it was important to knit together the academic aims of schools with the development of personal qualities and personal beliefs which might enable children to function in a society which was changing and under considerable pressure. Arnold thus encouraged better training for teachers.

This period also witnessed a massive growth in the range of bodies involved in the training and in-service training of teachers. When we arrive at the 1960s and 1970s, we find a field which is very accepting of *any type* of in-service education. It is a time when the whole plethora of educational activity which has occurred over the last 60 to 70 years comes to fruition in producing a wide choice of in-service training. Whilst it has been noted that the need for health and social education was recognized at an early stage, actual courses set up specifically for these topics do not seem to occur in the main until the 1960s. From there we seem to see a major increase in the number of courses and the number of people pressing for them.

Courses in Health and Social Education

Perhaps one of the major factors which prompted in-service training at a local level was the hysteria over certain types of problems which were being faced. Teachers in the 1960s recognized that they were now facing a different type of world, a world which was unlikely to be affected by war or undue economic strife but one where young people had more money, more freedom and what appeared to be changing values. It was a world where teenage groups found considerable uniformity in certain types of behaviour or in certain pop cultures. Around the early and mid-1960s teachers became very concerned indeed about some of the 'new' types of behaviour of young people. Local drug liaison committees were set up with the role of informing and supporting teachers. This was done by arranging various courses about drugs, and popularizing the taking of drugs as the 'new problem' of young people. Sometimes during these courses shock films were shown to teachers, who would hear from a police officer about the 'dreadful things' that were taking place.

As far as one can see, all this did was to isolate a new problem, to precipitate it and to make teachers feel that this was some type of expert field in which they were inexpert. They would hear an expert psychiatrist talking about drugs. They would be euphoric in the presence of the expert but would go away feeling more insecure about tackling that area within the curriculum than they were before they went (Cowley, 1968).

The natural progression from this was for the same expert who was once involved in talking to the teachers to be called into school to talk to the children. The same expert started to say what should be done in schools. One only has to look at some of the pressure groups operating in the drugs field around that time to see that it was easy for them to move from just saying what they witnessed in a counselling situation with drug takers to what they thought teachers should be doing. They became 'experts' over-night in education methodology and in health education. We have seen the same sort of 'training' continued today.

One major pressure on health education in-service training therefore comes from the needs of young people as perceived by teachers. It is essential that we recognize this as a pressure because it usually results in occasional courses being set up on certain topic areas. One questions whether education should alternate in a random way between one problem area and another.

The second source of pressure were the medical authorities. In the late 1960s they started to appoint many more health education officers to help to promote good health. The health education officer was often initially involved in going into schools, taking lessons for or with teachers or health visitors and trying to prompt activity. At that time this was perfectly acceptable because only a fairly small amount of health education was still being carried out in schools and many teachers believed this was not really their role.

Over the last five to ten years health education officers appear to have withdrawn from immediate contact with young people, leaving teaching to teachers. However, they were then left having to discover a new role for themselves. The role which has been established in very many areas has been that of 'trainers', and there is growing recognition among health education officers that training is a task requiring careful structuring and planning.

Another pressure for the provision of in-service training of teachers has come from national organizations. For instance the National Marriage Guidance Council has for many years been arranging various courses for teachers, training them particularly in counselling and group work skills. The Family Planning Association is another national organization which has been involved in in-service training. The Teachers' Advisory Council on Alcohol and Drug Education (TACADE) is a national organization which every year trains between 3000 and 4000 teachers in health education planning and co-ordination, and also specifically in the drug, alcohol, smoking and personal relationships areas of health education (TACADE, 1979).

Local education authorities provide another major source of in-service training. Most local education authorities have run some type of in-service training in health education, and some have been outstanding. Lancashire and Cleveland, for example, have well-organized programmes of education

in personal relationships, which look at the personal side of health education (Lancashire Education Authority, 1978; David and Cowley, 1980).

It seems that there are basically two forms of in-service training which
have developed over the last few years. In one approach, somebody decides
there is a need and organizes a course to fill that need. In the other approach,
somebody recognizes that teachers have a number of needs, but rather than
asking 'how do we put on a course to fulfil them?', instead asks, 'what *form*
of training may be *appropriate* and how should it be organized in order to
effect work practice of those who are taking part?' (Cowley, 1979*a*).

Different Forms for Different Aims

If a group leader in an in-service course has some specific aims, then one
form of training may not suit that particular aim. There are a whole range of
alternatives available.

Lectures

The emphasis in planning in-service work needs to be on the fact that those
who are present are adults and therefore have developed personal learning
styles. The lecture approach has been used widely in in-service education,
yet the lecture is most useful for conveying only certain types of messages.
In other words lecturing can be extremely useful for motivating people, for
giving them enthusiasm, for giving them a feel for a particular subject, for
giving them the opportunity to hear a large amount of information and
asking them to respond fairly vaguely to it. Lectures can have an euphoric
initial effect. People often feel they are sitting 'at the feet of an expert'. One
of the interesting side-effects of lectures is that they make people inclined to
invite another expert to actually do the job. For instance, those of us who
have been involved in lecturing know that teachers will at the end of the
lecture come and ask us to go into the school to talk to their own pupils. As
people hear a large amount of information, they can only recall a very small
amount of it. Very often they will then feel that they do not actually know
that particular field and so have to draw upon somebody else's expertise.
The overall findings from in-service research tend to indicate that we may
see very little effect upon *actual work practice* by the traditional lecture
approach, and we may need to move away from that towards a combination
of lectures and other types of learning experiences, where the lecture is
brought in only as the correct medium in a small number, in small parts of

courses (Barnes and Holloway, 1970; Thelen, 1971; Waynant, 1971; Eraut, 1972; Nagle, 1972; Safford, 1975; Stibbs, 1977).

The lecture/discussion sandwich

This method has been used to a large extent in health education work and yet it is not really the answer to the previously stated problem. Lectures followed by general discussion, as far as one can see, do not tend to have an immediate and influential effect upon work practice. It has been noted in a number of research studies (Neal and Mussenson, 1967; Neal and Radford, 1972; Barry, 1974; Coyle, 1974) that people comment on the time-wasting elements of discussions, where members may wonder where they are going, or may feel that a large amount of time is being spent on anecdotes rather than on getting to grips with the key issues which may then make them reflect on what they are doing in their everyday life. It has also been noted that the levels reached in general discussions are often not particularly deep and tend to remain superficial. There is one phenomenon which I particularly noted in the education of teachers in alcohol education, where one teacher would say, 'Ah, yes I was in the pub last night and there were a lot of young people there', the next would say 'Ah yes, all young people are getting problems with their drinking' and the next would say 'Lots of young people are becoming alcoholics'. This circular reaction tended to repeat itself as a phenomenon common to certain types of group discussion. People pick up anecdotes and a strong opinion leader in a group will swing the group possibly towards things which are not totally factual.

Research in in-service education has pointed towards the fact that the lecture-plus-discussion approach may have some effect on work practice, but this is likely to be a small one involving only a few of those actually attending the course. One would suspect that more developed methods are needed which relate better to the way in which adults actually learn.

Practical tasks linked to in-service education increase the effect

Some in-service education research has indicated that if people are asked to perform practical tasks in the middle of in-service work, if they are made to go back and look at their work practice, and if they are made to go back and try things out in the work practice, then it heightens the chance of in-service work actually having some type of long-term effect (Dalman, 1974; Safford, 1975; Hamilton et al., 1977). One particular form of training looked at the way in which the teacher increased or decreased the child's self-esteem (Cowley, 1979b). In a number of courses on pastoral care, this type of work has been developed with teachers constantly being referred back to look at their work practice. In a current Open University parenthood trials course, a considerable amount of in-service education requires teachers to be teaching in the classroom and reviewing the type of work they are actually doing (Cowley et al., 1980).

Practical tasks need conceptual reinforcement

There is a tendency in some in-service work, particularly when dealing with professional workers who are reluctant to think about theoretical issues, to stay at the level of only presenting to the audience a number of different practical examples to try out. Some research has indicated that to concentrate solely on teacher activities may be extremely limiting, because the effects only last as long as the training sessions which motivate this type of activity. Because people have a particular conceptual structure of the work in which they are involved, it would seem very necessary that, as they carry out their tasks, they are also able to conceptualize them and build them somehow into the way in which they view their work. In other words, if practical tasks form the basis of in-service training they also need conceptual reinforcement and that requires a very detailed and well-planned type of in-service education (Rubin, 1969a and b; Coyle, 1974).

This type of training has only received serious attention during the last two or three years. The method requires a person to have carefully worked out, step-by-step reasons why she carries out her work in a particular way. This is very true of health education, which often does not have the same carefully worked out rationale as, for instance, science education or mathematics education. The training begins with the trainer

Fig. 16.1

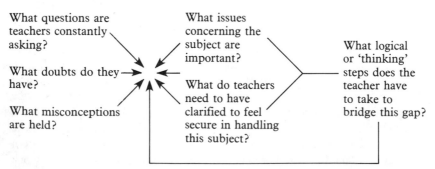

What questions are teachers constantly asking?

What doubts do they have?

What misconceptions are held?

What issues concerning the subject are important?

What do teachers need to have clarified to feel secure in handling this subject?

What logical or 'thinking' steps does the teacher have to take to bridge this gap?

analysing the conceptual steps which the trainee needs to experience. From that he then decides which steps will be necessary in taking people through logical argument to reach that position; this is illustrated in *Fig*. 16.1.

The author has been interested for a number of years in the idea of developing various small segments of learning, which could be put together into one- or two-hour learning sessions and which may suit a whole range of different types of adult groups. This type of modular approach can be developed in such a way that it can be evaluated and guidelines developed as to the most appropriate ways for slotting together such learning exercises. In the recent past some of these have been put together in the form of professional development workshops, written for the Health Education Council (Cowley, 1979*b*). The author and the Schools Council Health Education Project 13–18 team also worked together on a similar format (Cowley and SCHEP, 1979).

In the former case a manual, which is composed of some of these workshops, has been developed and is currently being used by a number of local education authorities. At this interim stage the workshops are put together in such a way that people have the opportunity of using a string of learning exercises and then evaluating for themselves the learning within the group. In the long term the approach undoubtedly would be to attempt to produce similar types of learning exercises but with substantial flexibility. Guidance will be given on the type of groups with which certain methods would work, and alternative methods of planning.

These workshops have attempted to use a number of findings from in-service education research. The SCHEP 5–13 training manual looked at the type of questions which seemed to be raised by teachers' groups in schools once they had some knowledge of the project materials themselves. The type of questions which arose were 'Should it be planned?', 'Why not leave some of this health education until 13 or 14 which may be a more appropriate age?', and such questions as 'I can't really teach that can I, if I smoke myself?' Many teachers were expressing similar doubts and questions concerning health education in schools. The particular project with which this style of in-service work was linked had very clear and declared aims as to what it wanted to see within schools. It hoped to see some type of planned programme; it hoped to see attention given to increasing children's self-esteem and the development of their relationships as an integral part of health education; it had the declared aim of being about good health, rather than about the problems. It therefore seemed important that in order to develop these central concepts of the project, an in-service training approach had to be developed which clarified and drew attention to these issues (Johnson, 1977).

These questions were looked at through the professional development workshops. The author of this chapter was commissioned to write these and to work with a development team to test them out with groups of teachers. As an extra training support a number of tasks and samples of reading were built into the workshop programme, which members had to complete prior to the group meetings. The whole programme was designed so that it could be carried out in a local education authority course, and then taken back into individual schools as school-based in-service education. In order to facilitate this the workshop manual contains various leaders' notes and support material, to allow a teacher to be able to take the full programme and to carry it out with the school's staff.

The initial stage of this training programme consisted of a dissemination through a network established by the disseminator of the Schools Council Health Education Project 5–13, but it is expected that the training programme will gain momentum and lead to a variety of usage in a variety of settings. A programme of the school-based in-service work is shown in Table 16.1.

In the development of the in-service training modules which accompanied the projects, one of the constant criticisms that has arisen is that the in-service training is fairly directive. It does set out to raise questions and clarify perceptions, and it is hoped that people following the programme will go away thinking about the promotion of good health rather than the promotion of problems.

It is interesting that this is an area which worries many people involved in health education, who feel that this type of training is manipulating or moulding people towards a particular end. I would certainly believe that one of the essentials of in-service education is that we accept that adult learners bring with them a large amount of experience and at the same time need to be given the opportunity to make their own decisions and choices for the type of work which they do. However, it is very obvious that if one presents a certain picture or a certain position to the person who is learning, their previous knowledge, attitudes and conceptualization will often prevent them from understanding what the communicator is saying. This particular style of workshop, therefore, is designed so that a teacher is taken through a series of learning exercises which are put together in such a way that they expect to challenge a person's conceptualization of a particular position. Undoubtedly they are to some extent directive, but the reason for

Table 16.1   Professional Development Workshop Manual: Programme

Question	Workshop	Task
STAGE I – CURRICULUM REVIEW		
What are we aiming to do with children aged 5–13? Do we plan it?	A Curriculum context ⟶	B Individual view questionnaire on health and health education
Isn't health education about teeth, hygiene and a few problems? Isn't it about telling people how to behave. . .?	C Health and health education	
Isn't health education just about giving information?	D Health education 5–13	
There are a lot of arguments against doing it!	E Health education – there are arguments against it	F Curriculum grids
STAGE II – CURRICULUM: KEY CONCEPTS		
Why is health education all about self-esteem		G Preliminary individual reading on self-esteem
Can it be effective?	I Self-esteem and identity	H Preliminary individual task – How do I as a teacher increase/decrease children's self-esteem?
How do we handle teaching about relationships?	K¹ Health education and relationships Pt. 1 K² Health education and relationships Pt. 2	J Preliminary task – Looking at classroom relationships
STAGE III – STARTING POINT FOR CURRICULUM DEVELOPMENT AND PLANNING		
Well, if we do develop it what have other schools done?	M Planning/co-ordination and development ⟶ N Working group meeting – further areas for development (carried out after fairly long break)	L Case studies reading – curriculum – parents Read results of F Allocation of areas for development

this is not in order to direct people towards certain end-products or positions but to direct people to *having* to consider the possibilities of certain positions or lines of thought. A number of research projects have suggested that teachers respond well to clear guidance and clear layout in in-service education (Neal and Mussenson, 1967; Cane, 1969; Schmuch and Miles, 1971; Lovegrove, 1972; Neal and Radford, 1972; Saskatchewan Department of Education, 1973; Barry, 1974; Lawrence et al., 1974; Renzulli, 1977; Cowley, 1978a). However, it would be impossible to think that most teachers would be able to be manipulated or moulded to accept a certain position purely because they had passed through an in-service course. The directiveness of this particular method, therefore, is aimed at developing conceptualization, rather than developing teachers with certain positions or practices.

The experience of those present must be built upon

One of the over-riding statements which seems to have come out of recent in-service educational research across the world, is that we must accept the fact that those attending are not young people; they are adults and therefore have a wealth of experience which they bring with them to the course. Unless we take due account of that experience and use it as the foundation for a course, it is very likely that they will not actually apply what they learn to their normal work setting.

The form of interactions can affect the learning that takes place

It is quite noticeable that on some courses people very quickly close up and will not join in either discussion or activities. It seems, therefore, that the way in which one arranges a group and gets the members to interact, the way groups are put together for certain types of learning exercises, the groups they are put into, the format of and the balance between different types of formal and informal activities, all have an immense effect on the type of learning that takes place, and therefore the effect that this may have upon work practice. In this type of small group work, it appears also that the introductory activity is crucial. For instance, if a group is split up into pairs and given a subject which does not make it interact easily, then it may very quickly deaden the whole of the group activity. On the other hand, if a group is kept together and given a very general subject which does not prompt any reasonable level of discussion or thinking, the rest of that discussion session may be endangered (Renzulli, 1977; Cowley, 1978b).

Factual training

Lectures may not be the most appropriate way of conveying knowledge to teachers because they may feel in the end that they do not retain enough information. One interesting scheme on which I worked attempted to analyse the types of myths which constantly come from teachers concerning certain areas of factual knowledge about health. It seemed to be that in a course of in-service work, it was not enough only to put over information; it was important at a very early stage to find out what people actually believed. It is a waste of time if people are given a large amount of information which they already have, or which they would seriously disagree with. What seems essential when deciding what information to impart to teachers is to find out initially what they actually know, then to devise some sort of training which attempts to correct wrong information, and then add further correct information in addition to what has already been covered. It is highly unlikely that this will be done just by talking about certain facts, and it is much more likely that teachers will need to study, to write, to fill in answers to certain factual questionnaires and so on, as part of the in-service work.

Affective training

Affective training is concerned with increasing teachers' sensitivity and awareness of teaching about emotions and the exploration of attitudes. We have found this particularly useful in the use of role play where people have to put themselves into another person's place and feel as the other person feels. This in turn helps them to relate these types of role-play exercises to the school situation. It seems, therefore, logical that exercises have to be conceived which make people express their attitudes and also explore and possibly change them. One way this has been attempted is to obtain the expression of attitudes before the learning event, so that people are 'pinned down' on the attitudes which they hold – this can be done by questionnaires. Members then go through a series of exercises which challenge these attitudes and at the end are able to compare the information which they have received with their previous and present attitudes.

Case studies, case records, role play, arguments and other types of exercises need to be developed as an integral part of the in-service training to enable group members to explore their own attitudes (Munger et al., 1963; Costin and Kerr, 1966; Rochester, 1967; McLeish, 1969; Crompton, 1971).

Sensitivity training

This is often seen as an important part of in-service training, and claims to affect people and make them more sensitive or aware of other people. Whilst undoubtedly this has been used extensively, we have to accept that this is only one part of the whole spectrum of what can be provided in in-service education. It has been noted that in some countries there has been a major move towards sensitivity training rather than towards increasing teachers' knowledge or conceptualization in health education. There are some practitioners who would suggest that sensitivity training may have quite a revolutionary effect upon teachers. Without daunting the prospects of those who are involved in that area, some research has also suggested that perhaps this type of work comprises only one small part of the in-service spectrum (Schmuch and Miles, 1971).

Strategies

One can very often look at an individual course and fail to recognize that it is part of a whole series of courses that have been taking place in one area at one particular time. The in-service educator needs to look at the strategies which are planned in the particular area from which teachers are coming. First, he must look at the long-term strategies. If, for instance, a person organizes a poor course, it is very easy for people to be immunized against further in-service education. It is very important that at an early stage in the planning of courses the right type of courses are planned for the right type of group. It has been a phenomenon in England that as health education was developed, firstly assistant teachers were taught about health education and then, as people recognized that headteachers might be blocking implementation, headteachers in turn were taught about health education. The Teachers' Advisory Council on Alcohol and Drug Education (TACADE) at one stage was working particularly with headteachers; it attempted to define much more clearly the needs of the headteachers' group and provide for them an *appropriate* form of in-service education. Further work on long-term strategies has been developed by a number of centres, and some have produced standard advertisements for making sure that people know exactly what they are coming to. Others have developed forms of contracting into in-service education, so that people are able to assess very clearly before they come what type of in-service training is to be provided (TACADE, 1978). The Social Biology Resources Centre (SBRC) in Melbourne has developed some interesting work in interviewing people before they attend a course (SBRC, 1978), while TACADE developed a system of producing advertisements so that the gaps between the adviser, the advertising personnel in the education office and the teachers could be minimized.

Evaluation

Evaluation is notoriously hard in the area of in-service education because it is extremely difficult to control all the variables which may also give rise to the development of a teacher's practice. Some evaluation has already been carried out into the type of professional development workshop technique which has been described earlier, but naturally this is only one of a whole range of techniques which can be used. The Schools Council Projects have had an evaluator working for them, and at present the general findings from the evaluation suggest that the development of in-service aids for curriculum review in health education seems to promote further thinking and further action (Stephens, 1979). A research project carried out into the effects of in-service education on headteachers pinpointed the necessity of looking at headteachers' positions prior to that particular in-service course and finding out what they already believed. The climate can change quite considerably and one can be battling with issues which are no longer important to the recipient group (Cowley and Hopper, 1980). Another research project currently being carried out into the workshop technique is a controlled evaluation comparing teachers who took part in that type of course with teachers who did not take part in any courses (Cowley, 1980a).

The advantage of the development of small modules of training is that they can be repeated. This then means that we can set up systems for evaluation, courses can be improved, re-evaluated and then made available for other people to take and to modify as they see fit, but with an awareness of the evaluation findings. We should be considering the form of each small learning exercise which is prepared as the part of any in-service course, and it may be advantageous if we can put some of those small pieces of training into modules which other people can use (Schmuch and Miles, 1971; Lawrence, 1974).

Evaluation can be in at least three forms:

1   *Monitoring in-service education*
    Post-course questionnaire to participants, tutors and others involved
    Possibly post-course interviews of selected participants.

2   *An evaluation 'proper'*
This is where various small aids are used for both pre- and post-testing to see the effects upon teachers. Examples of this are:
Pre-course interviews with tutors
Pre-course interviews with funders (e.g., LEA/voluntary body/ AHA)
Pre-course interviews with sample of course members
Pre-course questionnaire to course members
Observation of course
Post-course interviews and questionnaires as above.

3   *In-service research*
This is where a more rigorous research project is set up to look at the outcomes of an in-service course (Cowley, 1980*b*). It is necessary to choose the form of evaluation carefully to suit the particular training. There is little point in researching a course where there is very little chance of being able to control the variables affecting different groups. It would also seem at the same stage improper to produce a large training package which has not had some form of evaluation.

In-service training is likely to develop only to the degree that the trainers have a responsible attitude towards what is being done. In the past we have been fortunate to have a large number of people who put a considerable amount of effort into in-service work. What we need now is a serious recognition that health education cannot quickly jump onto the in-service education bandwagon. It is something which needs to be planned exceptionally carefully with long-term goals and evaluation in mind. Only in this way will we have some progress in the quality of in-service facilities rather than a massive increase in the quantity of such courses.

Summary

In this chapter the place of in-service education in the development of health education within schools is explored. The importance of careful planning of both the content and the form of in-service education is stressed, drawing upon research in this field. Various different forms of in-service provision are considered and their relative benefits and drawbacks suggested. In conclusion it is argued that more emphasis should be given to in-service training in this field of education.

References

Arnold, M. (1894) *Reports of Her Majesty's Inspector of Schools*. London, HMSO.

Barnes, P. and Holloway, S. (1970) 'Small and large group teaching in clinical dentistry'. *Br. Dent. J.*, vol. 129, no. 5.

Barry, E. (1974) 'In-service education for maths teachers'. *Sask. J. Educ. Res.*, vol. 4, no. 2, pp. 23–27.

Cane, B. S. (1969) *In-Service Training – A study of teachers' views and preferences*. Slough, NFER.

Costin, F. and Kerr, W. D. (1966) 'Effects of a mental hygiene course on graduate education students' attitudes and opinions concerning mental illness'. *J. Educ. Res.*, vol. 60, pp. 35–40.

Cowley, J. C. P. (1968) *Drug Education*. Stephen-Hughes Report. Unpublished.

Cowley, J. C. P. (1978*a*) 'Health education – in-service education of teachers'. *J. Inst. Hlth Educ.*, vol. 16, no. 3, p. 76.

Cowley, J. C. P. (1978*b*) *Training of Health Education Professionals – Strategies, philosophy and methods*. New South Wales, Australia, NSW Health Education Training Section, 10 July, 1978.

Cowley, J. C. P. (1979*a*) *In-Service Training of Professionals – It's not the same as just running courses*. London, 10th International Conference on Health Education.

Cowley, J. C. P. (1979*b*) *Professional Development Workshop Manual*. London, Health Education Council.

Cowley, J. C. P. (1980*a*) *Can We Provide Learning Situations that Develop Teachers' Concepts of Health Education?* MEd thesis, Nottingham University, School of Education.

Cowley, J. C. P. (1980*b*) 'In-service education of teachers: radical alternatives to traditional approaches'. *Int. J. Hlth Educ.*, vol. 22, no. 4, p. 227.

Cowley, J. C. P. and Daniels, H. A. et al. (1980) *Family Life/Child Development/Parenthood Education in Schools*. A trials in-service course. Milton Keynes, Open University, INSET Section.

Cowley, J. C. P. and Hopper, V. (1980) *The Development and Evaluation of a Seminar for Headteachers on Curriculum Planning*. Manchester, TACADE.

Cowley, J. C. P. and Schools Council Health Education Project 13–18 Team (1979) *Co-ordinators' Manual*. London, Schools Council.

Coyle, B. (1974) 'Teachers' view on in-service education'. *Curric. Rev. Bull.*, vol. 9, no. 4, pp. 154–156.

Crompton, C. E. (1971) 'Teachers' attitudes to educational controversies'. *Educ. Res.*, vol. 13, pp. 204–209.

Dalman, T. (1974) 'The two day workshop as an intervention technique for organisation development in catholic schools'. *Dialogue*, vol. 8, no. 2, pp. 25–38.

David, K. G. and Cowley, J. C. P. (1980) *Pastoral Care in Schools and Colleges*. London, Edward Arnold.

Eraut, M. (1972) *In-Service Education for Innovation*. Occasional Paper no. 4. London, National Council for Educational Technology.

Hamilton, D. et al. (1977) *Beyond the Numbers Game*. London, Macmillan, preface.

Johnson, V. (1977) 'Curriculum development in health education'. *J. Inst. Hlth Educ.*, vol. 15, no. 1, pp. 9–17.

Lancashire Education Authority (1978) *Pastoral Care and Education for Personal Relationships in Lancashire Secondary Schools*.

Lawrence, G. et al. (1974) *Patterns of Effective In-Service Education*. Tallahassee, Fla, Florida Department of Education, p. 17.

Lovegrove, W. R. (1972) 'Some problems involved in in-service education'. *Camb. J. Ed.*, vol. 2, no. 1, pp. 42–49.

McLeish, J. (1969) *Teachers' Attitudes – A study of national and other differences*. Cambridge, Cambridge Institute of Education.

Morgan, R. (1973) 'Innovation with man: a course of study'. *Forum*, Autumn 1973.

Munger, P. F. et al. (1963) 'Guidance institutes and the persistence of attitudes'. *Personn. Guidance J.*, vol. 41, pp. 415–419.

Nagle, J. E. (1972) 'Staff development – do it right'. *J. Read.*, vol. 16, no. 2, p. 125.

Neal, W. D. and Mussenson, D. (1967) 'The continuing education of teachers', in Richardson, J. A. and Bowen, J. (eds), *The Preparation of Teachers in Australia*. Melbourne, F. W. Cheshire, pp. 175–176.

Neal, W. D. and Radford, W. C. (1972) *Teachers for Commonwealth Schools*. A report to the Commonwealth Department of Education and Science on aspects of the organisation of careers and salaries in schools to be staffed by the Commonwealth Teaching Service. Melbourne, Advanced Centre for Educational Research, pp. 28–29.

Renzulli, J. S. (1977) 'Instructional management systems: a model for organising and developing in-service training workshops'. *Gift. Child Q.*, vol. 21, no. 2, p. 190.

Rochester, D. E. (1967) 'Persistence of attitudes and values of NDEA counsellor trainees'. *J. Counsel. Psychol.*, vol. 14, pp. 535–537.

Rubin, L. J. (1969*a*) 'A study of teacher retraining', in Watkins, R. (ed.), (1973) *The Role of the School in In-Service Education*. London, Ward Lock Educational.

Rubin, L. J. (1969*b*)*A Study of the Continuing Education of Teachers*. Santa Barbara, University of California, Centre for Co-ordinated Education.

Safford, P. L. (1975) 'Training teachers for drug abuse prevention – a humanistic approach'. *J. Drug Educ.*, vol. 5, no. 4, p. 335.

Saskatchewan Department of Education (1973)*Partnership for Professional Renewal*. Research, Planning and Development Branch.

Schmuch, R. A. and Miles, M. B. (1971) *Organisation Development in School*. Palo Alto, Cal., National Press Books.

Social Biology Resources Centre (1978) ISEC/78/4. Melbourne, Australia.

Stephens, M. (1979)*Evaluator's Notes*. Schools Council Health Education Project 13–18. Unpublished.

Stibbs, A. (1977) 'On the buses'. *Times Educational Supplement*, 7 January, 1977.

TACADE (1978) *Courses Designed to Offer a Structured Approach to In-Service Training*. Leaflet and supplementary materials. Manchester, TACADE.

TACADE (1979) Directors' Report. Manchester, TACADE.

Thelen, H. A. (1971)'A cultural approach to in-service teacher training', in Rubin, L. J. (ed.), *In-Service Education – Proposals and procedures for change*. Boston, Mass., Allyn & Bacon, p. 73.

Waynant, L. F. (1971) 'Teachers' strengths as a basis for successful in-service experiences'. *Educ. Leader.*, vol. 28, no. 7, pp. 710–713.

CHAPTER 17

EVALUATION OF HEALTH EDUCATION

Marilyn Stephens

Introduction

Wherever decisions about schools and their curricula are being made there is a role for evaluation to play. Evaluation, however, is not a popular business, especially for teachers whose workload seems doubled by an attempt to review or in some way develop or change a school's approach towards health education. At one time, when curriculum development in any area was (and to a certain extent still is) preoccupied by the task of reviewing resources for teaching, evaluation activities focused on the effects of changes in materials and methods. Moreover this information tended to be collected for and by 'outsiders', whose interests and audiences were schools in general rather than any one particular school. The researcher or outside evaluator has in the past been thought to be the person best qualified to look at the performance of schools and those within them, the teachers and others inside lacking the expertise and 'objectivity' required. This emphasis is shifting and must continue to do so. Teachers' unique positions and skills give them opportunities for evaluating their work, their students and their schools. Whether they can or not depends upon having the resources and time, as well as upon some knowledge of approaches and methods which are useful. The amount of technical knowledge demanded is not great and methods do exist or can be devised which are accessible to teachers (these will be discussed later), although gathering information will inevitably take time. Our belief has to be that this is time well spent and that teachers involved with such a complex and controversial area as health education ought to be spending some part of their time in evaluating their work. If Cinderella health education is to be invited to the curricular ball (and once there not to remain a wallflower), she must be able to withstand and flourish under all manner of evaluation processes. The greater the degree of participation by teachers in these processes, the more freedom they have to decide appropriate goals for their students and experiences through which these can be achieved. This chapter attempts to help teachers identify their evaluation problems in health education and to begin to work towards some possible solutions.

It may be necessary first to clarify what we mean by evaluation. Is it the same as assessment? Is 'Does it work?' the most important question an evaluator can ask? Until recently evaluation exponents tended to concentrate on evaluating the stated objectives of educational programmes, usually in terms of changes in student behaviour. We need to ask ourselves if data such as these about student behaviour give us a good basis for making decisions (such as course improvement or choosing between alternative projects) about an educational programme. Stenhouse (1975) adds to this by arguing that objective-type evaluations do not address themselves to understanding the educational process. Cooper (1976) gives a useful all-embracing definition of this wider role for evaluation: Curriculum evaluation is the collection and provision of evidence, on the basis of which decisions can be taken about the feasibility, effectiveness and educational value of curricula. It seems then that evaluation, in order to be aware of complex issues in education, to be relevant to the work of teachers and useful in terms of making decisions, needs to address itself to much more than the question, 'Does it work?'

The 'goal' or 'objective system of evaluation gives us some criteria against which we can compare the results of our measurement and hence the effectiveness of our course, innovation or whatever. However it is important to remind ourselves that 'goals' in health education, particularly for short-term classroom observation or measurement, may not always be seen in terms of behavioural change. Evaluation for health education in a wider sense may be more a study of processes, though outcomes are not ostensibly excluded. In addition there may be consequences of the course, innovation, etc., undergoing evaluation which were unintended. It is also important that any evaluation exercise makes room for collection of information about this and does not become too tunnel-visioned, checking always and only for alleged effects rather than looking for actual effects.

Gathering Information

Describing goals in health education

We need to be clear, realistic and honest about the intentions or goals of the health education activities. It is pointless and frustrating to embark on an 'Is it successful?' evaluation tack, without at first clarifying for yourself and involved colleagues what the intended outcome of the activities were and are. The original intentions (perhaps expressed at the early stages of planning a course, for example) may be too broad to be helpful, or they may have been changed by teachers working on the materials as they felt them to be inappropriate for their students. The whole business of describing goals in health education is particularly challenging and it is often difficult to break down any course into its component aims and objectives. We usually find it easier and have most practice in describing desirable course outcomes in terms of gains in knowledge and use of information (cognitive area) and in non-controversial performance skills (behavioural area). Health education is not at all straightforward in this respect; it is seen to be about values, attitudes and feelings (affective area) as well as about using information and in some cases behaving in a certain way.

The following extract is from the Schools Health Education Study, *Health Education – A conceptual approach to curriculum design*, and although the contexts and language used are American, it provides a useful and thorough breakdown of the cognitive, affective and action areas or domains with health education examples:

Classifications of Health Behaviour

– the ways in which individuals think, feel and act.

i. *Cognitive Domain*
    Those objectives which deal with recall or recognition of knowledge and the development of intellectual abilities and skills.
    a) Knowledge (of specifics, terminology, facts, ways and means of dealing with specifics, conventions, trends and sequences, classification and categories, criteria, methodology, universals and abstractions, principles and generalisations, theories and structures).
    b) Intellectual Abilities and Skills (comprehension, interpretation, application, analysis, synthesis, evaluation).

ii. *Affective Domain*
Those objectives which describe changes in interest, attitudes, and values, and the development of appreciations and adequate adjustments.
  a) Receiving (awareness, willingness to receive, controlled or selected attention).
  b) Responding (acquiescence, willingness to respond, satisfaction in response).
  c) Valuing (acceptance, preference, commitment).
  d) Organisation (conceptualization of a value, organisation of a value system).
  e) Characterisation by a Value or Value Complex (generalised set, characterisation).
Cognitive and Affective Behaviors – demonstration of these health behaviors is evaluated usually in a hypothetical rather than a life situation.
Example: Ability to analyze critically a health advertisement or to express attitudes about self-diagnosis and self-medication.

iii. *Action Domain*
Those aspects of health behaviors in which the individual actually applies knowledge and attitudes to a life situation.
  a) Observable Health Behaviours – those life health behaviours that can be observed and evaluated to some extent in the classroom setting.
      Examples: how a student relates to others, activities on the playground or in the school environment, personal appearance and grooming, and food selection in school cafeteria.
  b) Non-observable Health Behaviours – those health behaviours that cannot be observed systematically in a school setting and where information regarding the practice is derived often by inquiry of the student or others aware of his practices.
      Examples: smoking habits, nutritional practices, safety practices outside of the school environment, conduct on a date, use of alcoholic beverages, practices related to dental health, sleep, activity, and relationships within the family group.
  c) Dalayed Behaviours – those health behaviours that will not or cannot be practised in life situations until after the student reaches adulthood, is confronted with the problem, or is in a

position to assume greater responsibility for his own behavior. Examples: supporting health legislation, choosing a medical adviser, maintaining desirable weight throughout life, getting regular medical and dental check-ups, avoiding medical and health quackery, and using existing community health services.

Health education has already been described in this book as being about:

- giving information;
- clarifying values;
- building personal autonomy, i.e., knowledge and skills for making decisions;
- influencing behaviour to some defined end.

An overall aim with students could be 'the promotion of decision-making skills about health-related behaviour'. However, it seems more likely that the overall aim will be more directive in its suggestion of course outcomes, and will point to responsible decision-making skills and responsible behaviour (of certain kinds) in some areas of health education. In other words if the first aim of promoting decision-making skills was the order of the day for all aspects of health-related teaching, the success or otherwise of the teaching would be determined more by the clarity of thinking behind a decision or choice related to health behaviour, than by the behaviour itself. As well as being quite difficult to cope with for many involved with health education, it is unlikely that in some areas, for example drinking and driving, all choices of behaviour will be equally accepted by the teacher.

However, there does seem to be a growing concern for most areas of health education to be involved with the learning *processes*, namely how decisions are thought through and verbalized or acted out, rather than with actual choices of behaviour, or learning *outcomes*. Health *education* rather than health *instruction*? If, therefore, course outcomes are described in terms of responsible decision-making skills related to certain aspects of health behaviour, the evaluation must be related to these. Even if we wished to, we know that behavioural outcomes related to health would be almost impossible to monitor anyway due to access to appropriate situations outside school and to the long-term implications of much health education (for adult role, parenthood, etc.). There are no really satisfactory predictors of behaviour which we can monitor with confidence in school. Changes in values and attitudes, if measured, do not necessarily predict behavioural changes, although some links are evident.)However we can say that actions are partially determined by group expectations, an individual's perception of the importance of the action for his own well-being and other social considerations. Other similar sorts of arguments have pointed to the work in values clarification and simulated choice situations and role play as ways of strengthening the links between values, attitudes and behaviour.

Describing course goals

The Schools Council Health Education Project 13–18 offered a model or matrix to those schools working with them to help them plan courses in terms of content areas, school years (the third, fourth and fifth years were usually considered) and broad, long-term aims. Examples of two content areas or topics were given: personal health (body management and human biology) and relationships. Broad aims in each domain (cognitive, affective and action) were given as examples of overall goals for work with the three year groups. For each year some breakdown of course content was attempted. You will observe that the model is incomplete and does not attempt to tackle single lessons or activities. However, schools working with this model have found it to be a useful if obvious starter, and Table 17.1 shows one school's attempt to outline what health education might consist of in terms of content and long-term aims for the third, fourth and fifth years.

Describing goals for a particular lesson or activity

The Schools Council Health Education Projects team were reassured by the teachers with whom they were working in July 1978 at a writing workshop aimed at producing some health education teaching materials, by the fact that the simple, if frustrating checklist shown below was in great demand. The format is nothing new but serves as a useful reminder, leaving ample space for individual responses. The list attempts to help overcome the major difficulty of making the transition from a simple overall statement of aims (almost certain to be a conceptual statement) to more detailed specifications that are concrete and practical enough to be handled in a practical way.

Checklist for individual lessons

Aims

1.   The purpose or aim of this lesson or activity could be described as:

2. This lesson may be seen as existing alone (one-off), or rather as part of a course or a collection of multi-disciplinary contributions. If it is the latter, this lesson is contributing to an *overall aim* which could be described as:

Objectives

Health education activities are concerned with the following aspects, related to health behaviour or situations:
–   giving information, encouraging enquiry skills, etc.
                        cognitive component
–   exploring values, attitudes, feelings, etc.
                        affective component
–   practising and developing skills such as problem solving, decision making.
                        skills component.
Your lesson/activity may or may not include all these aspects. For the following you could fill in whichever are appropriate:
3. After this lesson/activity, I might expect students to *know*:

4. During and after this lesson I might expect or hope that students express (their own and others') *feelings and opinions* about:

5. During and after this lesson I might expect or hope that students express (their own and others') feelings and opinions about (see above) and these might/could/should be some of the following:

6. After this lesson (and perhaps as a result of many similar lessons) I might expect students to show an increased ability in the following *skills*:

7. Other objectives or comments about the purpose of the lesson:

Table 17.1   An outline of health education.

Examples of items within two content areas

YEARS
and
THEMES

5th year
'Me and the Community'

Adult exercise, Child care
Relationship of personal health
to occupation

Marriage and other long-
term relationships

4th year
'Me and others'

Adaptation to environment, physical
and mental stress

Others and same sex
Parents – authority
Loss and separation

3rd year
'Me Now'

Hygiene, exercise, effects of smoking,
alcohol, drugs, etc. Working of the body

Peer relationships, Parents
Situations for smoking, etc.

Content

PERSONAL HEALTH
BODY MANAGEMENT
HUMAN BIOLOGY

RELATIONSHIPS

Cognitive domain
Information
Knowledge
Understanding

1. Knows how the body works
2. Understands what the body needs to
   maintain health
3. Understands the link between behaviour
   and health

1. Understands the social skills involved in
   making and maintaining relationships in
   different social contexts
2. Develops some understanding of the nature
   of individual and group behaviour

Affective domain
Attitudes, feelings
Values
Self-concerns

1. Values the body and appreciates the need
   for its care
2. Accepts some responsibility for personal
   health

1. Becomes sensitive to the attitudes, beliefs
   and social needs of others and self

Action domain
Skills
Decisions

1. Chooses appropriate behaviour
2. Takes appropriate action for body
   maintenance

1. Acquires skills enabling them to manage
   themselves effectively in different social
   situations

Examples of aims for two content areas

Table 17.1 cont.

	Personal Health	Relationships	Food Selection	Growth and Development	Education for Parenthood	Community Health	Environment in which We Live	Safety and First Aid
Year 5 'Me and the Community'	Adult exercise Child care Relationship of personal health to occupation	Marriage and other long-term relationships	Nutrition and health (Stress and anxiety)	Social and emotional development (Contd)	Helping young people to cope	Voluntary organization National and community issues – abortion, etc.	Meeting needs of community e.g., leisure, living space	Leisure Road-driver education
Year 4 'Me and others'	Adaptation to environment Physical and mental stress	Relationships with others and same sex Parents ↔ Authority Loss and separation	Nutrition and health (Slimming and obesity)	Sexual development Changes accompanying Individual differences	Family roles Structures of one-parent families	Attitudes to physical and mental illness, etc. National and community issues Contraception, etc.	Effect of environment on physical and mental health	School/Work Principles of first aid
Year 3 'Me Now'	Hygiene, exercise Effects of smoking, alcohol, drugs Working of the body	Peer relationship Situations for smoking, etc. Parents	Nutritional needs of the body	Body changes at puberty Emotional and social changes accompanying development	Growth and development of young people	NHS roles and relationships to doctors and hospital staff	Health issues: litter, pollution, noise	Home Road traffic education

DOMAINS

Cognitive	Know how the body works. Understand what is needed for health. Link behaviour and health.	Understand social skills involved in maintaining relationships in different social contexts. Developing understanding.	Understand good diet and behaviour which leads to a good diet.	Aware of effect of puberty. Develop understanding of emotional changes.	Understand development and place in family structure.	How community health operates. Develop understanding of issues.	Understand effect on community of self and others.	Know how to care for self and others.
Affective	Values body and appreciates need to care. Accepts some responsibility for personal health.	Sensitive to attitudes and beliefs of self and others.	Develop sensitive attitude to nutrition.	Aware of individual differences.	Sensitive to problems of young people and needs.	Appreciate values involved.	Appreciate need for healthy environment.	Awareness of group attitudes to safety.
Action	Choose appropriate behaviour. Take appropriate action for body maintenance.	Acquire skills to manage social situations.	Ability to plan. Able to manage stressful situations.	Ability to cope with and understand changes.	Able to manage social situations involving young people.	Acquire social skills to manage rational decision-making.	Appreciate decision-making skill in managing environmental problems.	Acquire skills to manage social situations leading to danger.

Those for Whom the Evidence is Being Collected

Ideally those involved with the planning and teaching of health education activities in a school should be those most motivated to discuss and collect information about goals, teaching methods, problems and successes. Some schools have working parties or curriculum development teams which are primarily concerned with reviewing and developing health education, and evidence is often collected by and for such a group. However the audience is often much wider. Those schools working with the Schools Council Health Education Projects for 5–13 and 13–18-year-olds (with their own curriculum development teams) have been encouraged to consult other groups including the entire staff of their school, parents and other community figures such as social workers, doctors, etc., as they begin to review and plan health education for their school. It may well be that others outside the planning team are particularly interested in and concerned about the evaluation of health education in schools. It is as well to find out what these interests, worries, scepticisms and hunches are so that any communication about evaluation can be seen to bear these issues in mind. Information does need to be conveyed effectively and with evaluation findings this is often particularly difficult. There are often political and moral overtones.

It must be stressed that evaluation, particularly in health education, cannot and should not be expected to provide instant answers. It is unlikely that any information is ever wholly accurate or entirely valid. Test scores, for example, do not convey all the information needed for evaluation. Instead it is probably necessary to use less formal methods of gathering data and to accept the subjective element as the price to pay for the greater relevance of the information. If this is so, then we have to develop not only ways of handling these kinds of data but ways of communicating why these methods are more appropriate to those audiences who may well prefer test scores and conclusive statements. Any evaluation findings should be followed (and almost certainly are anyway) by negotiations, as different individuals and groups or audiences explore and interpret what has been gathered. Much will depend on how you intend to use the information and also on who collected it.

By Whom Is the Information To Be Collected?

We return to the earlier theme that the teacher actually planning and/or undertaking health education activities has a most important role to play in evaluation. However it is also important to consider the need for information about a subject to be drawn from as many points of view as possible, particularly if we feel it necessary to use less formal methods with their subjective elements. With this approach every piece of information is useful in building up the picture, none will suffice on its own and each will be interpreted for what it is. It may well be that an 'outsider' such as a researcher, curriculum developer, LEA adviser, etc., could play some part in this, or that ways could be devised so that colleagues join in for some sessions. In whatever way the evaluation tasks are shared, it is vital that the process is (and is felt to be by those involved) an 'inside-school based' activity where the information collected is seen to be extremely relevant and important for the school, its students and teachers, and the health education being taught.

Gathering Information From and About Students

'The customer is always right', says the adage. Who is the customer of curriculum development – the teacher, student or parent? For the moment we will concentrate on students as particularly important customers and summarize some ways in which information may be collected from and about them.

Student opinion and reaction

In working through materials we are usually very interested in eliciting an amalgam of opinion and reaction; not only what students think but also what they do. At secondary level questions such as 'How interesting did you find this piece of work?' and 'How long did it take you?' seem certain to arise.

Among the evaluation strategies proposed for use during the programme 'Man: A course of study' (Education Development Center, 1970) there is a pupils' opinion survey. This asks questions about reactions to the course, the activities which students found most hard, easy, most enjoyable, what has been learned most, and how students have perceived the demands of the materials. The questions are multiple choice ones and students are told how many answers they can tick. This example may be useful:

To do well in 'Man: A course of study', I have to: (tick *three* answers)

  – read well
  – be able to think of a lot of good examples

- memorise all the facts in the booklets
- ask questions
- take part in class discussions
- remember everything the teacher said
- agree with the teacher
- have my own opinion
- write well
- do extra projects
- be able to understand and remember films
- try to be as quiet as possible
- bring in extra information about the animals we are studying
- answer a lot of the teacher's questions
- other (what is it ....)

It is suggested in the teachers' handbook that the students fill in the form individually then discuss their response in groups. As far as the students are concerned the process is informal and provides a starting point for a useful discussion about how different people vary in their reactions to the work. For the teacher it may provide insights into the activities as seen from the student's point of view.

The younger the child the less his opinions are likely to be sought, understandably so. Teacher assessment of the reactions of children under eleven relies heavily upon methods of direct observation. It may well be that this is something on which to join up with colleagues, working out observation pointers together as a checklist for use as the teaching takes place.

Student opinion and reaction may, of course, be elicited in other ways such as one-to-one interviews, diaries or record books for the student to keep and informal group discussions. It may well be that it is less time-consuming to collect information about reactions and opinion (enjoyment, interest, etc.) together with information about attainment.

Student attainment

Attainment testing is unfashionable at present and, as has already been mentioned, should be viewed with particular caution for health education which is not a 'subject' that lends itself to the specification of precise, testable objectives. However, it may well be that once we have specified realistic short-term goals for our health education we would like to attempt some kind of monitoring of student progress towards these 'goals'. This information may help us reflect on the effectiveness of our teaching and should help improve both teaching and materials (in conjunction with other feedback, of course). Ways of gathering information about student attainment fall into three broad categories: standardized tests, criteria referenced tests and methods based on observation.

It is not difficult to see that standardized tests have the advantage of being quick to administer, but match up very poorly to the general purpose of our evaluation, particularly for health education. (A standardized test is one which has been given to a large number of children in controlled conditions and from the results of which 'norms' have been established for different groups of children. The result of giving the test to any child can therefore be compared with the average for a particular group.)

Criteria referenced tests give information about a student's performance in relation to a particular level of ability or skill which is the criterion. Items in these tests are usually devised so that the score can be represented as a degree of mastery, and are not designed to compare the individual performances of students. Criteria referenced tests can be and are, of course, produced by the teacher, and can be practical and differ little from the student's usual learning activities. Although these tests seem to 'fit the bill' much better than standardized tests, they do fall short in several aspects. They are restricted to a few concepts and skills, and would need to be multiplied many times if a reasonable range of objectives were to be covered. Even then mainly cognitive development and skills would be covered; attitudes, interests and personal characteristics may remain largely unexplored. However, at best, they do help a teacher to explore a student's thinking in an activity, and used occasionally help teachers to make decisions about learning opportunities. But they cannot provide the answer for gathering information about all students across a wide range of concepts, abilities, attitudes and interests. Tests should be seen as a supplement to other methods of providing information which are more flexible, less demanding of time and more wide-ranging.

Collecting information about students' progress or change in attitudes, values and feelings is particularly difficult, but particularly pertinent in health education. We are often looking for such long-term goals as:

- awareness of own values and those held by other important people
- awareness/insight into valuing process
- appreciation of peer group pressures and expectations
- awareness of risk-taking behaviour
- development of responsibility for oneself and other important people
- development of personal autonomy.

The techniques best suited to this type of evaluation are attitude scales, interviews and observations. However, it is often more relevant to ask students questions about situations (often involving people of a similar age-group), where the above components are all being explored in a realistic context.

The sorts of broad cognitive goals in which we are often interested in health education are:

- increase knowledge of health-related information —
- develop skills of inquiry, recall —
- increase concept development —
- higher order skills of analysis, synthesis and evaluation with health-related information, e.g., in survey work
- transference of information and cognitive processes to other settings, i.e., application, e.g., comparison of survey results of different age-groups.

Therefore one appropriate form of evaluation (in a classroom context) of student progress towards these 'goals' may well be to present the student with a 'problem' or situation involving some decisions about health-related behaviour. The student then attempts carefully to describe what one would do, or feel to be most appropriate for the people involved in such a situation. In this way the teacher can begin to explore how a student appraises the situation, what information is sought, what values are considered and how the consequences of decisions are appreciated. This would be a particularly challenging type of evaluation needing careful preparation and a great deal of sensitivity, particularly in view of the fact that the decisions finally suggested may not be deemed appropriate by the teacher, although the appraisal of the situation was thorough and used accurate information.

Methods involving observation

The examples have so far consisted of techniques which involve giving students special tasks to perform for the purpose of gathering information. They may produce data from somewhat artificial situations and do not allow for normal fluctuations in interest, etc. More wide-ranging methods are to be found in making use of the observations which teachers are all the time making of students' actions, responses and behaviours. The danger of observation being a merely personal reaction and providing data of little value to anyone else is great. If it is to be the basis of a useful method of gathering information, observation cannot remain totally unstructured. It requires a structure which comes from considering the goals of the students' work and from agreeing criteria which can be applied to interpreting children's behaviour in terms of progress towards the goals.

The Schools Council History, Geography and Social Science 8–13 Project has produced materials specifically aimed at helping teachers to observe and record students' progress. The items in their checklist are the project's objectives, which are grouped under the four broad headings of intellectual, social and physical skills and personal qualities (interests, attitudes and values). In the booklet *Evaluation, Assessment and Record Keeping in History, Geography and Social Science* (Schools Council, 1974), there is a discussion of the implications of each objective for teaching and learning and some hints about how to assess progress towards it. This example is for one of the social skills objectives:

General objective: to participate within small groups

What to look for:
- understands the need for rules in a group
- participates in deciding rules of the group
- can organise a group in such a way as to share roles and tasks among the members
- accepts the role of leader or follower as the situation demands
- appreciates the capabilities, qualities and sensitivities of other members of the group
- can put aside personal goals for the sake of the cohesion of the group.

Commenting on ways of gathering information about achievement of this objective, Cooper (1976) writes: 'As far as I can see, there are no ways in which the teacher can "test" for the quality of the child's social relationships by any paper or special test', and later, 'Certainly it would seem that observation would be the most useful tool in the teacher's attempt to assess this general objective. Since some children seem to show different characteristics inside the classroom and out (where perhaps the "model" student becomes a social outcast or a near-bully) the teacher should watch behaviour in as many different situations as possible.'

To summarize and pinpoint some of the features of an ideal method for gathering information from and about students, the following list may be useful. The method, or combination of methods used should have as many as possible of the following features:

- be as valid and reliable as possible
- ability to be used with and for students of varied abilities
- convenient and not too time-consuming for the teacher
- non-interference with normal working (where possible)
- capacity for providing information about the widest range of characteristics and behaviour
- ability to be carried out without causing anxiety or tension in students or teachers
- be essentially suited to the type of activities under scrutiny e.g., health education, and to the overall purpose of the evaluation exercise.

It is important here to restate that no one method of evaluation should ever stand alone. Student reactions and responses, and measurements of their attainment and records of observations, etc., are incomplete evidence without some additional back-up comment by the teachers involved with the activities under scrutiny.

Information From and About Teachers

There is a danger that when the time available for curriculum development and evaluation is limited, only one measure of 'output' is established, and this is all too often some form of student achievement. The point has already been made that if the purpose of evaluation is to review and improve a course, or number of activities, information must be collected from several sources. Achievement scores in themselves cannot totally assess the consequences of what teachers do in classrooms, as they in themselves cannot explain which factors in a given situation are the cause of learning or learning failure. We need also to devise ways of studying and collecting information about what is actually happening in the teaching situation. An 'outside' evaluator such as one working for a curriculum development project is likely to use a whole battery of teacher-directed techniques. Projects like the Schools Council Health Education Projects 5–13 and 13–18 commonly employ questionnaires, checklists, teacher diaries, group discussions, evaluation conferences and, most important, personal interviews. It is essential that a school-based team of teachers involved in curriculum development and evaluating from the 'inside', devises ways of collecting systematic feedback from those other teachers involved in the process. The crucial factor in deciding between success and failure of any curriculum development is the opinion teachers come to hold of its aims and objectives. It is to be hoped that some basic questions which place the feasibility of any development under scrutiny will be asked by the team within a school. These might include the following:

Are the aims the right ones to pursue?
Are the aims acceptable to our school and its teachers?
Is the content suitable for the target population of pupils and consistent with the aims?
Do the envisaged methods of teaching fit the content and aims?

Questionnaires and checklists

Early discussions where such intrinsic questions are asked are unlikely to produce immediate answers, but rather will give rise to some more specific key questions based on issues needing clarification and worries and interests of particular audiences. Teachers working on their own curriculum development are likely to be concerned about the effectiveness of materials and particular problems of classroom and student management. Instruments can be produced which pose questions on these levels, and although they may look crude can represent a delicate balancing of interests. Appendix V includes an example of an evaluation checklist devised for teachers working with some materials produced by the Schools Council Health Education Project 13–18. It may provide some useful hints as to the sorts of questions that seem to be important both to the writers and users of materials. Steadman (1976) suggests the following guidelines in order to minimize the inevitable shortcomings of the use of checklists and questionnaires:

1   Be sure the questions you ask are ones that teachers (i.e., your colleagues) can answer.
2   Observe the same kind of rules which govern the construction of an attitude scale; for example, at its most simple don't use four grades A–D for the expression of approval. Everyone will answer 'B'.
3   Consider carefully the sample or group of teachers from whom you draw opinion.
4   Arrange to cross-check opinions against the opinions of others, e.g., teachers' with students'.
5   Use more than one method of collecting information.

Teacher diaries

A diary will differ from a questionnaire or checklist in that it attempts to gain a more general but continuous picture of the teachers' involvement with a project or new materials or course. However, diaries can make heavy demands on teacher time. It may be, in the end, more productive to encourage a team of curriculum developers and users in a school to make notes in the margin of materials or activities under scrutiny, perhaps recording little more than the date and their reactions as the work progresses. This contemporary record can be easily amplified in discussions between the teachers involved. It is essential that some sort of teacher record is kept of reactions as work progresses, as it is unlikely (if unfortunate) that meetings will be frequent enough for memory only to suffice. Projects such as SCHEP 5–13 and 13–18 relied heavily upon such feedback, and found it immensely useful when rewriting the projects' materials.

Using observers to collect data

It may well be that a curriculum development team within a school is in a position to and wants to use either 'inside' or 'outside' observers to collect information about teaching activities. Techniques such as observation and interaction schedules may well be used (Cooper, 1976; Steadman, 1976). It is important that the data should be collected in a form which the teacher concerned can use. In order to ensure this, it is necessary for the teacher to insist on certain procedures and observation techniques, and of course a post-observation conference or discussion.

Group discussions

In briefly summarizing how information might be collected from and about teachers, the assumption is made that several colleagues will be working together with both the time and opportunity to meet regularly to plan, develop their curricular ideas, adopt some level of evaluation and discuss their findings. It is vital that any evaluation data are *used* and not just filed away. The interpretation of findings and negotiations about their implications are of great importance if involvement and motivation are to be maintained. Future evaluation attempts may well be undermined if the information collected is not seen to be carefully reviewed and used to help make decisions about the developing curricula.

As well as the purpose of evaluation being directed at a course, materials, etc., it may well be that you would wish an evaluation to help you make broader curriculum decisions about health education. Questions such as

'What exactly *is* health education?', 'What are the needs of young people?', 'Are there special teaching skills required?', are also likely to be bearing down on you if you are reviewing and developing health education (and related areas) in your school. In many ways the whole process of curriculum review is one of evaluation in its broader sense. This way of evaluating or reviewing a curriculum in order to plan and develop health education for a particular school has been attempted by the Schools Council Health Education Projects 5–13 and 13–18, in conjunction with the Teachers' Advisory Council on Alcohol and Drug Education (TACADE). This chapter has tended to concentrate rather on the more specific evaluation of what has been planned and implemented. However, it seems that planning and implementation are helped enormously in terms of clarity, quality and commitment if these broadly philosophic issues are discussed, in a structured way, by a curriculum development team.

Describing the Curriculum Context

Information gathered in the ways described earlier is not alone in affecting decisions about curricula. Whether or not a course or proposed development in health education is 'successful' and activities become part of what a school plans for with future commitment, will depend on many other factors. These may well be shaped by organizational and historical issues. If an evaluation purpose is to look at long-term success in this way, then some sort of consideration and description of the curriculum context of the health education development is needed. For example, health education is likely to involve some level of co-operation between departments, using as it does a wide variety of teacher skills and knowledge, and this co-operation may affect the outcomes of any integrated studies-type approach. Previous experience with similar types of curricular development in the field of humanities, religious education and human biology may well affect both teacher and student enthusiasms and the quality of work. It is therefore important to ask: 'What are the organizational and historical factors likely to impinge upon the development of health education in this school?', 'What might the effect be?', 'How can we monitor and describe what happens?'

Concluding Remarks

The practical constraints limiting a full review, development and evaluation of any aspect of the curriculum are all too apparent and painful. The most obvious ones are time, lack of resources (both human and material) and lack of apparent expertise. Although some of the methods outlined here are already part of a teacher's everyday repertoire, extra time will probably be needed to make notes and records. It is unlikely that all aspects of the health education activities under scrutiny can or should be evaluated. Choices will need to be made, based on agreed priorities. For example, perhaps one or two particularly difficult or sensitive areas would benefit from a careful and thorough evaluation. Some teachers may feel that a detailed look at student responses about several areas is a better way of spending the available time, or that they ought to concentrate on collecting information about and from teachers, at least at first. Obviously questions about overall success, improvements, etc., will depend upon a broad base of information collected over a period of time, and a plan for this will need to be devised. In formulating such a plan it is important to bear in mind the following four questions:

For what purpose is the evaluation intended?
For whom is the 'evidence' being collected?
Who is to collect (or might collect) the information?
What are the practical constraints (time, deadlines, number of colleagues involved, etc.) which seem particularly pertinent?

One of the main values of evaluation is that it provides a forum for acknowledging and debating values in education. Nowhere is this debate needed more than in areas related to social education. Choices about what to evaluate and how to do it are not at all straightforward, and it is hoped that the preceding chapter has helped to clarify some of the more important issues. The kinds of activity described are not new, but familiar events and activities are often the hardest to examine critically. If teachers choose to include evaluation within their role, further help will be needed and this chapter attempts only to serve as a starting point for a more detailed investigation of techniques and ways of evaluating health education in schools. If health education itself is an immensely complex process, how can its evaluation be any less so?

Summary

Evaluation is not popular and is often seen as the domain of an expert, but teachers are encouraged in this chapter to see evaluation in schools as everybody's business. The participation of teachers is particularly vital within the complex goals of health education.

It is suggested that evaluation should provide information to help teachers make decisions about educational programmes, rather than measuring success or failure in terms of stated objectives or goals. These goals in health education are explored fully. Definitions are examined closely and emphasis laid on the more recent view that processes matter perhaps more than outcomes. Some practical examples of ways of describing course goals are outlined, including a model from SCHEP 13–18. In addition, ways of gathering information from and about students and teachers are summarized, and the importance of asking teacher colleagues the right questions is emphasized with some examples.

The chapter concludes by recognizing the enormous practical constraints which prevent a full evaluation of health education in schools. Choices will need to be made on agreed priorities and a plan devised, bearing in mind the following four key questions:

For what purpose is the evaluation intended?
For whom is the 'evidence' being collected?
Who is to collect (or might collect) the information?
What are the practical constraints which seem particularly pertinent?

References

Cooper, K. (1976) In *Curriculum Evaluation Today – Needs and implications*. Schools Council Research Studies. London, Macmillan.

Education Development Center (1970) 'Man: A course of study', in *Evaluation Strategies*. Cambridge, Mass., Education Development Center, p. 46.

Schools Health Education Study (1967) *Health Education – A conceptual approach to curriculum design*. St Paul, Minn., 3M Education Press.

Schools Council (1974) *Evaluation, Assessment and Record Keeping*. Schools Council History, Geography and Social Science 8–13 Project. Glasgow and Bristol, Collins and ESL Bristol.

Schools Council (1975) Schools Council Health Education Project 5–13. London, Nelson.

Schools Council (1977) Schools Council Health Education Project 13–18. Southampton University and Fforbes-Hamilton Ltd.

Steadman, S. (1976) In *Curriculum Evaluation Today – Needs and implications*. Schools Council Research Studies. London, Macmillan.

Stenhouse, L. (1975) *An Introduction to Curriculum Research and Development*. London, Heinemann.

APPENDIX I
A SELECTION OF AGENCIES OFFERING
RESOURCES FOR HEALTH EDUCATION

ASSOCIATION FOR IMPROVEMENTS IN THE MATERNITY SERVICES (AIMS)
10 Stonecliffe View, Old Farnley, Leeds LS12 5BE. Tel: 0532 634580

The Association for Improvements in the Maternity Services (AIMS) is a pressure group consisting of consumers and professionals who are concerned about present standards of maternity care. They receive, in return for a £3.00 annual subscription, a quarterly newsletter containing feedback from conferences and meetings, reports of current developments in maternity services and paediatrics, write-ups of campaigns on the maternity unit closure and home birth fronts and accounts of personal experiences.

Members living close to one another often form a group and campaign for improvements in their own area. AIMS gives information about all aspects of the maternity services and support and advice to parents seeking to register a complaint.

AIMS leaflets are available on a variety of subjects including 'Home Birth', 'Leboyer Deliveries' and 'Hospital Checklist'. A resource list is available from the Hon. Secretary.

BOULTON-HAWKER FILMS LIMITED
Hadleigh, Ipswich, Suffolk IP7 5BG. Tel: 0473 822235

Boulton-Hawker Films Ltd have been producing and distributing 16mm educational films for schools since 1946. Their current catalogue lists over 200 films including 30 titles dealing with health education. Amongst the subject areas covered are alcohol (its use in society and effect upon the human body), smoking and drug taking, sexually transmitted diseases (how they affect the human body and how they can be treated), family planning, vasectomy, eating habits and dieting, and psychological stress. There are also a number of films available which are concerned with human biology and sex education. Subjects dealt with include the working and functions of the human body, human heredity and growth, adolescence and childbirth (from conception to delivery and parents' adaptation to a newborn baby).

A free catalogue is available on request from Boulton-Hawker, together with details of how the films may be purchased or obtained on hire. Video cassettes are also available.

BRITISH DIABETIC ASSOCIATION, YOUTH DEPARTMENT
10 Queen Anne Street, London W1M OBD. Tel: 01-323 1531

The department exists to service the educational requirements of diabetic children, their parents and 'educators' (i.e., teachers, nurses, dieticians), together with meeting the increased need and demand for information on diabetes in children.

At present the main functions of the department are:

1 Two-week holidays for children aged 6–8, 7–9, 9–12, 11–14 and 10–15.
2 One- or two-week adventure holidays and trips abroad for 13–18-year-olds.
3 Evening meetings for parents of newly diagnosed children.
4 Parent/child weekends.
5 Foreign penfriends and exchanges.
6 Careers advice.

These events are spread throughout the UK and are always attended by adequate numbers of medical, dietetic and lay staff for purposes of supervision and education.

Further plans include:

1 Expansion of items 1–5 above.
2 Surveys into the employment of diabetics.
3 Possible day courses for in-practice teachers and paramedical staff.

BRITISH EPILEPSY ASSOCIATION AND EPILEPSY RESEARCH FUND
Crowthorne House, Bigshotte, New Wokingham Road, Wokingham, Berkshire RG11 3AY. Tel: 034-46 3122

The British Epilepsy Association (BEA) is the national voluntary organization representing the interests of 300,000 people with epilepsy in the United Kingdom, at least 100,000 of whom are children and young people. Their condition varies greatly from one individual to another and the BEA's primary role is to create a climate of opportunity in which people can achieve their potential as individuals, and not as bearers of inappropriate labels. The BEA offers direct advice and welfare services, a comprehensive education and training service, and promotes self-help Action for Epilepsy Groups nationwide. For schools a multimedia range of health education material including films, tape/slide sets, photo packs and printed material is available. For more details contact the Education Department at the above address. The BEA also produces a resource list which is updated at regular intervals.

BRITISH LIFE ASSURANCE TRUST FOR HEALTH EDUCATION (BLAT)
BMA House, Tavistock Square, London WC1H 9JP. Tel: 01-388 7976

The BLAT Centre for Health and Medical Education exists, as its name suggests, to promote the further education of the medical profession and the general public in the field of preventive medicine and health.
　　Working mainly through the medium of educational technology, BLAT seeks to promote this further education by encouraging individuals and institutions to introduce new ideas and materials into their teaching. Its activities cut right across the traditional boundaries of preschool, primary, secondary, higher and further education. The research and teaching functions of BLAT have resulted in a large number of publications in the form of books, journal articles, conference papers and learning materials. Facilities available include a film library, an information library, an audiotape recording and duplicating service, a photographic service, a printing service and guidance in the preparation and design of visual and audiovisual materials. BLAT, a World Health Organization Collaborating Centre, is a creation of the British Life Assurance Trust for Health Education which was founded in 1966 by the British Medical Association, the Life Offices' Association and the Associated Scottish Life Offices.

Resource lists

1   *Medical Films* is a catalogue listing over 800 16mm films available for hire from the BMA/BLAT film library, together with films which have received the British Life Assurance Trust's Certificate of Educational Commendation or are award winners in the BMA film competition. Each entry lists the technical details, information on the intended audience and educational purpose, a synopsis of contents and a critical review. Full details from the BMA/BLAT Film Library, BMA House, Tavistock Square, London WC1H 9JP.

2   *Information* is a bimonthly abstracting and current awareness journal giving details of publications, research work, educational software and hardware, and general news in the field of health and medical education. Annual subscription £3.00; enquiries to the Information Officer/Librarian.

3   Lists of audiovisual materials on specific health or medical topics can be compiled on request to the Information Officer/Librarian.

BRITISH NUTRITION FOUNDATION
15 Belgrave Square, London SW1X 8PS. Tel: 01-235 4904

The British Nutrition Foundation aims to inform opinion leaders, including educational bodies and the media, and through them advises the general public on matters relating to food, nutrition and health. This is achieved through seminars, conferences and the publication of a wide variety of books and leaflets. It also produces a food and nutrition resources kit for teachers.

The BNF *Nutrition Bulletin* is published three times a year and is aimed at the non-specialist who wants an up-to-date overall view of nutritional topics. The Foundation also examines developments in nutrition research and opinion, encourages further research where needed and offers advice to industry and government on relevant food and nutrition policies.

A book list and audiovisual list are available.

BRITISH RED CROSS SOCIETY
9 Grosvenor Crescent, London SW1X 7EJ. Tel: 01-235 5454

The British Red Cross is an independent voluntary organization. Its two main aims are training and voluntary service to the community, within the fields of first aid, nursing and welfare. It operates through local offices in England, Wales, Scotland, Northern Ireland, the Channel Islands and the Isle of Man, whose addresses are listed in the local telephone directories. Details of training courses available to the public may be obtained from these offices.

BROOK ADVISORY CENTRE
233 Tottenham Court Road, London W1P 9AE. Tel: 01-580 2991; 01-323 1522

There are branches in Bristol, Birmingham, Cambridge, Coventry, Edinburgh, Liverpool and London providing help and advice about birth control, pregnancy testing, counselling and referral and help with emotional and sexual difficulties to young people. Branches can also provide advice and speakers to various groups and educational establishments. The Sex Education Resource Centre, 15–17 Bayswater Avenue, Bristol BS6 7NU (Tel: 0272 313362) and the Education and Publications Unit, 10 Albert Street, Birmingham B4 7UD (Tel: 021-643 1554) both provide educational material. The Education and Publications Unit provides a catalogue of such material, available free on request.

CAMERA TALKS LIMITED
31 North Row (Park Lane), London W1R 2EN. Tel: 01-493 2761

Camera Talks Limited has produced a great number of programmes for health education in schools, colleges and universities. These consist of 35mm filmstrips, slide sets accompanied by cassette tapes which are impulsed for synchronization with the slides and printed commentaries.

About 150 of these programmes are available on health education, sex education and allied fields. All of them may be sent to professional people on an approval basis (sale or return). All enquiries should be made by telephone or letter to Camera Talks Limited at the above address.

CATHOLIC MARRIAGE ADVISORY COUNCIL
15 Lansdowne Road, London W11 3AJ. Tel: 01-727 0141
18 Park Circus, Glasgow G3 6BE. Tel: 041-332 4914

You do not have to be married or a Catholic to talk with one of the Catholic Marriage Advisory Council's counsellors; they are pleased to help anyone who wants to discuss relationships. Counsellors work at many local centres throughout the country; ask the London Headquarters for the address of a centre near you. The experience of those counsellors who regularly visit schools to talk with pupils about sex, love and personal relationships is made available to teachers through the CMAC Service for Teachers. This service includes a curriculum for secondary schools, a resource list, lesson notes on family planning and pupils' leaflets for CSE files and 'O' level projects. There is a correspondence service for teachers who write in about individual school courses, and a display of books in London. Courses and workshops are arranged for teachers in many localities. A resource list is also available.

CENTRAL FILM LIBRARY
Bromyard Avenue, Acton, London W3 7JB. Tel: 01-743 5555

The Central Film Library is one of the main distributors of 16mm documentary films and video cassettes for non-theatrical screenings on education, training and general information. Material is on hire and free loan within the United Kingdom. Titles on health and social studies include a recent series of antismoking 'trigger' films designed to provoke class discussion; all are free to the borrower, involving return postage only, and range in length from 8–34 minutes. Other useful films are available on sex education, obesity, hygiene, the blind and teaching the deaf. A catalogue is obtainable for £1.50, post free.

CONCORD FILMS COUNCIL LIMITED
201 Felixstowe Road, Ipswich, Suffolk IP3 9BJ. Tel: 0473 76012

Concord Films Council Ltd is a non-profit making registered charity operating a 16mm film library. It also acts as a distributor for pre-recorded video cassettes and other audiovisual aids. The Council specializes in the distribution of material concerning contemporary social issues and has a wide range of films on health education topics. It acts as the distributor for both the sale and loan of material produced by many organizations includ-ing the Health Education Council.

Concord produces a catalogue bi-annually listing over 2000 items avail-able for hire, many of which are also available to purchase. The 1980–1981 catalogue costs £1.50 and teachers can obtain supplements of new titles updating this for an additional £1.00. Special listings, including one on health education, are available free on request. Also available are lists of other media resources, including video cassettes.

COUNCIL FOR THE EDUCATION AND TRAINING OF HEALTH VISITORS (CETHV)
Clifton House, Euston Road, London NW1 2RS. Tel: 01-307 3456

This is a statutory organization responsible for the education and training of health visitors. The prerequisites for entering the profession include state registration as a nurse and obstetric qualifications. A syllabus is published by CETHV and includes preparation in health education, principles of teaching and learning and some teaching practice.

Many health visitors are responsible for the health care and some of the health teaching provided in their local schools. Provision is therefore made within the further education programme to develop this special interest.

More recently CETHV has issued guidelines and criteria for courses in school nursing, and is scrutinizing the training provision for state registered nurses working in schools. Course lists relating to further education and short courses are published annually, in April/May, and can be obtained from the above address.

Two films are available on loan, free of charge, from Guild Sound and Vision Film Library. The most recent, *One Step Ahead*, shows some aspects of health teaching in schools.

EDUCATIONAL FOUNDATION FOR VISUAL AIDS (EFVA)
254 Belsize Road, London NW6 4BY. Tel: 01-624 8812

The prime function of EFVA is to assist in providing the education service with a range of audiovisual teaching materials and audiovisual equipment, and to provide local authorities lacking their own facilities with the means of maintaining and repairing the equipment.

The Foundation's Training Department, also housed at the National Audiovisual Aids Centre, offers a wide range of courses for all personnel involved in training. These courses cover the use of all media, including the latest TV and video equipment, slide-tape and projected aids.

EDUCATIONAL PRODUCTIONS LIMITED
Bradford Road, East Ardsley, Wakefield, West Yorkshire WF3 2JN.

Educational Productions Ltd publish a range of audiovisual aid resources in health and hygiene, child care and nursing, and physical education. These resources range from inexpensive wallcharts to books, slide sets and film-strips. The materials are listed in their home economics and physical education catalogues which are available free of charge from the above address.

FAMILY PLANNING ASSOCIATION (FPA)
Margaret Pyke House, 27–35 Mortimer Street, London W1A 4QM. Tel: 01-636 7866
2 Claremont Terrace, Glasgow. Tel: 041-332 9144

The FPA runs, in conjunction with the Health Education Council, the Family Planning Information Service for the public and relevant NHS staff, distributing over 100 different leaflets and other publications free of charge (DHSS funded) and providing a personal enquiry service by visit, letter or telephone, and an information centre on family planning matters (a number of FPIS leaflets, etc., are widely used in schools).
    The FPA national office, education unit and regional offices also provide a wide range of courses for members of many professions (including teachers) to enable them to handle the personal relationships side of their work. FPA policy is to enable teachers to handle personal relationships in education themselves, though some schools still request help from speakers from FPA regional offices and (providing the time is available and the approach is considered appropriate) the FPA provides such assistance.
    The FPA still has some 20 private clinics, but the great majority of its 1000 clinics were transferred to area health authorities in 1976, and the Association's main work is now in information and education as outlined above.

GATEWAY EDUCATIONAL MEDIA
Waverley Road, Yate, Bristol BS17 5RB. Tel. 0454 316774

Gateway Educational Media produce and distribute 16mm sound films, 8mm loop films, 35mm filmstrips and filmstrip/cassette learning packages. They also market a useful range of filmstrip and slide viewers. They have a number of titles on health education, covering anatomy and nutrition and the 1978 BISFA Gold Award Winner *The Human Eye*. Gateway also distri-bute films produced by Indiana University including titles on psychology and social problems. Write for a free catalogue, specifying particular interests.

GENERAL DENTAL COUNCIL
37 Wimpole Street, London W1M 8DQ. Tel: 01-486 2171

The Council is the statutory body of the dental profession. For many years it has carried out a dental health education programme which is designed to appeal mainly to schools and colleges of education and provides a wide variety of dental health education material including children's posters, leaflets, films, slides and models, etc. A number of the items are either free of charge or on free loan. A catalogue is available.

GIBBS ORAL HYGIENE SERVICE
Dental Health Education Consultants, Hesketh House, Portman Square, London W1A 1DY. Tel: 01-486 1200

Gibbs Oral Hygiene Service was founded in 1952 on the initiative of leading members of the dental profession and is financed by Elida Gibbs, a Unilever company. It is a comprehensive dental health education service and can provide the expertise based on experience for any dental health education exercise. Its major objective is to present dental health in an imaginative way so that all audiences will find it an interesting topic. The full range of services consist of:

1 Complete range of imaginatively produced booklets, leaflets and posters for all age-groups.
2 Project kits for infant and junior schools.
3 Textbooks and slide packs for tutors.
4 Ten 16mm films for all age-groups.
5 Free lecture service for all health and teaching personnel responsible for promoting dental health.

For further details of this service write for a free catalogue.

GUILD SOUND AND VISION LIMITED
Woodstone House, Oundle Road, Peterborough PE2 9PZ. Tel: 0733 63122

One of the world's largest distributors of educational, sponsored and training film and video programmes, Guild Sound and Vision Limited distributes over 7000 titles, including those of the Open University, ILEA, BBC Enterprises, film libraries and others.

Additionally they operate Guild Television Service providing TV entertainment for British personnel overseas; a training production and consultancy service; and an audiovisual equipment hire service. A resource list is available.

HEALTH EDUCATION BUREAU
7 Ely Place, Dublin 2. Tel: Dublin 762393/4

The Health Education Bureau was set up in 1975 by the Government acting on a report by the Committee on Drug Education. Its field of activity was very limited because of financial restrictions until January 1978. Since then a full staff has been appointed and the promotion of health education using formal and informal delivery methods has been increased.

The Education and Training Division is mainly responsible for the initiation, development and implementation of health education programmes in schools.

In primary schools a series of kits on selected health topics is currently being developed. In secondary level schools, a pilot programme is currently examining

1   Organization of health education in the curriculum,
2   Development of suitable materials and
3   Teacher training needs.

An assessment of health education practices and attitudes among school pupils, teachers and parents is planned for the future.

The division has produced its first newsletter for schools, entitled *School News in Health Education*. It is also active in promoting health education in teacher training colleges and further education institutions generally.

For information about resources and other details regarding the organization write to the above address.

HEALTH EDUCATION COUNCIL
78 New Oxford Street, London W1A 1AH. Tel: 01-637 1881

The Health Education Council is a government supported body, based in London. The Council supports curriculum development in schools, organizes in-service training and provides free resource lists on the teaching of a variety of topics. A new resources centre at 71–75 New Oxford Street provides a reference collection of audiovisual aids, teaching material and a library.

HEALTH EDUCATION INDEX

Published by B. Edsall and Co. Limited, 36 Eccleston Square, London SW1V 1PF.

The *Health Education Index* is the most complete resource reference in health education which classifies in more than 150 categories, from over 500 sources, over 9000 different items of every kind of health education material, including leaflets, booklets, film strips, slides, tapes, tape cassettes, video cassettes, films, overhead projector transparencies, models, flannel graphs, wallcharts, teaching kits and over 300 posters illustrated in miniature.

In addition to classifying, describing and pricing this range of material, it also lists selected books for junior school health education in its fullest sense, by looking further afield than health education text books, to enable teachers to introduce health education side by side with mainstream education. The selection is grouped under 'Social and Emotional Development', 'Caring for Oneself' and 'Physical Growth and Development', for the 5–8 years infant and lower junior group and the 8–12 years upper junior and lower secondary group respectively. Each title is briefly annotated and the price and source given.

Appropriate official and unofficial reports are listed under subject headings, and there is a comprehensive descriptive listing of voluntary organizations relevant to health education and concerned with physical, emotional, environmental and social health.

The index is revised approximately every two years. It is the most comprehensive source book available.

INSTITUTE FOR THE STUDY OF DRUG DEPENDENCE (ISDD)

Kingsbury House, 3 Blackburn Road, London NW6 1XA. Tel: 01-328 5541/2

The ISDD was established in 1968 as an independent non-profit making, interdisciplinary centre. It houses a collection of literature on all aspects of the non-medical use of drugs excluding use of alcohol and tobacco, ranging from scientific reports to material from the underground press. ISDD's facilities are available to any enquirer by post, telephone or personal visit. Opening hours are 9.30 to 5.30, Monday–Friday. The ISDD's Evaluation and Research Unit was established in 1972 and has carried through a programme of research aimed at evaluating existing methods, and developing and testing fresh approaches in drug and alcohol education and in-service training. The Unit has also carried out sociological research into alcohol in teenage culture (*Standing Their Round*, HEC, 1980), and has interests in relation to solvent sniffing problems and the theoretical bases of health and social education. A resource list is available.

INSTITUTE OF HEALTH EDUCATION
14 High Elms Road, Hale Barns, Cheshire. Tel: 061-980 8276.

Membership of the Institute of Health Education is open to professional workers with a background in medicine, teaching and education, nursing, community medicine, public and environmental health, sociology, public relations and related fields, who are on the staffs of local authorities, national organizations, government departments, universities, colleges and schools. Corporate membership is open to professional associations, royal colleges, government departments, local authorities, national organizations and educational establishments who are interested in health education and welfare.

Members are actively encouraged to exchange information and views and the Institute provides a comprehensive information service. In addition to the quarterly journal, regular newsletters with information on new materials, audiovisual media and techniques are produced. Frequent meetings are held in various parts of Britain at which speakers who are eminent in their field are invited to present papers of interest to health educators and at which health education issues are actively discussed. The publications of the Institute are free to members; the Institute's journal is available to non-members on subscription.

THE KRAFT KITCHEN
Kraft Foods Limited, St George's House, Bayshill Road, Cheltenham, Glos. GL50 3AE. Tel: 0242 36101

The Kraft Kitchen produces a range of leaflets covering various aspects of nutrition. Up to twenty copies of any of the leaflets can be obtained free of charge. A small charge is made for larger quantities. A guide giving details of the leaflets available can be obtained from the above address.

LEVERHULME HEALTH EDUCATION PROJECT
University of Nottingham, Block C, Cherry Tree Buildings, University Park, Nottingham NG7 2RD. Tel: 0602 56101, Ext. 3383

Most school-related work is caried out by Dr C. Anderson. The Project's special interests include what happens to health education curriculum proposals in actual classrooms, and conversely what classroom characteristics a proposal would have to take account of to be really practical; a guide to in-service training based on classroom analysis; and a criticism of curricular experiments in the 'soft' area of the curriculum. A publications list is available.

Other members of the project have worked on topics concerned with children, mothers and the area health authority services, which have some relevance for schools.

MANCHESTER REGIONAL COMMITTEE FOR CANCER EDUCATION
Kinnaird Road, Manchester M20 9QL. Tel: 061-434 7721

In addition to directing a comprehensive programme of educational talks about cancer to adults in the Northwest region, the Committee has interested itself in the cancer education of older children. Research among secondary school children resulted in the production of a resources pack, *Quest*, for their teachers. Subsequent work in the field of education has involved similar work in teacher training establishments and more recently in the field of further education.

NATIONAL ASSOCIATION FOR MATERNAL AND CHILD WELFARE
1 South Audley Street, London W1Y 6JS. Tel: 01-491 2772

The primary object of the Association is the furtherance of education in matters connected with maternal and child welfare. Conferences are held annually in London and other cities. Matters arising will be dealt with and research into particular problems may be undertaken.

Membership is open to regional, area and local health, education and social services authorities, together with other public or local authorities which may exercise full delegated powers in these fields in the United Kingdom, such as community health councils, teaching hospitals and university departments of child health.

Favourable rates for the supply of publications produced for the Association are available to all affiliated bodies. Overseas contacts are maintained.

Those concerned with health education may find the Association useful in the following ways: publications and suggested syllabuses for use in schools, colleges, clubs, groups of young people, etc; advisory service – parentcraft education (boys as well as girls); examinations at different levels in child care and development (graded certificates of instruction are awarded to successful candidates). A list of publications is available.

NATIONAL CHILDBIRTH TRUST (Education for Parenthood)
9 Queensborough Terrace, Bayswater, London W2 3TB. Tel: 01-229 9319/9310

The National Childbirth Trust (NCT) organizes classes for preparation for childbirth and has branches all over the country. It trains antenatal teachers, promotes breast-feeding and through its branches organizes post-natal support for new parents.

Many parents attending antenatal classes express the wish that something with the same interest in, and care for, the individual as a potential parent had reached them earlier in their educational lives. The Education Committee of the NCT seeks to promote education for parenthood in schools and colleges by making the baby and its needs more important and relevant, so that young people may appreciate what is involved in being born, giving birth and in being parents. Birth education is therefore encouraged by the provision of resource lists of books and visual aids, and study days for teachers in London and the regions.

NATIONAL CONFEDERATION OF PARENT-TEACHER ASSOCIATIONS (NCPTA)
43 Stonebridge Road, Northfleet, Gravesend, Kent DA11 9DS. Tel: 0474 60618

The NCPTA exists to help schools of all kinds to establish happy relationships between home and school. The membership subscription covers public liability insurance for all Association activities, supply of the Home and School Council Working Papers as published, newsletters three times a year, conferences and discussion and other activities.

NATIONAL COUNCIL ON ALCOHOLISM
3 Grosvenor Crescent, London SW1X 7EE. Tel: 01-235 4182

The National Council on Alcoholism was established in 1962 as a voluntary organization but its major source of funds is the Department of Health and Social Security The Council:

1   provides a national and public focus for problem drinking;
2   maintains and co-ordinates the work of local councils on alcoholism;
3   helps both statutory and voluntary organizations in planning appropriate services for people with drinking problems;
4   provides policies and programmes in the fields of primary prevention.

Its task is to create in the general public a greater awareness of the social, economic and health problems which arise from excessive or inappropriate drinking patterns.

NATIONAL DEAF CHILDREN'S SOCIETY
45 Hereford Road, London W2 5AH. Tel: 01-229 9272/6

The main work of the Society consists of advice and guidance on welfare and education, financial help for holidays, advice on special equipment, bursaries and information and publicity. Support is given to regional groups throughout the country.

NATIONAL MARRIAGE GUIDANCE COUNCIL
Herbert Gray College, Little Church Street, Rugby, Warwickshire CU21 3AP. Tel: 0788 73241
58 Palmerston Place, Edinburgh EH12 5AZ.

The Council co-ordinates the work of 150 local marriage guidance councils, many of whose counsellors may be helpful in educational discussion work. The Council has a bookshop and publications list.

NATIONAL SOCIETY FOR THE PREVENTION OF CRUELTY TO CHILDREN (NSPCC)
Junior Section, 1 Riding House Street, London W1P 8AA. Tel: 01-580 8812

Sets of information sheets for students aged 15+ are available from the Society covering all aspects of the NSPCC's structure and case work. Individual copies of these packs are sent free of charge but a charge of 50p per copy is made for bulk orders of six packs or more. Simplified information packs are available for 7–11-year-olds.

The NSPCC can arrange for speakers and film shows on the Society's work for groups of students undertaking courses in parenthood and allied subjects. A list of available films is included in the information pack for older pupils as well as a list of the Society's publications and publicity material.

The Society's information service is aimed at explaining to children in practical terms problems, both emotional and material, which parents may face in bringing up their children and the case work help available to such parents.

ROYAL ASSOCIATION FOR DISABILITY AND REHABILITATION
25 Mortimer Street, London W1N 8AB. Tel: 01-637 5400

The Royal Association for Disability and Rehabilitation works to relieve, rehabilitate and generally assist disabled people. It promotes understanding of the treatment of disability and a fuller knowledge of the causes of disablement and of the ways in which these may be eliminated or reduced. It also promotes the education, welfare and rehabilitation of disabled people and their integration within the community. The Association encourages research into the causes, prevention, treatment and cure of disabling diseases and conditions.

ROYAL COLLEGE OF MIDWIVES
15 Mansfield Street, London W1M OBE. Tel: 01-580 6523

The Royal College of Midwives, governed by a national council, is the only professional organization and trade union specifically for midwives. The aim of the College is to 'advance the art and science of midwifery and to maintain high professional standards'.

The Education Department offers a variety of post-certificate courses for midwives including short residential and non-residential ones preparing midwives for their role in the preparation of parents for parenthood, and for teaching in health education programmes in schools. The College also co-operates with the media in the preparation of teaching aids in this field.

ROYAL SOCIETY FOR THE PREVENTION OF ACCIDENTS (RoSPA)
Cannon House, The Priory, Queensway, Birmingham B4 6BS. Tel: 021-233 2461

RoSPA is the largest and most comprehensive safety organization in Europe and is concerned with safety on the road and in the home, in all occupations from factory to farm, in leisure pursuits including water safety, and is actively engaged in safety education in schools and colleges. In addition, it is concerned with such engineering and enforcement matters as have a bearing on its work. Representatives of official organizations involved in such matters serve on RoSPA's committees while RoSPA, in its turn, is represented on government committees, the committees of the British Standards Institution and those of research and educational bodies. RoSPA is a completely independent professional body with a wealth of voluntary expertise at its disposal, embodied in its national committees. Most of the Society's income derives from subscriptions, although the Government makes grants for specific activities, and money is earned from the sale of goods and the provision of services, notably training.

A full list of publications, posters, films, etc. is available direct from RoSPA.

SCHOOLS COUNCIL FOR THE CURRICULUM AND EXAMINATIONS
160 Great Portland Street, London W1N 6LL. Tel: 01-580 0352

The Schools Council is an independent organization funded by central and local government. It sponsors school-based research leading to improved teaching methods and changes in the curriculum. It monitors and makes recommendations to the government on examinations. The Council is representative of all educational interests (including teachers, parents, employers, trade unions, examining boards, further and higher education, local authorities, DES, etc.) and provides a national forum for public debate on curricula and examinations.

The following resources are obtainable from the Schools Council Project Information Centre at the above address:

- Profile on Health Education Project 5–13
- Profile on Health Education Project 13–18
- *Project Profiles and Index* (£4.50) – a loose-leaf directory of all the Council's projects. Subscribers also receive a bimonthly bulletin *Link*, which contains updated information on the various projects.

SCOTTISH HEALTH EDUCATION UNIT
Woodburn House, Canaan Lane, Edinburgh EH10 4SG.

The Scottish Health Education Unit is concerned with health education in Scotland. It produces posters and leaflets for the public on a wide variety of health subjects and interests. It organizes campaigns to increase awareness of health, runs a library service and funds research.

SOCIAL MORALITY COUNCIL
23 Kensington Square, London W8. Tel: 01-937 8547

The Council provides an advisory and development service in the field of social and personal education. The administrative and development office is at the above address while the resource and information centre is at St Martin's College, Lancaster. The first of a series of regional field officers has been appointed in the Southwest, based with the Devon Local Education Authority in Exeter.

Three of the Council's current projects are:

1 Community learning and service in collaboration with Community Service Volunteers.
2 The hidden curriculum and school management in collaboration with the Industrial Training Service.
3 Moral education across the curriculum with the Subject Teaching Association.

The Council has a particular interest in the work of the Schools Council Moral Education Project.

THE SPASTICS SOCIETY
12 Park Crescent, London W1N 4EQ. Tel: 01-636 5020

The Spastics Society is the world's leading organization for the care, treatment, training and education of children and adults who suffer from cerebral palsy (spasticity). It was founded in January 1952 by a group of parents who were concerned about the neglected needs of their disabled children. It covers England and Wales, and now has 190 affiliated local groups.

Since its inception, the Spastics Society has established over 60 national schools and centres to cater for the wide variety of needs among spastic children and adults.

A leaflet describing the aims and achievements of the Society in more detail is available from the Information Department at the above address.

STEP MANAGEMENT SERVICES
Federation House, 2309/11 Coventry Road, Sheldon, Birmingham B26 3PB. Tel: 021-742 4296

The Schools Traffic Education Programme (STEP), in co-operation with road safety departments, provides a wide range of traffic education materials for secondary schools, including:

- teachers' courses (free);
- teachers' reference manual (free);
- resources and project material (free);
- assisted purchase of a training moped;
- classroom materials such as films and film hire service, slide/tape packs, playground training aids, textbooks, teaching packs, work sheets and overhead transparencies;
- course structure outlines for CSE examinations;
- one-year and two-year non-examination courses;
- post-examination courses.

A resources catalogue is available on request from the above address.

TEACHERS' ADVISORY COUNCIL ON ALCOHOL AND DRUG
EDUCATION (TACADE)
2 Mount Street, Manchester M2 5NG. Tel: 061-834 7210
6 Tourney Road, Bournemouth BH11 9SX. Tel: 02016 77801

TACADE is a national educational organization comprising two separate
units: the Teachers' Advisory Council on Alcohol and Drug Education and
the Health Education Development Unit. The Council develops in-service
teacher training courses in health education, with specific reference to
alcohol and drug education. It provides courses, material for use in the
classroom, back-up resources for teachers and a loan scheme for more
in-depth work in related areas. TACADE also provides speakers and a
reference and study facility in Manchester. The Council publishes *Monitor*,
a termly bulletin which is widely distributed to schools.

TENOVUS CANCER INFORMATION CENTRE
90 Cathedral Road, Cardiff CF1 9LN. Tel: 0222 42851

The Centre's publications include surveys of opinion and attitudes of the
public and of GPs on cancer, and various leaflets and posters on smoking
and advice on the early detection of women's cancers. The Cancer Information Pack for Schools is designed for the 13–14-year-old age-group and
consists of an illustrated teacher's book, a set of overhead transparencies,
slides, fact sheets and work cards dealing with the causes, diagnosis and
treatment of cancer.

The Centre has an extensive film library from which 16mm films suitable
for professional purposes and for the lay public on various cancer education
topics may be borrowed. In addition, a lecture service is available in the
Southeast Wales area. A resource list, film catalogue and reading list are
available from the above address.

TRANSPORT AND ROAD RESEARCH LABORATORY (Department
of the Environment, Department of Transport)
Old Wokingham Road, Crowthorne, Berkshire, RG11 6AU. Tel: 03446
3131

TRRL carries out research to help in formulating, developing and implementing government policies relating to roads and transport, including
their interaction with urban and regional planning in the fields of highway

engineering, traffic engineering and safety, and transport.

Safety research involves studies in the abilities of road users, perception and decision-making skills, motivation, behaviour in accidents and normal behaviour. There are also studies to make methods of improving road user behaviour more effective; these include training, education, publicity and enforcement.

Digests of published reports are available from the TRRL Library at the above address.

APPENDIX II

HEALTH EDUCATION COURSES

(This information was kindly supplied by the Health Education Council.)

The following master's degree, diploma and other courses on health education and related subjects are currently available in the United Kingdom.

Postgraduate Degrees

Two courses are currently offered:

1 *Master of Science (Health Education)* in the Faculty of Education, at Chelsea College, London University.
2 *Master of Science* in the Faculty of Medicine, at the University of Manchester (Department of Community Medicine).

Postgraduate Diploma in Health Education

There are two diploma courses available as professional training:

1 *Diploma in Health Education* at Leeds Polytechnic (Health Education Department), validated by the University of Leeds School of Medicine.
2 *Diploma in Health Education* at the Polytechnic of the South Bank (School of Nursing and Community Health Studies), validated by the Council for National Academic Awards (CNAA).

Other Relevant Postgraduate Diploma Courses

These include:

1 *Diploma in Education* at the University of London Institute of Education. This is a course in the method and practice of teaching health education, and includes an option entitled 'Education, Health and Welfare'.
2 *Diploma in Professional Studies (Health Education)* at Kingston Polytechnic, validated by the CNAA. This is also a course in the theory and practice of health education for teachers.
3 *Diploma and/or MA in Rural Social Development* at the University of Reading School of Education. This course is relevant for health educators working in developing countries.

Health Education Certificate Courses

A large number of these courses are available at polytechnics and colleges. They are usually held one day per week for one year and are aimed specifically at members of the health services.

APPENDIX III

CURRICULUM MATERIALS FOR USE IN HEALTH EDUCATION PROGRAMMES

Active Tutorial Work (Lancashire County Council and Blackwell)
Books 1–4
Books 5–6 (in preparation)
A useful source of materials on health education, personal and social education, careers and study skills for use in the tutorial period in secondary schools.

The Health Education Council have sponsored a national dissemination scheme with a field officer offering in-service training for use with the work, which in turn is based on developmental group work concepts associated with Dr. Leslie Burton of Swansea University.

Alcohol Objectives Workshop (TACADE)

This is a ready-made course designed to help teachers to assess the needs of children vis-à-vis alcohol and to design an educational programme for different age-groups.

Breakaway Series (Hulton Educational Publications 1973–1977)

Of special interest are:
Book 1: *People with Problems*
Book 2: *Finding a Job and Settling Down*
Book 5: *Keeping the Peace.*

There are fifteen books in the series and thirty topics in each book, each of which is given double-page treatment. On the left, a strip cartoon treatment of topics such as 'Boredom', 'The Drug Addict', 'The Unmarried

Mother', 'The Lonely Teenager', 'Under Stress'; with further reading and 'Things to Do' on the right-hand page.

Checkpoints, John Foster (General Editor) (Edward Arnold)

These are very useful booklets on many topics, for average and below-average pupils aged 14–16. Information, discussion points, writing and project work are included.

The Childwall Project – Design for Living (E. J. Arnold, 1972–1974)

This is a social studies course for children of average and below-average ability structured to occupy half-a-day per week of their last two years in school. It is an integrated course in the sense that concepts and techniques of many disciplines are introduced when the pupils require them to explore a particular problem.

Each theme is subdivided into topics. Materials within the kit, often a tape recording, provide the 'impact' necessary to motivate the pupils to investigate the background to a topic. The next section of each topic, entitled 'enquiry', is where skills and concepts are acquired. Finally, the pupils re-assess the problem with the benefit of their newly acquired knowledge.

Each theme is produced as a self-contained kit with material for the teacher and twenty pupils. Additional pupils' materials are available only in packs of ten.

1 *Responsibilities of Adulthood*
2 *Understanding Children*
3 *The World of Work*
4 *Living Today*
5 *The World Around Us.*

Connexions (Penguin)

The seventeen titles include:
Break for Commercials
Disaster
Fit to Live in
For Better, for Worse
His and Hers
The Language of Prejudice

Shelter
Violence
Work.
These are magazine-style topic books suitable for non-academic pupils.

Dilemmas, David Walker (Edward Arnold)

Short plays on moral and social problems.

Enquiries, W. J. Hanson (Longman)

This is a useful series of books on fundamental social topics for students aged 14–17.

Family Life/Child Development/Parenthood Education in Schools (Open University)

This project is part of the Open University's in-service education of teachers section. It is producing a wide range of pupil and in-service aids related to the above themes and overlapping with health education.

The in-service education of teachers section is planning to increase its contribution to health, social and personal education in schools.

General Studies Project (Longman/Penguin)

This is intended for 16–18-year-old post-'O' level students, although it can be adapted for use with younger and less academic students. Annual subscription covers catalogue of 100 study units, and 350 vouchers for further copies of units. Units are catalogued under eleven themes, including Environment, Family, Population, Science and Responsibility.

Good Health (Collins Educational)

An integrated course for 9–13-year-olds.
1   Our Bodies
2   Our Safety
3   Our Families
4   Our Lives.

The quality of life as it relates to the health of the individual, the family, the community and the environment is the keynote of the project. Each unit comprises ten copies of the work book, twenty-eight different cards and a teacher's guide.

Health Education Council Project 12–18: *Living Well* (Cambridge University Press, 1977)

Directed by Peter McPhail, this provided excellent discussion and teaching material on personal relationships and health topics.

Mind Out, Jane Moran (Edward Arnold)

Plays and pages of facts on problems of alcohol, smoking, gambling, drugs, crime and sex.

Open to Question, Richard Nicholson (Edward Arnold)

A series of discussion starting points for pupils aged 14–18. The approach is open-ended and the material is in the form of newspaper articles, interviews, advertisements and photographs.

Problem Page, Sue Porter (Edward Arnold)

Resource material in areas of ethics and human relationships, covering problems at school, at home and with the opposite sex.

Professional Development Workshop Manual (Health Education Council, 1979)

This manual forms the basis of school-based in-service education for schools catering for children in the age-group 5–13. It concentrates upon health education, but raises questions which are central to curriculum review generally. It is available through regionally appointed trainers, associated with the Schools Council Health Education Projects.

The Root of the Matter, H. R. H. Davies (Edward Arnold)

The thirty topics for fourth- and fifth-year pupils are on a wide range of problems relevant to the world today.

Schools Council Health Education Project 5–13 (Nelson, 1977)

This is based on a very wide interpretation of health, encompassing not only hygiene and physical health and development, but also many emotional, social and environmental facts of human life.

The project provides excellent and strongly recommended material in three parts:

1 *All About Me* for ages 5–8, a teachers' guide.
2 *Think Well* for ages 9–13, a set of eight teachers' guides.
3 Pupils' materials.

Schools Council Health Education Project 13–18

This project, which in 1980 began moving into a dissemination phase based on Southampton University, has produced aids for in-service education of teachers in health education in schools for the age-group 13–18. It is also concerned with developing materials for this age-group.

Schools Council Home and Family Project 8–13

Home Economics in the Middle Years, Teachers' Guide (Faber, 1979).

Schools Council Integrated Studies Project (OUP)

Pupil and teacher materials are available for the three units:

1 *Exploration Man*
2 *Communication with Others*
3 *Living Together*.

Schools Council Moral Education Project 5–13 (Longman, 1978)

Schools Council Moral Education Project 13–18 (Longman, 1972)

Teachers' guides and pupil materials.

Schools Council/Nuffield Humanities Curriculum Project (Heinemann Educational, 1971)

The Family
Relations between the Sexes
Poverty
People and Work
Law and Order
Living in Cities
Education
War and Society.
The project is for pupils aged 14–16. The method of using this project is

as important as the material, which is not aimed at lower ability pupils.

Situations (Blackie)

Situations 1 (Fourth-year pack)
Situations 2 (Fifth-year pack)

This is English material based almost entirely on social situations. Developed by the serving teachers of the North-West Curriculum Development Project, Situations is intended for fourth- and fifth-year students. The 'situations' of the title are not topics, but open-ended teaching units. Pupils are encouraged to interpret accurately a scene, emotion or event presented by literature, slides, photographs, taped songs, sound or speech, and to compare it with their own experience. The early situations concern mainly adolescents; the fifth-year course moves towards a more objective study of adult relationships.

Thinkstrips (Longman)

These are comics based on social and health topics to help teenagers to imagine the situations they will meet and the decisions they will have to make. Designed especially for less academic 14–16-year-olds, but suitable for all abilities. They provide points for discussion and suggestions for projects and activities including role play. Some examples of titles are: 'It's your round' (drink); 'It'll never be the same' (parenthood); 'It's only fair' (personal relationships).

You and Your Parents, You and Your Environment (Macmillan Education)

These are two kits in the Viewfinder series; they aim to encourage pupils to see themselves in relation to their families and to the wider community to which they belong. The kits contain teacher's notes, pamphlets, case studies and 'view charts' on which pupils can record their opinions and reactions. They are designed to be used with pupils of average and below-average ability and could well form a basis on which teachers and pupils could build their own collection of material.

APPENDIX IV

A REVIEW OF GOVERNMENT REPORTS CON-CERNED WITH HEALTH EDUCATION

(By kind permission of the Teachers' Advisory Council on Alcohol and Drug Education, 2 Mount Street, Manchester.)

Over the last few years a growing number of government reports, White Papers and memoranda have pointed towards the need for health education, to an extent not witnessed before. Some of the recommendations in these publications have constantly referred to the place and the importance of health education in schools. This appendix aims to summarize some of the major references made to health education in schools and, secondly, comments on a number of general themes running through these publications.

Preventive Medicine

In the 1976–1977 parliamentary session the House of Commons Expenditure Committee produced its first report on preventive medicine,[1] which was followed by a government White Paper, *Prevention and Health*, presented to Parliament in December 1977.[2] The Report made the following recommendations:

'Health education should begin as early in the life of the individual as possible. However, the teaching at home must be supplemented by more and better teaching at school, supported by more effective community service.' (para. 80 and rec. 4, para. 309)

'Pupils at both primary and secondary school should undertake a period of physical exercise, whether a team game or not, at least once a week.

Wherever this is not the norm we strongly commend it to the authorities responsible for curricula.' (para. 260 and rec. 50, para. 309)

'Children should be treated as first priority for preventive programmes.' (para. 301 and rec. 58, para. 309)

'Health education should be taught (to teachers) in refresher courses.' (para. 83 and rec. 6, para. 309)

All of these recommendations were supported by the government in the 1977 White Paper.

The following recommendations were put forward by the Select Committee and are still under discussion or partly approved of by the government:

'We are, however, concerned that a large number of teachers attend family planning and other courses at their own expense because their Education Authorities are not prepared to sponsor them. We recommend that teachers should be sponsored for such courses.' (para. 82 and rec. 5, para. 309)

'Health Education should form a more important part of the basic training of teachers.' (para. 83 and rec. 6, para. 309)

'There should be more sex education in schools, with particular emphasis on the importance of responsible and loving relationships, provided that the views of the parents have been considered in this context.' (para. 174 and rec. 33, para. 309)

'. . . more resources should be devoted to an intensive campaign for dental health education, particularly in schools.' (para. 228 and rec. 37, para. 309)

'The relevant Government Departments (i.e. the DHSS and the DES) should actively promote the practice of physical exercise.' (para. 260 and rec. 47, para. 309)

The White Paper[2] mentions that the document *Education in Schools* (Green Paper, Cmnd. 6869) and the first report of the Select Committee on Violence in the Family both stress the need for education in parenthood for both boys and girls. It stresses that the gains from a preventive approach to health include gains for the individual, for the health services, for the health professions and for the economy (para. 258).

The White Paper goes on to say:

'Education and guidance on healthy living are necessary both at home and at school to counteract some of the undesirable pressures to which the younger generation is subjected.' (para. 46)

'Teachers of many subjects can contribute to sex education. They can often plan together a balanced programme appropriate to the needs of each age group. In-service courses, in which teachers can discuss changing health and social needs and perhaps come to terms with their own feelings about them, are valuable. The Departments (DHSS and DES) therefore hope that as resources permit, Local Education Authorities will seriously consider allowing teachers to attend suitable in-service health education courses.' (para. 179)

Violence to Children

The report from the Select Committee on Violence, entitled *Violence to Children*[3] states:

'We believe, as our predecessors did (the Select Committee Report *Violence in Marriage*) that much more should be done in the school curriculum to ensure that all pupils receive some education in the skills of parenthood. By this we do not mean simply abstract instruction in the physiological mechanisms of conception and childbirth, but learning about what young children are really like . . . . We recommend that the Government, whether through the DHSS or the DES, should ensure that education for parenthood is available for boys and girls of *all* levels of intellectual ability.' (para. 60)

Violence in Marriage

The Select Committee on Violence in the Family, in its report *Violence in Marriage*,[4] recommended that much more attention be given within our schools and further education system to the problems of domestic conflict (para. 16).

DES Circulars

In 1977 the DES circulated all LEAs and training establishments with a memorandum on health education.[5] This brings to the reader's attention the handbook *Health Education in Schools*, and quotes from the Green Paper *Education in Schools*:

'Education for good, healthy and happy personal relationships begins in the home, but through childhood and adolescence young people will be greatly influenced by teaching and example at school.'

The memorandum lists those available reports which refer to health education, and states that these have implications for both teachers and their trainers. It continues by listing the following curriculum development projects:

- *Living Well*, Health Education Council Project 12–18
- *All About Me* and *Think Well*, Schools Council Health Education Project 5–13
- Schools Council Health Education Project 13–18
- *Health Education*, Schools Council Working Paper no. 57.

The need for collaboration between education and health services is stressed in the memorandum, and it is accepted that individual LEAs will respond to the need for health education in their own way.

In the DES circular on the curriculum, *Local Authority Arrangements for the School Curriculum*,[6] it is important to note that questions are posed about the following specific aspects of the curriculum:

'*Section B. Curriculum balance and breadth*
B5 How do the authority help secondary schools provide for 1) moral education, 2) health education, 3) careers education, 4) social education through community links etc. whilst giving adequate attention to the basic educational skills? What part is played by the idea of a core or protected part of the curriculum?
B6 How do schools promote racial understanding?'

Nutrition Education

In the 1977 report *Nutrition Education*,[7] the following is stated:

'We identified teachers as one of the key groups with influence in imparting nutrition education. The role of teachers is only one part of the total contribution to nutrition education made by schools and other educational establishments.' (para. 3.6.1)

'It is also important that a good example be set by schools in all other aspects of school life (for example in school tuckshops or vending machines).' (para. 3.6.6)

'In order to provide the best nutrition education in schools, it is clearly desirable that teachers, particularly of Home Economics and the biological sciences, should be properly equipped.' (para. 5.5.2)

Drug Misuse

In the DES report *Drug Misuse Among Children of School Age*,[8] it is stated:

'Those responsible for the school curriculum should consider the inclusion of education about the right use of drugs and the danger of experimentation and misuse in the context of general health and social education. (rec. 1)

a) LEAs should encourage schools . . . to review and define their policies and attitudes on such matters as:
The development of a system of pastoral care designed to ensure a continuing awareness and concern for the welfare of the individual.

b) LEAs should consider the desirability where necessary of initiating co-operation with other local statutory services, the police and voluntary bodies concerned with the welfare of young people, and of ensuring that the support services available to the community at large are linked with the support services within the school.'

The Court Report

The Court Report[9] refers to health education thus:

'We warmly welcome the tendency, especially in secondary schools, for the nexus of topics connected with health education to be taken as a serious subject of study and discussion by senior teachers whose experience of life is as important to their success as their mastery of fact. We have been impressed by the quality of the teaching materials created by the Schools Council project on Health Education for children aged 5–13.'

'We urge that society should not leave the job solely to the schools.'

'Attention to improving an individual's general ability to cope with life is the chief issue and should in any case be a primary objective of schools.'

'Emphasis should be placed on skills in interpersonal relationships, in communication and in helping children to understand themselves and the world around them.'

Alcoholism

The report of the Advisory Committee on Alcoholism[10] states:

'1. Health education designed to alert people to the dangers of alcohol and to discourage excessive drinking should be encouraged and expanded.' (rec. 1)

'2. At school a child will be increasingly influenced by his peers as well as by his teachers. Here the form and content of education about drinking can be structured with a view to countering, where appropriate, accepted attitudes.' (p. 6)

Health Education in Schools

Health Education in Schools[11] discusses health, the health services, biology and health education, communicable diseases, pollution, toxic materials, accidents, dental health, drugs, alcohol, smoking, sex education, mental health and health education in schools.

The recent discussion paper produced by the Department of Education and Science, *A Framework for the School Curriculum*,[12] stresses that health education is one part of the overall role of the school in the personal and social education of its pupils and in their preparation for adult and working life:

'Schools contribute to the preparation of young people for all aspects of adult life. This requires many additions to the core curriculum in areas such as craft, design and technology; the arts; including music and drama; history and geography (either as separate subjects or as components in a programme of environmental and social education); moral education, health education, preparation for parenthood and an adult role in family life; careers education and vocational guidance; and preparation for a participatory role in adult society.'

The HM Inspectors' report[13] which was published at the same time also made similar suggestions:

'Religious education, the study of personal relationships, moral education, health education, community studies and community service could all contribute to personal and social development. . . .'

Concluding Remarks

From these publications some general points emerge which perhaps could be summarized as follows:

1 At a time when the prevention of ill health rather than the treatment of ill health is being emphasized, schools are regarded as very important areas for health education.

2 Health education is very different today from what it was ten or twenty years ago, and now incorporates material relevant to good social relationships, identity and parental roles.

3 Schools should not feel that they have little influence. They may be regarded as only one agency among many doing the same health education work, but they are seen as crucially important in this work if other agencies are to succeed.

4 On a number of occasions quality rather than quantity in health education is mentioned. Basic skills are a part of health education and do not conflict with the teaching of it. (It has been suggested that health education facilitates good learning by attempting to rectify factors which affect learning.)

5 The combined influence of all agencies is expected to have effects.

6 There is a great need for the prevention of ill health, and children are a crucial group to educate.

7 If education is to have breadth and relevance, health and social education should not be used to replace academic areas. The curriculum should be balanced in such a way as to incorporate health/social education for

children of both sexes and all ability ranges.

8 In-service training is essential in this area of the curriculum.

References

1. Expenditure Committee (1977) *Preventive Medicine*. Vols. I–III. First Report 1976–1977. London, HMSO.
2. DHSS, DES, SO and WO (1977) *Prevention and Health*. Presented to Parliament, December 1977. London, HMSO.
3. Select Committee on Violence in the Family (1977) *Violence to Children*. Report 1976–1977. London, HMSO.
4. Select Committee on Violence in the Family (1975) *Violence in Marriage*. Report 1974–1975. London, HMSO.
5. DES and Welsh Office (1977) *Health Education in Schools*. Joint administrative memorandum DES 15/77, WO 8/77. London, HMSO.
6. DES and Welsh Office (1977) *Local Authority Arrangements for the School Curriculum*. DES 14/77, WO 185/77. London, HMSO.
7. British Nutrition Foundation, DHSS and Health Education Council (1977) *Nutrition Education*. Joint report. London, HMSO.
8. DES and Welsh Office (1977) *Drug Misuse Among Children of School Age*. London, HMSO.
9. Committee on Child Health Services (1977) *Fit for the Future* (The Court Report). Vol. 1. London, HMSO.
10. DHSS (1977) Advisory Committee on Alcoholism: *Report on Prevention*. London, HMSO.
11. DES (1974) *Health Education in Schools*. London, HMSO.
12. DES (1980) *A Framework for the School Curriculum*. London, HMSO.
13. HM Inspectorate (1980) *A View of the Curriculum*. Matters for Discussion Series no. 11. London, HMSO.

Further Reading

DHSS (1976) *Prevention and Health: Everybody's business*. London, HMSO.

Scottish Education Department (1974) *Health Education in Schools*. Curriculum Paper 14. London, HMSO.

Scottish Education Department (1977) *The Structure of the Curriculum in the Third and Fourth Year of the Scottish Secondary School*. London, HMSO.

APPENDIX V

SCHOOLS COUNCIL HEALTH EDUCATION PROJECT 13–18 EVALUATION CHECKLIST

Unit 1 Pressure Points

Please complete this sheet if you have used the unit with students.
Where appropriate, please refer to page numbers and specific parts of the unit, as this will add enormously to the value of your feedback.

Organization of feedback
Please complete the following details:
1   Age/Year of students:

2   Size of group:

3   Comment about ability:

4   Context of group, e.g., unit taught as part of social studies, with tutor group, biology group, etc.

5   Time taken to complete work, e.g., 2 × 40 mins, 1 × 80 mins, etc.

6   Your own teaching background specialism:

7   Do you take part in the Health Education Workshops?

8   Other comments, e.g., about physical conditions/setting if appropriate:

Teacher notes

The aims of this particular piece of work are described in the Teacher Notes. Please comment after each question.

9 Are the intentions of the work clear?

10 Do they seem to be important for this age-group?

11 How would you summarize the intentions of your own teaching of this unit? It may well be that you have decided to redirect the aims to suit a different purpose.

The Teacher Notes contain instructions and suggestions for organizing the teaching of this unit, e.g., divide class into single-sex groups, etc.

12 Are these suggestions for management useful and clear? Please comment and refer to any suggestions that are unhelpful or inadequate.

13 Please describe any changes that you made to these suggestions and/or describe those you think would improve the existing notes.
Changes made:

Possible changes:

14 This unit has been written as an introductory piece of work for students aged 13–16 years. It attempts to form a base from which different types of health behaviour can be explored. It has been written to be used by teachers of varied subject backgrounds. Please comment on these and any other aspects of the Teacher Notes.

Student material

Please comment about the general practicalities of using the materials with students.

15 Could they read it?

16 Could they understand it, i.e., in terms of vocabulary, sentence structure, etc.? (Please give details.)

17 Please describe any changes (not already given in no. 13) that you have made to the student materials, and/or describe those you think would improve the existing suggestions.
Changes made:

Possible changes:

18 Describe your student's general reaction to the work, e.g., in terms of involvement, interest, discussion and other activities stimulated, etc.

19 The Teacher Notes describe the overall aims of the unit more specifically. How successful has the work been in achieving these outcomes with your students? For example, one general aim is described as: 'To look at the way behaviour alters in different contexts, and the way it is seen differently by those involved.'
Please comment, and where possible give an example to illustrate your view.

Use of other resources

20 You may have decided to use additional material or resources. If not already given in nos. 13 or 17 (changes, etc.) please describe them and their use here.

Possible future use of materials

21 What value, if any, might these materials have for you in the future? It may well be that you already have access to similar or better ideas, or feel that this unit is not particularly important or relevant. Please comment.

Presentation/format

22 Please comment generally about the presentation and format of the materials. Include any suggestions for improvement (if not already given in nos. 13, 17 or 20). In particular we would welcome comments about how the materials could be improved to be made as readable as possible.

Other comments

23

We should be grateful if you would also add your name, but please feel under no obligation to do so.

Name: Thank you for your help.

APPENDIX VI

BIBLIOGRAPHY

The editors acknowledge the help of the Health Education Council and the Schools Council Health Education Project 13–18 in the compilation of this bibliography.

General

Anderson, D. (1979) *Health Education in Practice*. London, Croom Helm.

Dalzell-Ward, A. J. (1976) *A Textbook of Health Education*. London, Tavistock.

David, K. and Cowley, J. (1980) *Pastoral Care in Schools and Colleges*. London, Edward Arnold.

Department of Education and Science (1977) *Health Education in Schools*. London, HMSO.

Department of Education and Science (1978) *Health Education in the Secondary School Curriculum*. Working paper supplement to *Curriculum 11–16*. London, HMSO.

Department of Education and Science (1979) *A Framework for the Curriculum*. London, HMSO.

Department of Education and Science (1979) *Special Educational Needs*. Report of the Committee of Enquiry into the Education of Handicapped Children and Young People (The Warnock Report). London, HMSO.

Department of Health and Social Security (1976) *Fit for the Future* (The Court Report). Report of the Committee on Child Health Services. London, HMSO.

Department of Health and Social Security (1976) *Prevention and Health: Everybody's business*. London, HMSO.

Draper, P., Best, G. and Dennis, J. (1976) *Health, Money and the NHS*. London, Guys Hospital.

Dubos, R. (1970) *Man, Medicine and Environment*. Harmondsworth, Penguin.

Faulder, C. et al. (1976) *The Woman's Directory*. London, Virago.

Gatherer, A. (ed.) (1980) *Is Health Education Effective?* London, Health Education Council.

Hopson, B. and Hough, P. (1975) *Exercises in Personal and Career Development*. London, Careers Research and Advisory Centre.

Howe, G. (1976) *Man, Environment and Disease in Britain*. Harmondsworth, Penguin.

Illich, I. (1977) *The Limits of Medicine*. London, Calder and Boyars.

Inner London Education Authority (1977–1979) *Good for You*. Health Education Curriculum Units 1 and 2. London, ILEA, Learning Materials Service.

Inner London Education Authority (1978) *Health Education: Guidelines to materials*. London, ILEA, Learning Materials Service.

Lea, M. V. (1975) *Health and Social Education*. London, Heinemann.

Levitt, R. (1976) *The Reorganized National Health Service*. London, Croom Helm.

McKeown, T. (1976) *The Role of Medicine*. Oxford, Oxford University Press.

Open University (1980) *The Good Health Guide*. London, Harper & Row.

Schools Council (1977) *Health Education in Secondary Schools*. Schools Council Working Paper 57. London, Evans/Methuen.

Scottish Education Department (1974) *Health Education in Schools*. Scottish Education Department Curriculum Paper no. 14. London, HMSO.

Scottish Health Education Unit (1979) *Annotated Bibliography of Health Education: Research completed in Britain from 1948–1978*. Edinburgh, Scottish Health Education Unit.

Sutherland, I. (1979) *Health Education – Perspectives and choices*. London, Allen & Unwin.

Tones, B. K. (1979) *Effectiveness and Efficiency in Health Education*. Edinburgh, Scottish Health Education Unit.

Willis, M. and McLachlan, M. (1977) *Medical Care in Schools*. London, Edward Arnold.

Winstanley, M. (1980) *A Guide to Better Health*. London, Hutchinson.

Alcohol

Aitken, P. P. (1979) *Ten- to Fourteen-Year-Olds and Alcohol: A development study in the central region of Scotland*. London, HMSO.
Carnana, S., Cowley, J. and Rutherford, D. (1978) *Teaching About Alcohol and Drinking*. Manchester, TACADE.
Hawker, A. (1978) *Adolescents and Alcohol*. London, Edsall.
TACADE (1977) *Alcohol: Basic facts*.
TACADE (1977) Drug and Alcohol Consultancy Pack.
TACADE (1979) *Alcohol Education*. Advice Leaflet no. 1.

Counselling

Hamblin, D. (1974) *The Teacher and Counselling*. Oxford, Oxford University Press.
Milner, P. (1974) *Counselling in Education*. London, Dent.

Dental Health

Health Education Council (1978) *The Scientific Basis of Dental Health Education*. London, Health Education Council.

Drugs

Dorn, N. (1977) *Teaching Decision Making Skills About Legal and Illegal Drugs*. London, Health Education Council.
Dorn, N. and Thompson, A. (1978) *Planning Teaching About Drugs, Alcohol and Cigarettes*. Rev. ed. London, Institute for the Study of Drug Dependence.
TACADE (1976) *Guidelines for Parents*.
TACADE (1977) Drug and Alcohol Consultancy Pack.
TACADE (1980) *Drugs: Basic facts*.

Human Development

Department of Health and Social Security (1977) *Reducing the Risk: Safer pregnancy and childbirth*. London, HMSO.
Diagram Group (1977) *Child's Body: A parent's manual*. London, Paddington Press.

Diagram Group (1977) *Man's Body: An owner's manual*. London, Paddington Press.

Diagram Group (1977) *Woman's Body: An owner's manual*. London, Paddington Press.

Evans, M., Rice, W. and Cowley, J. (1979) *Parenthood Education in Schools*. Manchester, TACADE.

Open University (1979) *The First Years of Life*. London, Ward Lock.

Open University (1979) *The Pre-School Child*. London, Ward Lock.

Mental Health

Argyle, M. (1979) *Social Skills and Mental Health*. London, Methuen.

Payne, J. (1978) *All in the Mind*. Oxford, Oxford University Press.

Wilson, J. (1968) *Education and the Concept of Mental Health*. London, Routledge & Kegan Paul.

Nutrition

Department of Health and Social Security (1978) *Eating for Health*. London, HMSO.

Relationships and Sexuality

Campaign for Homosexual Equality (1978) *Homosexuality, A Fact of Life*. Teachers' Guide.

Cossey, D. (1978) *Safe Sex for Teenagers*. London, Brook Advisory Centre.

Dallas, D. (1972) *Sex Education in School and Society*. Slough, NFER.

Farrell, C. (1978) '*My Mother Said . . .*' Study of the way young people learned about sex and birth control. London, Routledge & Kegan Paul.

Rogers, R. S. (1974) *Sex Education: Rationale and reaction*. Cambridge, Cambridge University Press.

Safety

Department of Education and Science, *Safety Handbooks*, nos. 1–6.

Smoking

Baric, L. (1979) *Primary Socialisation and Smoking*. London, Health Education Council.

Royal College of Physicians (1977) *Smoking or Health*. London, Pitman Medical.

AUTHOR INDEX

References in italics are to bibliographic details

SUBJECT INDEX

Note: h.e. = health education; p.e. = physical education; r.e. = religious education

The Harper Education Series has been designed to meet the needs of students following initial courses in teacher education at colleges and in University departments of education, as well as the interests of practising teachers.

All volumes in the series are based firmly in the practice of education and deal, in a multidisciplinary way, with practical classroom issues, school organisation and aspects of the curriculum.

Topics in the series are wide ranging, as the list of current titles indicates. In all cases the authors have set out to discuss current educational developments and show how practice is changing in the light of recent research and educational thinking. Theoretical discussions, supported by an examination of recent research and literature in the relevant fields, arise out of a consideration of classroom practice.

Care is taken to present specialist topics to the non-specialist reader in a style that is lucid and approachable. Extensive bibliographies are supplied to enable readers to pursue any given topic further.

Meriel Downey, General Editor